# Fitness
## Through
## Aerobics • Step Training • Walking

### Fourth Edition

## Karen S. Mazzeo
Bowling Green State University

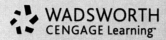
**WADSWORTH**
CENGAGE Learning

Australia • Brazil • Japan • Korea • Mexico • Singapore • Spain • United Kingdom • United States

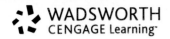

**Fitness Through Aerobics • Steps Training •
Walking, Fourth Edition**
**Karen S. Mazzeo**

Publisher: Peter Adams

Acquisitions Editor: Nedah Rose

Assistant Editor: Colin Blake

Technology Project Manager: Donna Kelley

Marketing Manager: Jennifer Somerville

Marketing Assistant: Michele Colella

Marketing Communications Manager: Bryan Vann

Project Manager, Editorial Production: Kelsey
McGee

Creative Director: Rob Hugel

Art Director: Lee Friedman

Print Buyer: Rebecca Cross

Permissions Editor: Roberta Broyer

Production and Composition: Glyph International

Photo Researcher: Ella Avetissian

Interior Images: Jeffrey L. Hall

Cover Designer: Denise Davidson

Cover Image: Step Aerobics Class © Peter
Barrett/CORBIS

For product information and technology assistance, contact us at
**Cengage Learning Customer & Sales Support, 1-800-354-9706**
For permission to use material from this text or product,
submit all requests online **www.cengage.com/permissions**
Further permissions questions can be emailed to
**permissionrequest@cengage.com**

Library of Congress Control Number: 2005937326`

ISBN-13: 978-0-495-01271-9

ISBN-10: 0-495-01271-8

**Wadsworth**
20 Davis Drive
Belmont, CA 94002
USA

Cengage Learning is a leading provider of customized learning solutions
with office locations around the globe, including Singapore, the United
Kingdom, Australia, Mexico, Brazil, and Japan. Locate your local office at
**www.cengage.com/global**

Cengage Learning products are represented in Canada by Nelson Education, Ltd.

To learn more about Wadsworth, visit **www.cengage.com/wadsworth**

Purchase any of our products at your local college store or at our preferred
online store **www.cengagebrain.com**

Printed in the United States of America
2 3 4 5 6      18 17 16 15 14

# Contents

## Dedication

To my soulmate of 40 years, *Sir Richard.*

Thank you for your constant support regarding all the "hats" I wear—writing, consulting, and teaching. With your "mass knowledge on all subjects" and humor, we make a great team!

**Saint Karen**

## Acknowledgments

Special appreciation to the following individuals who have shared their time and superior talents in this endeavor:

Steve Albrecht
Laura Ware Babbitt
Renee Barnes
Todd Belknap
Dr. Bonnie Berger
Colin Blake
Dr. Glenna G. Bower
Dr. Richard W. Bowers
Dr. Kathy Browder
Elaine D. Bryan, M.S.
Ruth Marie Carver
Mary Beth Chambers
Karen Cohn
Sandra Craig
Dr. Lynn Darby
Kay Deidrich

Peggy S. Dominque
Toni Eckert
Philip H. Goldstein
Jeffrey L. Hall
Peter Holmes
Sylvia Hom
Lara C. Houk
Virnette D. House
Rob Huffman
Linda Jerome
Carin Peirce Johnson
Dr. Vanya C. Jones
Tammy Kime-Sheets, R.D., M.Ed
Ben Kolstad
Craig Learner
Kirpal Singh Mahal

Lauren M. Mangili
Richard A. Mazzeo
Kelsey McGee
Dick Michaels
Bethany Peppers
Deaudre Perry
Steve Rogers
Nedah Rose
Carrie Robinson Sanderson
Jonathan Sigalet
Sid Sink
Shane Sockrider
Mona Tiwary
Jennifer Villani
John Virostek
Angela Wines

Appreciation to the following for granting permission to use copyrighted materials:

Kenneth Cooper, M.D., M.P.H., and Bantam/Doubleday/Dell
National Center for Nutrition and Dietetics of the American Dietetics Association
Oregon Dairy Council
Werner W. K. Hoeger, Ph.D., and Wadsworth, Cengage Learning
Tammy Kime-Sheets, M.Ed., R.D.

A special thank you to the following, for equipment, clothing, facility usage, memberships, or research:

- Hydropedes™ Insoles, Dick Michaels and Renee Barnes, Owners, 300 E. Grace St., Barstow, CA 92311 (800) 743-0845, Fax (760) 256-4414, www.hydropedes.com for gel insoles.

- Doug Jackson, M.Ed., CSCS, ACE, Fitness 21 Express™, 1474 Coral Ridge Drive, Coral Springs, FL 33071 (954) 755-9121, www.personalfitnessadvantage.com for research.

- Polar Heart Rate Monitors® Sylvia Hom, Polar Electro Inc., 1111 Marcus Ave., Lake Success, NY 11042 (516) 364-0400, Fax (516) 364-5454 sylvia.hom@polar.fi, polarusa.com for heart rate monitors.

- SPRI™ Products, Inc., 1600 Northwind Blvd. Libertyville, IL 60048 (800) 222-7774 www.spriproducts.com and staff Craig Learner, Toni Eckert and Kay Diedrich for rubber resistance tubing, Xerball®, logoed shirts, and fitness text.

- St. Julian's Fitness Inc., Tom and Shane St. Julian, Owners, 1096 North Main Street, Bowling Green , OH 43402 (419) 354-5060 for facility usage and memberships.

- The Kerr House International Health Resort and Spa, Laurie Hostetler, Owner Director, 17777 Beaver St., Grand Rapids, OH 43552 (419) 832-1733 www.thekerrhouse.com, info@thekerrhouse.com

- Walk4Life, Inc.™, Ruth Marie Carver, Owner, 12137 Rhea Drive, Plainfield, IL 60544 (888) 422-1806 www.walk4life.com for pedometers, shirts, research, and visuals.

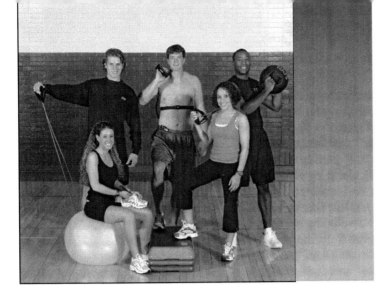

# Introduction

*You alone are the Captain of your ship*
*You alone control the choices*
*No one, and nothing else*
*can do it for you . . .*

*Fitness Through Aerobics • Step Training • Walking, Fourth Edition,* a total fitness textbook, presents the latest research using easy to understand descriptions and illustrations. Opportunities are present to apply what you learn by completing the Goal-Setting Challenges and Exercises at the conclusion of each chapter.

This *Fourth Edition* helps individuals like you understand the principles and techniques involved in aerobics, strength training, and flexibility exercise. It also helps you in structuring a training program that will work for you, for the rest of your life.

The aerobic fitness activities mentioned here—aerobic dance (also called aerobics), step training (which uses a 4"–12" step bench), and fitness walking (performed at a pace equal to 14–20 minutes per mile)—are three very popular methods of achieving and maintaining physical fitness.

To provide an informed basis from which to begin making your physical fitness choices, two forms, entitled, "Student Information Profile" and "Student Physical Activity Readiness," are provided within the Introduction. The student is directed to fill out these forms and submit them to the instructor for review, *prior to* the first workout session. The pages of this text have been perforated to ease this bookkeeping process. This hold-harmless documentation ensures that

each student's readiness to begin a workout program has been identified.

Chapter 1 gets you started thinking "fitness" by providing the definitions, criteria, principles, objectives and assessment skills for monitoring various heart rates. New to the *Fourth Edition* are various pieces of state-of-the-art fitness equipment you'll want to consider incorporating into your program, like how to use the Polar® F11™ Heart Rate Monitor, instead of relying solely upon self-monitoring.

Chapter 2 includes a discussion on motivation, and its three component parts, plus suggestions on how to empower yourself if you're not motivated to do something. You are given the opportunity to improve your motivation by understanding how you perceive, store, and retrieve images through eye-accessing cues, and, by updating your self-talk to include *present tense* thinking. Both of these elements are key to your long-range improvement in attitude and motivation concerning fitness. Concluding Chapter 2 are four steps for setting powerful goals. You are referred back to these four steps (in Chapter 2) at the conclusion of each chapter of the text, where ideas for goals to set and methods to monitor their progress are offered.

All physical fitness programs must be built upon a foundation of safety, efficiency, and comfort.

Chapter 3 mentions possible program challenges and then gives numerous solutions like wearing the amazing Hydropede™ insoles to ensure *foot comfort* for your workouts and all day long.

Chapter 4 continues the safety theme by presenting body positions to use in conjunction with exercise, since proper postural alignment (good positioning, especially of the spine and joints) underlies all physical movement. This chapter, therefore, marks the point at which your participatory fitness program must begin.

Chapter 5 establishes where you are today through testing procedures that enable you to label your starting point as 'physically fit' or 'lacking physical fitness.' You are then able to establish specific goals and have a measured standard against which to continuously monitor your progress. You're encouraged to keep a Fitness Journal throughout the course, using the sample form that is provided at the conclusion of Chapter 5, to guide the recording process.

Within a workout hour, there are four program segments. Chapter 6 details the principles and techniques involved in the first program segment preceding any other form of exercise—the warm-up. It concludes with a self-evaluation instrument, Exercise 6.1, Fitness Course Self-Assessment Check Sheet, located at the conclusion of the chapter. As the course and text progresses, each participant can self-assess the skills presented within each segment.

Chapters 7, 8, and 9 present three cardiovascular training options: aerobics, step training, and fitness walking, respectively. Chapter 7 covers the principles of building, sustaining, then lowering heart-rate intensity through the kinds of impact and other criteria used. A wealth of basic aerobics step and gesture techniques are presented, and how to apply creative variation to these techniques.

Chapter 8 presents step (bench) training principles and basic techniques for safe, efficient, and varied movement. Included are the directional approaches, steps, patterns, and variations, concluding with the opportunity to create your own patterns.

The exercise movements in Chapters 6, 7, and 8 are all photographed using a "mirrored" method. A movement described and visualized as using the *left* foot/arm/side of the body is actually the *right* foot/arm/ side of the model (see Figure I.1). Thus, you do not have to reverse the direction of what is pictured and what you perform. You simply do the movement on the *same side of the body* as you see it photographed and described.

Chapter 9 presents the third aerobic option, fitness walking. This chapter has been significantly expanded to encourage the use of a high quality pedometer like the DUO® Walk4Life™ that can measure one's total activity time and steps taken in a day, and can continue to log up to 1,000,000 steps before resetting itself. Complete details to add this motivational tool to your exercise program are given. Directions for using the currently popular Elliptical Trainer conclude the chapter.

With so many aerobic possibilities from which to choose, lifetime adherence to cardiovascular exercise becomes more of a reality for participants in the course.

Chapter 10 targets the third program segment, strength training. The principles and techniques use a variety of resistance—your body weight as the resistance, 1–4 lb. hand-held weights, Spri™ resistance bands, tubing, the Xerball® medicine ball, and a stability ball, alone, or with the step bench. The vast research included here helps you to understand the importance of developing more lean weight in order to further "build the furnace" with which to "burn the extra calories" one consumes.

Chapter 11 completes the four key program segments with the principles and techniques for cooling down and stretching properly to increase flexibility. A 12-position yoga routine provides transitional exercise movement from the intense workout state, to the relaxation techniques performed resting on the floor that complete your session.

The principles of stress management are presented in Chapter 12, followed by relaxation techniques, the revitalizing touch needed in all physical fitness programs. You're given the opportunity to construct an individualized relaxation technique through a seven-step process.

Chapter 13 focuses on your diet and current nutritional concerns. New to the *Fourth Edition* is the latest food guide pyramid system entitled *MyPyramid.* It was developed by specialists in the fields of nutrition and exercise, and promoted by the U.S. Government. It is an individualized eating system that you can easily access via the Internet. To this comprehensive nutritional program, the *Fourth Edition* adds specifics for nutrient density eating, a fluid replacement pyramid, nutrition fueling athletic performance, the 2005 Dietary Guidelines for Americans to follow, and how to read food labels. Eating behavior problems and possible solutions are given. An assessment monitoring your food and beverage intake for several days establishes an awareness of your consumption. Accurate goal setting can then follow.

The discussion of positive weight management in Chapter 14 includes assessment of body composition using the 3-site skinfold technique or the Body Mass Index (BMI), and an understanding of the weight wellness mindset. A powerful mental training tool entitled "Eating Management Panel with One Large Dial" provides a creative strategy for eating (using quantified internal cues) to avoid the problem eating extremes of starving or stuffing oneself.

This chapter concludes with the "10 Rules for Successful Weight Loss." These principles have been found to be the most crucial guidelines for those people serious about fat weight loss. They require you to consciously *make the best choices* all day, every day. The text closes with relevant web sites you'll want to check out if you need more details on a topic that has been presented here, or simply motivation to *use* what you have already learned.

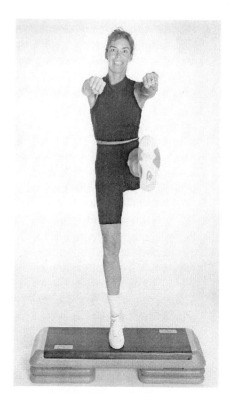

**FIGURE I.1**    Mirrored Method of Photography

Cues:  Step up *L*, kick *R* leg, waist high.

# *Student Information Profile*

Please fill in the following information, remove from the textbook, and give to your instructor:

Name _____ Level: F/So/J/S/Grad/Other

Address_____ Phone _____

Email Address _____ Student I.D. No. _____

Recommended Ideal Weight _____ Age _____ Height _____ Weight _____

Rate Your Fitness Level:    SUPERIOR/EXCELLENT/GOOD/FAIR/POOR/VERY POOR—PRECOURSE

Previous class or instruction in course: _____

Sports in which you participate weekly: _____

Reason(s) for taking this course content: _____

Did anyone recommend this course or instructor? _____ If so, whom? _____

Physical limitations:_____

Activity that you would especially like instructor to cover:_____

Heart rate:  Resting _____ Training Zone _____–_____

List any drug you take (that may alter your heart rate): _____

Do you desire to: (circle) Gain lean weight / Lose fat weight / Stay same weight

Do you smoke?_____ If so, number of cigarettes per day: _____

Indicate your alcohol consumption: Never/Daily/Others _____

List your interest in music, favorite song, favorite artist: _____

Other interests: _____

If age 35 or older, or have specific limitation: I have my doctor's written permission to participate.

Doctor's name and phone number: _____

**I have read and understand the responsibilities for participants and the instructor.**

_____        _____
Signature                                                                                        Date

© Wadsworth, Cengage Learning, Karen S. Mazzeo

# *Student Physical Activity Readiness*

Name_____  Email address _____

Address _____

Phone (Home) _____ (Cell) _____ Age _____ Height _____ Weight _____

**This questionnaire is part of the necessary prescreening for fitness testing and participation in exercise. If you respond "Yes" to any question, your instructor will want to talk to you further.**

|  | YES | NO |
|---|---|---|
| 1. Has your doctor ever said that you have heart trouble? | _____ | _____ |
| 2. Do you frequently have pain in your chest or heart, especially when exercising? | _____ | _____ |
| 3. Do you often feel faint or have spells of severe dizziness? More so with exercise? | _____ | _____ |
| 4. Has your doctor ever told you that you have high blood pressure? | _____ | _____ |
| 5. Have you ever been told that you have a heart murmur? | _____ | _____ |
| 6. Has a doctor ever told you that you have a bone or joint problem, such as arthritis, that has been aggravated by exercise or might be made worse by exercise? | _____ | _____ |
| 7. Do you have diabetes mellitus? | _____ | _____ |
| 8. Are you over age 35 and unaccustomed to vigorous exercise? | _____ | _____ |
| 9. Are you taking any medications or other drugs that might alter your response to exercise? | _____ | _____ |
| 10. Are you pregnant? | _____ | _____ |
| 11. Do you smoke? | _____ | _____ |
| 12. Have you had surgery recently, are you obese, or do you have special limitations? | _____ | _____ |
| 13. Do you have an at-risk cholesterol reading? | _____ | _____ |
| 14. Do you have an abnormal resting ECG? | _____ | _____ |
| 15. Do you have any family history of coronary disease before or by age 50? | _____ | _____ |
| 16. Is there a good physical reason not mentioned here why you should not follow an activity program? | _____ | _____ |

If you answered YES to any question, please provide a brief explanation (use a separate sheet if necessary).

**I have answered the above questions to the best of my knowledge.**

_____                    _____
Signature                                                    Date

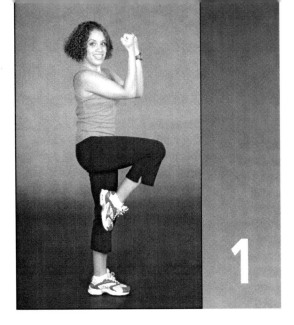

# Aerobic Exercise:
## The Way to Fitness

*"We've engineered activity out of everyday life."*[1] *This comment was made by one of the top fitness-research professionals today. Does this describe you? If so, it is time to take charge. You have the power to change, and become the best you can be!*

**F**itness is one of life's positive choices. Making the decision to engage in the physical fitness activities that follow—aerobics, step training, fitness walking, strength and endurance training, and flexibility training—is the important first initiative toward achieving a meaningful, active, and healthy lifestyle. Incorporating a variety of physical activity into your life regularly provides the foundation and basis for a long life of quality rather than just existing and "putting in time" in life.

However, if true fitness is the goal you seek, the "use it or lose it" philosophy is a core belief that you must accept. This text will provide you with the knowledge base from which to "use it" wisely—safely, efficiently, timely. Knowledge is not power, though. The *application* of knowledge is power, and the all-important application of knowledge rests on your shoulders, in your hands, and through your feet. It must be triggered by your mind and fueled by your will. Ideas to facilitate this triggering and fueling will be given throughout the text so you will develop the mental training to go along with the physical conditioning.

## A Commitment to Fitness

Achieving physical fitness requires a commitment and dedication to personal excellence. Shortcuts are few, but pleasurable alternatives are many. Once you have achieved physical fitness, you must maintain your fitness for a lifetime. Fitness is a journey—a continual process—not just one destination.

Write a personal commitment to fitness at the onset of this course as described on page 11, Goal-Setting Challenge, #3. Maintaining fitness is a lot easier than achieving it initially. You also will discover that the less physically fit you are, the longer you will take to become fit.

The learning process begins by first understanding the basics, which requires a common language that communicates the essentials of achieving fitness. The process of learning and engaging in fitness, and then achieving and maintaining fitness for a lifetime is powerful and rewarding.

---

**The total physical fitness journey requires:**

- making a commitment to fitness
- seeking valid information
- establishing your starting points
- setting reasonable and challenging goals
- monitoring your daily progress
- making self-disciplined choices continually

---

The five basic elements of physical fitness are:

1. *Aerobic fitness* (cardiovascular and respiratory)
2. *Flexibility* (ability to bend and stretch)
3. *Muscular strength and muscular endurance* (thickening muscle fiber mass to enable individuals to endure a heavier workload)
4. *Good posture* (holding body in proper position for safety and efficiency)
5. *Body composition* (maintaining proper fat-to-lean weight ratio).

## *Definitions*

Total physical fitness is a *positive state of well-being allowing sufficient strength and energy to participate in a full, active lifestyle.* According to the American Medical Association, *physical fitness* is "the general capacity to adapt favorably to physical effort. Individuals are physically fit when they are able to meet both the usual and unusual demands of daily life, safely and effectively without undue stress or exhaustion."

The term *aerobic* means *promoting the supply and use of oxygen.* All body cells require oxygen to exist. The body's demand for oxygen increases when engaging in vigorous activity that produces specific beneficial changes in the body. Working out aerobically can refer to any exercise mode as long as certain basic criteria are met.

Within the last decade or so, the exercise mode of *aerobic dance,* generalized then to the term *aerobic exercise dance,* has evolved into the currently preferred term *aerobics.* These terms are used interchangeably. *Aerobic* is an adjective, and *aerobics* is the noun denoting a mode of activity.

## *Healthy Lifestyle Choices*

Factors that enhance the ability to perform well during physical conditioning workouts include eating nutritionally, maintaining proper body weight, relaxing, and getting adequate sleep. The positive effects and benefits of exercise require a balance in *biochemical functioning*—energy intake, energy expenditure, and energy rejuvenation. These factors are introduced here and are expanded in later chapters.

## Eating

To provide the fuel needed to produce the energy required for all aerobic exercise and to ensure proper body regulatory functions, growth, and repair, participants should eat a well-balanced diet. This diet provides all the nutrients needed to stay well, to be able to perform well, and to maintain proper weight.

Regarding how much to eat and the time of day for eating, food intake should generally follow a *25–50–25 rule:* 25% of intake for breakfast, 50% for lunch, and 25% for the evening meal. Incidentally, weight control is easier for those who exercise either before breakfast or 1½ hours after the heaviest meal of the day.[2]

Participants should refrain from eating for 1 or preferably 2 hours before participating in aerobic activity and, instead, eat afterward. More blood (and oxygen) is needed in the digestive tract to digest food. When exercising, as much as 100 times more oxygen is needed in the working muscles (arms and legs) than when at rest. The body has great difficulty increasing blood and oxygen to two major body systems (digestive and skeletal muscle) at once.

## Relaxing and Sleeping

Reflective relaxation and adequate sleep are important restorative mechanisms. Aerobic exercise takes a great deal of energy, and the body's way of restoring energy is through relaxation and sleep, which help restore the ability to concentrate and to maintain a positive attitude. Physiologically, relaxation and sleep help by lowering the body temperature and the heart rate, which in turn lower the body's demand for oxygen and nutrients, thereby conserving while restoring the body's supply of energy.

## *A Total Physical Fitness Conditioning Program*

A total physical fitness conditioning program consists of five basic elements, as visualized in Figure 1.1: aerobic fitness, flexibility, muscular strength and endurance, good posture, and body composition. A well-rounded fitness conditioning program involves all five components.

## Aerobic Fitness

Because the basis of true fitness is the condition of the heart, blood vessels, and lungs, aerobic fitness is essential to physical fitness. By engaging in aerobic exercise dance (or any other aerobic activity, such as step training or fitness walking), the heart gradually strengthens and develops a greater capacity to pump more oxygenated blood to the body with fewer contractions. Exercised hearts are stronger and beat slower.

Highly trained and conditioned endurance athletes have resting heart rates as low as 30 to 32 beats per minute—admirably low. With regular, stimulating exercise, the heart becomes a more efficient pump. It pumps more blood with each stroke, and with a more efficient stroke volume, the heart can function with less effort. By getting your heart into

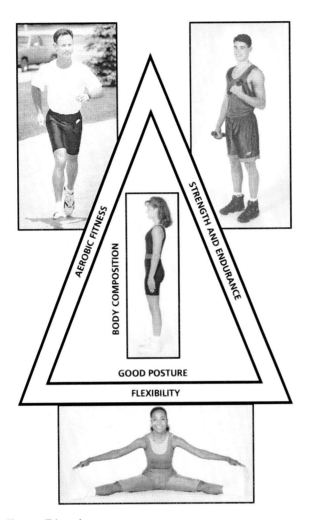

**Figure 1.1** Fitness Triangle

greater the range of movement, the more the muscles, tendons, and ligaments can flex or bend.

Muscles are arranged in pairs. One muscle's ability to shorten or contract is related directly to the opposing muscle's length or stretch. Flexibility is maintained or increased by movement patterns that stretch the muscle slowly and progressively beyond its relaxed length. The stretch is performed to a point at which the person feels tension developing in the muscle, but not to a point of pain.

## Muscular Strength/ Muscular Endurance

*Muscular strength* is the *ability of a muscle to exert a force against a resistance.* Strength activities increase the amount of force that muscles can exert, or the amount of work that muscles can perform. Activities such as weight training can develop strength in the skeletal muscles.

*Muscular endurance is the ability of muscles to work strenuously for progressively longer periods* without fatigue. It is the capacity of a muscle to exert a force repeatedly, or to hold a static (still) contraction over time.

Muscular strength and endurance activities do not provide increased oxygen to condition the heart to function more efficiently.[8] Their primary target is skeletal muscle.

*Note:* In addition to providing physical fitness to the heart, blood vessels, lungs, joints, and skeletal muscles, the *bones* can be kept physically fit, too. According to the American College of Sports Medicine (ACSM), in its published position stand on physical activity and bone health,

> Weight bearing physical activity, particularly those with moderate to high bone-loading forces, have a beneficial effect on bone health throughout the age spectrum.[9]

Therefore, many of the active exercises presented throughout the text can keep yet another key health

condition, you are practicing preventive medicine. You may be lessening the risk for a coronary heart attack 5, 10, 15, 20 years from now. And if you do have a heart attack, your chances of surviving are far greater if your heart, lungs, and blood vessels are in good condition.[3]

*Fitness* is incredibly important as a determinant of health and longevity. Is it possible to be *fat* and fit? The data show that *unfit* men are twice as likely to die young as fit men, *even among the fat group.* The fat, fit group had a *better* chance than the thin, unfit group.[4]

A person can exist without big, bulging muscles or without the perfect figure or with a head cold, but not very long without a good heart and lungs. Unfortunately, more than

40% of all people who have a first heart attack do not receive a second chance to change their habits or to develop an aerobic program. They die.[5] Nearly half of all deaths in the United States each year are attributed to heart-related diseases.[6] If only we could establish a lifestyle pattern priority early in life to counteract this overwhelming statistic!

Simply by choosing more active behaviors over more sedentary ones adults can burn calories and build fitness. Remember to walk the dog every day, even if you don't have one![7]

## Flexibility

*Flexibility* is defined as *the functional range of motion of a given joint and its corresponding muscle groups.* The

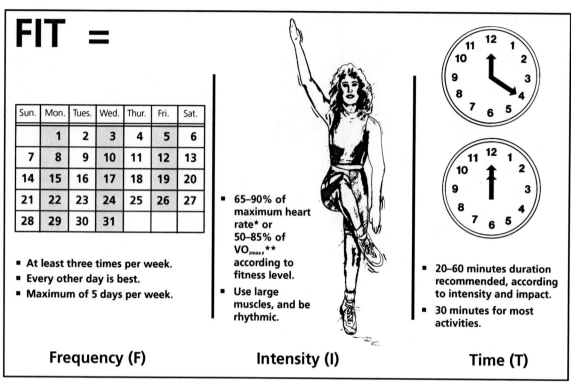

**FIT =**

At least three times per week.
Every other day is best.
Maximum of 5 days per week.

**Frequency (F)**

- 65–90% of maximum heart rate* or 50–85% of VO$_{2max}$,** according to fitness level.
- Use large muscles, and be rhythmic.

**Intensity (I)**

- 20–60 minutes duration recommended, according to intensity and impact.
- 30 minutes for most activities.

**Time (T)**

\* Maximum heart rate = highest heart rate for a person, related primarily to age and used to determine intensity.
\*\* VO$_{2max}$ = maximum oxygen uptake, the maximal amount of oxygen the body is able to utilize per minute of physical activity.

**Figure 1.2** The FIT Formula

component in shape, that we might not initially think about keeping fit.

## Posture/Positioning

Proper positioning of the body when performing any type of physical exertion promotes a safe and efficient workout. Once the basic mechanics are put into practice, this fitness component becomes integral to every move.

## Body Composition

An individual's total body weight is composed of fat weight and lean weight (fat-free weight). Keeping an appropriate ratio between these two weights is important for the entire body's best functioning and helps prevent obesity and its attendant health risks. This fitness component is managed by establishing a proper diet and exercise plan that promotes an ideal recommended weight. If you aren't beginning your program

at your ideal recommended weight, you can refer to the guidelines in Chapters 13 and 14 that detail how to achieve ideal weight.

In summation, of the five components involved in developing a total physical fitness conditioning workout program (your *prescription exercise plan*), aerobic fitness training is considered the most important. The remainder of this chapter takes a detailed look at the research and general principles to follow, including modes of activity and monitoring techniques. Aerobic exercise modalities and techniques and the other four physical fitness components are explained more fully in later chapters.

## *Aerobic Fitness Training*

*Training* refers to muscle stimulation. *Aerobic training uses the FIT formula (see Figure 1.2) and is accomplished*

*by any exercise that is performed regularly using a frequency minimum of three times per week (F), requires a steady supply of oxygen (I), and demands an uninterrupted work output from muscles for an extended time (T).*

Activities such as aerobics, step training, and fitness walking significantly increase the oxygen supply to all body parts, including the heart and the lungs, through continuous, rhythmic movement of large muscles and connective tissue. This type of movement conditions the body's oxygen transport system (heart, lungs, blood, and blood vessels) to process the use of oxygen more efficiently. This *efficiency in processing oxygen* is called *aerobic capacity* and depends on your ability to:

- Rapidly breathe large amounts of air.
- Forcefully deliver large volumes of blood.
- Effectively deliver oxygen to all parts of the body.

The *training effect*, or total beneficial changes that usually occur, consists of:

- Stronger heart, sending more oxygenated blood to all tissues of the body.
- Production of more blood cells.
- Slower resting heart rate.
- Expanded blood vessels.
- Improved muscle tone.
- Lower blood pressure through improved circulation.
- Stronger respiratory muscles.
- Regulation of the release of adrenalin.
- Increased lung capacity.
- More regular elimination of solid wastes.
- Lower levels of fat found in blood.
- Strengthening of muscles and skeleton to protect them from injury later in life.
- Deterring osteoporosis by increasing bone density.
- Increased sensitivity to insulin and lowered blood sugar levels in mild, adult-onset diabetes.
- Improvement in the way the body handles cholesterol, by increasing the proportion of blood cholesterol attached to high-density lipoprotein (HDL), a carrier molecule that keeps cholesterol from damaging artery walls.

In short, aerobic capacity depends upon efficient lungs, a powerful heart, and a good vascular system. Because it reflects the conditions of these vital organs, *aerobic capacity is the best index (single measure) of overall physical fitness.*

Aerobic capacity is what is measured, quantified, and labeled in a physical fitness stress test, performed either in a laboratory (called a laboratory stress test) or on a

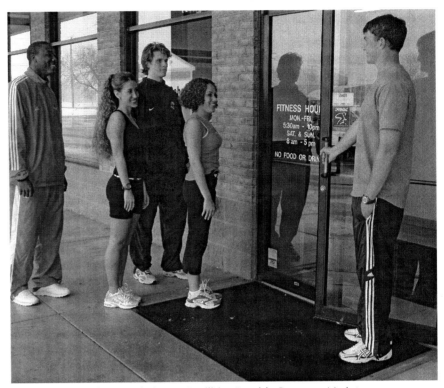

**Figure 1.3** Professional Fitness Facilities Provide Program Variety

premeasured distance such as a track (called a field stress test). You are given the opportunity to test your aerobic capacity in Chapter 5, using either method.

Aerobic exercise dance, step training, fitness walking, or any aerobic activity conditions the heart muscle by strengthening it through a principle called *progressive overload*. The heart will pump more blood with each beat, and it also will have longer rests between each beat, thereby lowering the pulse rate.

Aerobic exercise overloads the heart by causing it to beat faster during the workout session, making a temporarily high demand on the cardiovascular and respiratory systems. Over time, as you become more fit, the heart eventually will adjust to this temporarily high demand, and soon it is able to do the same amount of work with less effort. By overloading the heart with any vigorous aerobic exercise, your aerobic capacity will increase and you can achieve a desirable training effect.

## Aerobic Exercise Alternatives

Whether you have a class, or go to a professional fitness facility[10] to work out alone or with friends (see Figure 1.3), you can obtain the needed variety in your aerobic fitness program by participating in any of the following alternative exercises:

- Aerobic exercise dance (aerobics)
- Bench/step training
- Cardio kick boxing
- Cross-country skiing
- Cycling
- Elliptical trainer
- Jogging/running
- Jumping rope
- Rowing
- Skating (ice/roller/in-line)
- Sliding
- Spinning
- Stair climbing
- Swimming
- Ultimate frisbee
- Walking/hiking (moderate to fast pace-walk)

## Aerobic Criteria

For an exercise to be labeled "aerobic," the movements must meet the five following criteria, according to the American College of Sports Medicine:

1. *The exercise must use the large muscles of the body* (arms and legs). Exercise gesture and step patterns found in aerobic exercise dance and bench step movements are excellent choices.

2. *The exercise must be rhythmic.* One-two-one-two, accompanied by a steady beat of music, using either a fast or slow tempo, is suggested.

3. *The exercise must be done a minimum of three sessions per week.*

   - The suggested guideline is 4 days a week or every other day.
   - Some key researchers recommend 5 days as a maximum. Beyond this, injuries to the musculoskeletal system from overuse are 10 times more likely to occur. Novices to physical fitness conditioning need at least 2 days off per week.
   - For those whose athletic status requires more workouts or days per week, the body will reveal maximum frequency. A sudden elevated resting heart rate in the morning signifies the day(s) not to work out. This is a built-in body signal, and it can be seen/heard/felt readily simply by monitoring the resting heart rate daily. Upon arising in the morning, this heart rate is monitored for 1 full minute.

4. *The exercise must be performed continuously for 20–60 minutes.*

   - Duration depends upon the intensity and the impact (see Chapter 7) of the activity.
   - Lower intensity and lower impact activities, such as fitness walking (see Chapter 9) should be performed over a longer time period (40–60 minutes).
   - Because high-impact activities such as running and jumping

generally cause significantly more debilitating injuries to exercisers, shorter workouts (20 minutes) are recommended.

   - The Cooper Institute recommends that all adults should accumulate 30 minutes of at least moderate physical activity, at least five times a week. This equates to three, 10-minute walks, or going about a mile and a half at a rate of 3–4 miles per hour. One could also jog, do aerobics or simply do vigorous household chores . . . It doesn't matter what you do, as long as you're moving and spending the energy.[11]

   - *Moderate* rather than high-intensity exercise seems most likely to be associated with psychological well-being.[12] . . . Although as little as 5 minutes of walking can be mood elevating, there is general agreement that a minimum of 20–30 minutes of exercise is needed to generate the psychological benefits.[13]

   - Additional psychological benefits are associated with exercising longer than 30 minutes. For example, 40–50 minutes is needed to attain the positive-addiction state where the mind spins free.[14]

   - Another reason to exercise regularly is that (in nonpsychiatric populations) the mood benefits appear to last for 2–4 hours after exercise.[15]

5. *The exercise must maintain the heart rate in a specific target heart rate training zone,* the individualized safe pace at which to work or exercise aerobically. This reflects intensity and is explained scientifically as one of the following:

   - 65–90% of your maximum heart rate *or*
   - 50–85% of your maximum oxygen uptake ($VO_{2\ max}$) or heart rate reserve.

*Maximum heart rate (MHR)* is the highest safe heart rate for an individual and is related primarily to age. *Maximum oxygen uptake* ($VO_{2\ max}$) is the maximal amount of oxygen the body is able to utilize per minute of physical activity. *Heart rate reserve (HRR)* is the difference between the maximal heart rate and the resting heart rate (RHR).

## Intensity

Frequency and time duration of workouts are easy to determine, but the amount of exertion (intensity) during the workout to keep it safe while making fitness gains continually can be more of a challenge to determine, especially for the novice. Because they lack guidance or instruction, most new exercisers, therefore, do not monitor intensity (heart beats per minute) when elevating their heart rate, during cardiovascular training.

To improve your health and fitness, you *must* have a way of determining how hard you should exercise, and then *use it* during your workout. Your heart rate intensity can be measured and monitored in one of several ways (see Figures 1.4, 1.5a,b, 1.6):

- By far the easiest and most accurate way to monitor one's cardiovascular intensity level (beats per minute) is through the use of a heart rate monitor (see Figure 1.4).

- Calculate your target heart rate (THR) training zone using the Karvonen formula (detailed as Exercise 1.3, at the end of the chapter), then maintain that training zone during the aerobic portion of your workouts. This monitoring is accomplished by taking your pulse during your aerobic workout (see Figure 1.5a and b) and is suggested for the novice, who does not have access to a heart rate monitor.

- Using the Borg scale for ratings of perceived exertion (RPE) (see Figure 1.6). This shows a high correlation with heart rate and other

## *Monitoring Intensity*

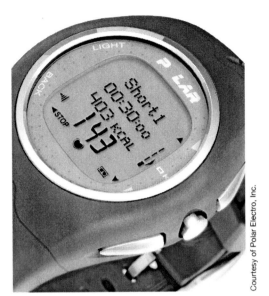

**Figure 1.4** Using a Polar®F11™ Heart Rate Monitor

Courtesy of Polar Electro, Inc.

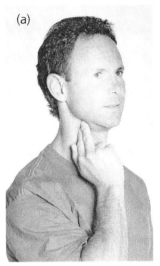
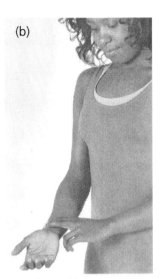

(a) Taking the carotid pulse

(b) Taking the radial pulse

**Figure 1.5** Taking the Pulse

When you exercise below this level, the exercise stimulus is only marginally conducive to the development of cardiovascular/respiratory endurance.

| | 0.5 | 1 | 2 | 3 | 4 | 5 | 6 | 7 | 8 | 9 | 10 |
|---|---|---|---|---|---|---|---|---|---|---|---|
| **WHAT IS FELT** | "Very, Very Light; Just Noticeable" | "Very Light" | "Light (Weak)" | "Moderate" | "Somewhat Hard" | "Heavy / Strong" | | "Very Hard" | | | "Very, Very Hard; Almost Maximum; Exhaustion." |

**Warm-Up Phase**

**3–5 ACSM Recommended "Aerobic" Range**

**Cool-Down Phase**

**PHASE OF PROGRAM**

For aerobic fitness, if you can sing here, you need to work harder.

Feel as if you could maintain the intensity for a long time while thinking, talking with a partner, or enjoying the class or scenery.

"Peak aerobic dance-exercise, step training, or fitness walking."

Pulse races and it becomes difficult to say more than a few words for a prolonged time. There is a sense that this level of intensity cannot last.

The end of a competitive race or sprint interval.

Source: "Physical Bases of Perceived Exertion," by Gunnar Borg, in *Medicine and Science in Sport and Exercise* 14 (1982). Used by permission.

**Figure 1.6** Borg Scale Ratings of Perceived Exertion

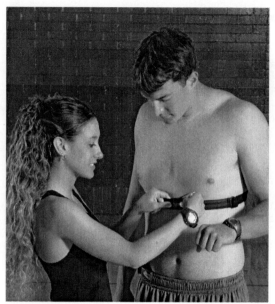

**Figure 1.7** Wet and Wear the Polar®WearLink™ Coded Transmitter Around the Chest Area

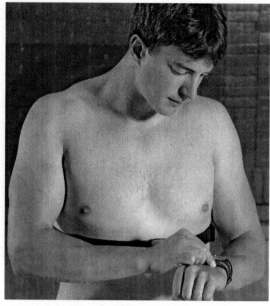

**Figure 1.8** Polar®F11™ Heart Rate Monitor Requires the User to Input Personal Data

metabolic parameters, according to ACSM guidelines. RPE monitoring is suggested only for individuals who already have become accustomed to taking a heart rate pulse.

■ Using the talk test (see Chapter 9 opening figure). This easy and practical method is best used *in conjunction with* the THR and RPE for monitoring exercise intensity.

## Methods of Monitoring Your Target Heart Rate

Here are details specific to each of the four methods of monitoring your heart rate intensity presented in this text:

### 1. Using a Heart Rate Monitor

The best way to ensure that you are achieving your target heart rate (THR) (also called training zone) while you exercise aerobically is by wearing a heart rate monitor. Here are several points to consider when purchasing and using a heart rate monitor:

✔ Look for a model that tells you when you're in, or out of, your THR / training zone with an audible signal, in addition to visually

displaying your exercising heart rate.

✔ Look for the additional features that will help you reach your total fitness program goals. For example, if you are closely monitoring your weight, look for a heart rate monitor unit that also tracks the amount of calories you burn during your workout session. To be able to calculate this information, the exerciser must input personal data variables into the unit.

The gold standard for heart rate monitors is produced by Polar® Electro, Inc. (see Figures 1.4, 1.7, 1.8) and their state-of-the-art model is the Polar®F11™ Heart Rate Monitor. To use the Polar®F11™, the exerciser must wet and then wear the Polar® WearLink™ Coded Transmitter that comes with it. The electrode areas of the strap detect your heart rate, so the strap needs to be placed around your chest, as shown in Figure 1.7. The detachable connector (in Figure 1.7, the young woman's fingers are on it, snapping it into place) transmits your heart rate signal to the wrist unit, which looks exactly like a watch. This heart rate monitor model requires the user to input the following personal variables (see Figure 1.8):

height, weight, age (actually, your birth date), sex, and the activity level (intensity) you choose to begin working at ~ top, high, moderate, or low. Note: You can change the data (settings) you enter, or, if another person uses your heart rate monitor, his or her data can be input and tracked, replacing yours.

This two-piece unit acts as a "computerized personal trainer" tracking such items as your fitness testing results, your recommended exercise program in detail, goals to set, calories burned, long-term logging of exercise data entered and a multitude of other exciting fitness program possibilities. Check the owner's manual for full details on how to use it, or investigate its capabilities at Polar® Electro Inc.'s web site.[16]

### 2. Taking Your Pulse

If you do not own or have access to a heart rate monitor, the second way to calculate appropriate exercise intensity is using the target heart rate training zone method. To use this method, you first must know how to take your pulse accurately. The pulse equals heartbeats per minute and can be felt and counted at one of six pulsation points. Select the area from which you can best obtain a pulse, using your index and second fingers. The two places used most often to count the pulse are the neck near the carotid artery and the wrist near the radial artery. Both are shown in Figure 1.5.

1. The carotid artery, located in the neck, is usually easy to find. Place your index and middle fingers below the point of your jawbone and slide downward an inch or so, pressing lightly. When you use the carotid artery pulse-monitoring method, apply light pressure, as excessive pressure may cause the heart rate to slow down by a reflex action.

2. The radial artery extends up the wrist on the thumb side. Place your index and middle fingers just below the base of your thumb. Press lightly. Count the number of pulsations, or beats, for 60 seconds. The total is the number of heartbeats per minute. To count correctly, you must count each beat you feel.

Having gained the skill of pulse taking, you can establish your *resting heart rate*. This number is used to establish your target heart rate training zone (see Exercise 1.3, #3 at the end of the chapter).

**Monitoring Resting Pulse Rate**
A true *resting heart rate* (RHR) is not taken in a class but, instead, when you have been at complete rest, preferably upon awakening after sleeping for several hours.

Keep a clock or watch with a second hand next to your bed. When you awaken (without an alarm clock ring), take your pulse for 1 full minute and record that number on Exercise 1.1, as your RHR. Do this on five consecutive mornings, then determine an average (add all RHRs and divide by 5). This is a rather accurate determination of your resting heart rate.

It should be noted here that normally healthy individuals should find that exercise is a positive outlet

---

## Exercise 1.1
## RHR Average

**Week 1:**

Day 1: _____

Day 2: _____

Day 3: _____

Day 4: _____

Day 5: _____

Sum total:_____

÷ 5:_____ RHR average

Record this average RHR at the end of this chapter on Exercise 1.2 Heart Rates Part I, Week 1: _____, at the bottom left.

---

for stress. Stress affects you even as you sleep (through a constant rapid heart rate), a time when the heart ideally should take a break and slow down for 6 to 8 hours.

One of the two visible signs of improvement in heart and lung fitness is a lower resting heart rate. Because the RHR is the basic thermometer of fitness, after a 10- to 15-week fitness course you and your classmates may experience:

- An average –3 heartbeats per minute resting heart rate decline.

- An average –10 heartbeats per minute by smokers who quit (or change their consumption significantly) during the course and as much as a –24 heartbeats per minute decline.[17]

---

***Unusual stress and illness sharply elevate the resting heart rate.***

---

Continue to monitor your RHR for the entire course on the same form, Exercise 1.2 Part I, recording your last reading also at the bottom of the page. Figure any change that has occurred during the course, to complete the exercise. Has your RHR lowered?

**Determining Target Heart Rate Training Zone** Now place your average RHR figure in the formula for determining your target heart rate (THR) training zone on Exercise 1.3 #3. The other variables figured into the formula are current *age*, and *lifestyle* (represented as a percentage of maximum heart rate).

| If you are: | Use: |
|---|---|
| ■ a nonathletic adult | 50% to begin |
| ■ sedentary | 60–69% |
| ■ moderately active | 70–75% |
| ■ very active and well trained | 80–85% |

Using Exercise 1.3, #1 and #2, record your age and the selected percentage range from above that describes your lifestyle. Figure the Karvonen equation. The result is your target heart rate, the safe exercise training zone for you. Record your target heart rate now, on Exercise 1.2 Part II in the space provided.

**Taking a Count After an Aerobic Interval** As you begin an aerobic fitness program, you will want to monitor your pace several times during the workout hour so you can learn constant endurance pacing. Mentally remember your readings, and record them at the end of class on Exercise 1.2, Part II.

When you take a pulse rate during the learning process and find that your pace is *below* your established training zone, increase your intensity. If you have a pulse rate *higher* than your established training zone, lower your intensity.

To become familiar with your own response to various intensity levels so you can regulate yourself better, ask yourself, "How do I *feel* when I get this pulse?" Focus not only on your pulse count but also on what feelings and conditions the number relates to, so you can begin to recognize the signals your body sends. This also will help prepare you to use the RPE monitoring method of intensity, which, as you become a more advanced exerciser, will be a more practical method than counting your heartbeats per minute.

Continuing at a pace that is too intense will prove to be an anaerobic exercise program. Anaerobic activity is basically stop and start, in which the heart is not kept at a constant, steady pace for 20 to 60 minutes. *Anaerobic* describes an activity that requires all-out effort of short duration and does not utilize oxygen to produce energy. This type of exercise quickly uses up more oxygen than the body can take in while engaging in the exercise, causing an oxygen debt. This in turn causes lactic acids (waste products) to accumulate in the muscles, which leads to exhaustion.

In this case, slow down, walk around, find your pulse, and count it for either 6 or 10 seconds. Each of these counts has been found to be a scientifically accurate measurement for aerobic activity pulse rates. Taking a timed count of greater than 10 seconds immediately after aerobic exercise will tend to be inaccurate because the heart rate slows down to a *recovery pulse* rapidly.

---

*Taking a 6-second count is easy. All you do is add a zero to the pulse you feel, and record that number. You must begin and end exactly with a timer.*

---

You or your instructor will determine whether you will count for 6 or 10 seconds. Immediately following the aerobic exercise segment, count your pulse and multiply the number you get times 10 if using the 6-second count, or times 6 if using a 10-second count. Each of these methods will equal heartbeats per minute and will be in your training zone.

Table 1.1 lists target heart rate counts for individuals who wish to attain fitness using the ideal aerobic range for most people (60%–75% of heart rate reserve). Locate the column across the top that is closest to your age and the row down the left side reflecting a figure closest to your resting heart rate. The box where the column and row intersect is *your 10-second target heart rate training zone.*

As your cardiovascular and respiratory systems become more fit and efficient, work (exercise) will become easier and you will have to increase the intensity of your activities. Techniques for increasing and decreasing the intensity of your workout will be explained in Chapters 7–9.

## Table 1.1 Target Heart Rate Training Zones*

| | | 15 | 20 | 25 | 30 | 35 | 40 | 45 | 50 | 55 | 60 | 65 | 70 | 75 | 80 |
|---|---|---|---|---|---|---|---|---|---|---|---|---|---|---|---|
| | 90 | 27–29 | 26–29 | 26–28 | 25–28 | 25–27 | 24–26 | 23–26 | 23–25 | 22–24 | 22–24 | 21–23 | 21–22 | 20–22 | 20–21 |
| | 85 | 26–29 | 26–29 | 25–28 | 25–27 | 24–27 | 24–26 | 23–25 | 23–25 | 22–24 | 22–24 | 21–23 | 21–22 | 20–22 | 20–21 |
| | 80 | 26–29 | 25–28 | 25–28 | 24–27 | 24–26 | 23–26 | 23–25 | 22–25 | 22–24 | 21–23 | 21–23 | 20–22 | 20–21 | 19–21 |
| | 75 | 26–29 | 25–28 | 25–28 | 24–27 | 24–26 | 23–26 | 23–25 | 22–25 | 21–24 | 21–23 | 20–23 | 20–22 | 19–21 | 19–21 |
| | 70 | 25–29 | 25–28 | 24–27 | 24–27 | 23–26 | 23–25 | 22–25 | 22–24 | 21–24 | 21–24 | 20–22 | 20–22 | 19–21 | 19–20 |
| | 65 | 25–28 | 25–28 | 24–27 | 23–26 | 23–26 | 22–25 | 21–24 | 21–24 | 21–23 | 20–23 | 20–22 | 19–21 | 19–21 | 18–20 |
| | 60 | 25–28 | 24–28 | 24–27 | 23–26 | 23–26 | 22–25 | 21–24 | 21–24 | 20–23 | 20–22 | 19–22 | 19–21 | 18–21 | 18–20 |
| | 55 | 24–27 | 23–27 | 23–27 | 23–26 | 22–25 | 21–24 | 21–24 | 21–24 | 20–23 | 20–22 | 19–22 | 19–21 | 18–20 | 18–20 |
| | 50 | 24–28 | 23–27 | 23–26 | 22–26 | 22–25 | 21–25 | 21–24 | 20–23 | 20–23 | 19–22 | 19–21 | 18–21 | 18–20 | 17–20 |

*Column header: Your Age. Left side label: Your average Resting Heart Rate per minute.*

*The numbers in the squares represent pulse beats counted in 10 seconds.

By using the target heart rate training zone, you automatically compensate for increased fitness and still maintain the same training effect. Thus, your heart rate will increase during vigorous aerobic activity and should return to normal (pre-activity heart rate) within a short time after the workout. As a rule, the faster it slows down (recovers from exercise), the more physically fit you are, for recovery heart rate improvement is another indication of increased fitness level.

### 3. Ratings of Perceived Exertion: Borg Scale

The third method for monitoring intensity utilizes the psychophysical Borg scale for ratings of perceived exertion (RPE),[18] as shown in Figure 1.6. This scale is based on the finding that, while exercising, a person has the ability to accurately assess how hard the body is working. This is basically a judgment call and *is more appropriate when used by individuals who have been exercising for a while.* The untrained exerciser typically reports a higher RPE than an athlete at the same exercise heart rate.

RPE seems to correlate strongly with other workload indicators, such as ventilation, oxygen consumption, and muscle metabolism. Participants tune into the overall sensation of effort exerted by their entire body rather than one factor such as local calf or hamstring exhaustion, panting, sweating, or body temperature. When used along with heart rate monitoring, RPE is useful for the novice, who may not be aware yet of how exercise is supposed to feel.

You might begin to make mental notes to yourself during the workout hour concerning your ratings of perceived exertion. After the workout, immediately record what you felt for each phase of the workout, expressed as numbers from 0 to 10 on Exercise 1.2, Part III, at the end of this chapter. Begin to notice the correlation be-

tween target heart rates achieved and how ratings of perceived exertion feel.

### 4. Talk Test

A fourth and less formal method for determining aerobic intensity, the *talk test*, is based on the premise that, while exercising, the participant should be able to hold a conversation (see the Chapter 9 opening figure). If the participant can gasp out only one or two words at a time, the exercise intensity probably is anaerobic and should be adjusted to allow for two- to three-word phrases. Because the accuracy of the talk test varies within any given population, it is best utilized in conjunction with the THR and the RPE for monitoring exercise intensity.[19]

### Which Method Is Best?

The experts do not agree on which is better, THR or RPE. Some claim that only THR methods are accurate. Others believe that RPE combined with the talk test are more practical. Because all the methods are useful and none is consistently ideal, a good solution is to *use a combination of all three*. Once a participant has developed a good understanding of the heart rate/RPE relationship, heart rate can be monitored less frequently and RPE can be used as a primary means of measuring exercise intensity, with the talk test as an informal supplemental backup measure.[20]

### Duration of Time Variable

The duration of an exercise session (20–60 minutes for cardiovascular fitness goals) is a variable element determined by the *intensity* and *impact* of your movement. (Impact is discussed fully in Chapter 7.) Once you have established your safe exercise zone, intensity is an easy choice to make; it is reflected by heartbeats per minute and is the result of using the upper or lower end of your training zone

(Exercise 1.3). It is one of the small choices you must make personally and continually during each workout, according to:

- what phase of the workout you're in
- any limitations (illness, injury, etc.) to your program.

Intensity is experienced directly as the beats per minute (BPM) you see on the heart rate monitor, or count, as your pulse; or it is the RPE "feeling sense" of 3, 4, or 5, which quantifies how hard you *feel* you're working. Working at heart rates beyond your established safe THR zone, or an RPE of 6–7+, will result in heart rates beyond your safe zone of intensity to use during endurance exercise.

Therefore, it is helpful to monitor the intensity you're using at least twice during the aerobic segment of each workout session, by taking your pulse or quantifying your RPE. These numbers can be recorded at the conclusion of each class session, on Exercise 1.2, Heart Rates: Parts II & III, at the conclusion of this chapter.

Of course, if you're using a heart rate monitor, you can just follow the logging of data directly onto your programmed wrist unit (watch).

## *Summary*

"With life expectancy on the rise ~ it's now 78.2 years for a 50 year-old man and 82.1 years for a 50 year-old woman . . . [people] could be faced with decades of ill-health, if they don't make changes."[21] Enjoy making the changes *you* need to make, in order to be fit for life!

# *Goal-Setting Challenge*

Fitness is a choice, as is understanding how to apply what you learn. With these beliefs in mind:

✓ 1. Review each heading presented in Chapter 1. What question(s) come to mind regarding the information contained under those headings? Write down each point in question, on the space provided below.

_____

_____

_____

_____

_____

_____

_____

_____

_____

_____

_____

_____

_____

_____

✓ 2. Set an "assertiveness goal" for yourself to ask the instructor to more fully explain the above concept(s) at your next class meeting and to provide other recommended resources to read that will help clarify the point(s) you do not understand. This will facilitate your taking ownership for your learning. Record this as your Chapter 1 Aerobic Exercise Program Goal, following the four steps presented in Chapter 2, Exercise 2.3, then recording it in a Fitness Journal that you develop or purchase.

✓ 3. As part of this goal, state that you are purchasing a *daily planner* schedule book and set a goal to *make a date with yourself* to work out consistently, regarding **F**requency, **I**ntensity, and **T**ime duration (your **FIT** formula), practicing all that you are learning. Then, *keep every scheduled date* with yourself! If you work better with contracts and written commitments, write out a commitment to fitness and ask a best friend to be a witness, signing and dating your commitment.

## Part II: Target Heart Rates

Record 6-second or 10-second heart rate counts for the two aerobic intervals that you monitor in class. Were you over or under your target heart rate training zone?

| Week | I | | II | | III | | IV | | V | | VI | | VII | | VIII | | IX | | X | |
|------|---|---|---|---|---|---|---|---|---|---|---|---|---|---|---|---|---|---|---|---|
| Class | 1 | 2 | 1 | 2 | 1 | 2 | 1 | 2 | 1 | 2 | 1 | 2 | 1 | 2 | 1 | 2 | 1 | 2 | 1 | 2 |
| -1- | | | | | | | | | | | | | | | | | | | | |
| -2- | | | | | | | | | | | | | | | | | | | | |

**Aerobic Intervals**

My THR for 1 minute is: _____ - _____ .

## Part III: Ratings of Perceived Exertion

What did you feel during the various segments of your workout hour?

| 0.5 | 1 | 2 | 3 | 4 | 5 | 6 | 7 | 8 | 9 | 10 |
|-----|---|---|---|---|---|---|---|---|---|----|
| very very light | very light | light (weak) | moderate | some-what hard | heavy/ strong ("flow state") | hard | very hard | | | very very heavy almost maximum |

| Week | I | | II | | III | | IV | | V | | VI | | VII | | VIII | | IX | | X | |
|------|---|---|---|---|---|---|---|---|---|---|---|---|---|---|---|---|---|---|---|---|
| Class | 1 | 2 | 1 | 2 | 1 | 2 | 1 | 2 | 1 | 2 | 1 | 2 | 1 | 2 | 1 | 2 | 1 | 2 | 1 | 2 |
| Warm-Up | | | | | | | | | | | | | | | | | | | | |
| Aerobic Segments | | | | | | | | | | | | | | | | | | | | |
| Cool-Down | | | | | | | | | | | | | | | | | | | | |
| Relaxation | | | | | | | | | | | | | | | | | | | | |

## *Exercise 1.2  Heart Rates*
## Part I: Monitoring Your Resting Heart Rate

**NOTE:** Take your resting heart rate at the first possibility in the morning, before arising. Use the first two fingers at thumb side of wrist, the carotid artery in neck, the temple area, or other pulse point. Make comments within the graph.

| Week | II | | III | | IV | | V | | VI | | VII | | VIII | | IX | | X | |
|------|---|---|---|---|---|---|---|---|---|---|---|---|---|---|---|---|---|---|
| Class | 1 | 2 | 1 | 2 | 1 | 2 | 1 | 2 | 1 | 2 | 1 | 2 | 1 | 2 | 1 | 2 | 1 | 2 |
| 90 and above | | | | | | | | | | | | | | | | | | |
| 85 | | | | | | | | | | | | | | | | | | |
| 80 | | | | | | | | | | | | | | | | | | |
| 75 | | | | | | | | | | | | | | | | | | |
| 70 | | | | | | | | | | | | | | | | | | |
| 65 | | | | | | | | | | | | | | | | | | |
| 60 | | | | | | | | | | | | | | | | | | |
| 55 | | | | | | | | | | | | | | | | | | |
| 50 | | | | | | | | | | | | | | | | | | |
| 45 | | | | | | | | | | | | | | | | | | |
| 40 | | | | | | | | | | | | | | | | | | |
| 35 and below | | | | | | | | | | | | | | | | | | |

**Twice-Weekly Resting Heart Rate**

Resting H.R.   Week 1: _____   At Finish: _____   (−)Loss/(+)Gain: _____

# Exercise 1.3 How to Figure Your Target Heart Rate Training Zone

Three basic factors enter into figuring your estimated safe exercise zone. These must be established first:

1. Current age: _____.

2. How active is your lifestyle? _____% MHR.

   If you are: *(Choose one and place on the line above:)*

   - Non athletic adult: use 50% of your maximum heart rate.
   - Sedentary: use 60–69% of your maximum heart rate (but only for the first 2 or 3 weeks).
   - Moderately physically active: use 70–75% of your maximum heart rate.
   - Active and well-trained: use 80–85% of your maximum heart rate.

3. Your average resting heart rate (figured on Page 9)._____

Now place your numbers in the Karvonen formula:

A.      220          – _____ = _____ **Estimated Maximal Heart Rate (MHR)**
   **(Index number)**      **(Your age)**

B. _____ – _____ = _____
        **MHR**              **Resting HR**          **Heart Rate Reserve**

C. _____ × . _____ = _____ + _____ = _____ *
   **Heart Rate Reserve**   **Lower-end lifestyle**                    **Resting HR**
                            **activity range** (i.e., #2 above)

   _____ × . _____ = _____ + _____ = _____ *
   **Heart Rate Reserve**   **Higher-end lifestyle**                   **Resting HR**
                            **activity range** (i.e., #2 above)

*Range of your target*

**This means in 6 seconds (1/10th of a minute), my heart beats:**

   _____ – _____

This range is your estimated safe exercise zone. Keep your heart rate working in this range while you exercise aerobically for approximately 30 minutes of each session. Remember, refigure as you "age," as you can reclassify your lifestyle percentage, or as your resting heart rate declines markedly.

---

For example: Chris is 20 years old, a moderately active person (70–75% range), with a resting heart rate of 62.

A. 220 – 20 = 200  Estimated Maximum Heart Rate

B. 200 – 62 = 138 Heart Rate Reserve

C. 138 × .70 =  96 + 62 = 158*
   138 × .75 = 104 + 62 = 166*   ) Target heart rate training zone

If Chris keeps working (aerobically exercising) at the range of 158 to 166 heartbeats per minute, the heart will be working safely toward the training effect.

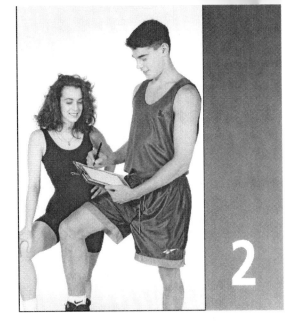

# Motivation and Goal Setting

**2**

*Finding the courage to change
is no more difficult
than learning to make
one small choice at a time.*

Shad Helmstetter

To develop a mindset for enjoying living a fitness lifestyle, you first must become *aware* of how you make the choices you're currently making and, more specifically, what internal resources you're using to make these choices. Even though you can directly experience the results of your choices, you probably are unaware of the internal process you used to lead you to make your choices.

Awareness of this internal process is essential to making new, more positive choices, for making all subsequent changes last a lifetime, and more important, for enjoying the journey. The end result is that your mindset, or thinking, changes!

## Taking Risks

Taking risks and embarking on something new requires courage. Changing your physical fitness status is one such situation. Being open to identifying your medical history to yourself and to others is difficult. Taking the risk of receiving pretesting results you don't really want to know (because you have a feeling they are not what you're going to want to hear) is hard to do. Being open to

suggestions on how to significantly change an unhealthy lifestyle that has become quite comfortable takes a significant act of courage and determination.

You have enrolled in this fitness course, so celebrate the decision you have already made—that first, small choice. You're on your way! The first step is behind you. If you approach becoming fit with an "eating-the-elephant-one-bite-at-a-time" mindset, you can digest each bite easily and it can become a part of you. This proactive, planned approach combined with consistent practice can become a lifestyle change that lasts.

Individuals who have a quick-fix, get-fit/lose-fat-in-a-few-weeks mindset and a need for instant results usually become impatient with their progress. They will do too much too soon, incur injuries, or lower their resistance and choke on the big bite of change they're trying to take all at once.

Which is your mindset, proactive or reactive? If it is the latter, *reframing* it (thinking about it differently) as a methodical, planned approach provides you with the opportunity to experience lasting results. Successes come continually

when change is a one-small-choice-at-a-time process instead of a one-big-end result. Celebrate your decision to change, and feel good about this one small choice. Then have patience with yourself, stay open-minded to ideas presented for you to consider, and enjoy the *process* of change that now is about to happen within you.

## Moving Out of Your Comfort Zone

Define to yourself: What are the reasons that have moved me out of my comfort zone and motivated me to take that first step, that one small choice, toward fitness? This is accomplished internally by forming *visual* pictures in your head, listening to what you're *saying* to yourself, or connecting with how you *feel* about your physical fitness status. Do you see/hear/feel/taste/smell (experience somehow) that you:

- Can't keep up and are out of breath while trying to accomplish everyday physical tasks?
- Choose to look better cosmetically and be more attractive to yourself and others?

- Have a physical ailment that you know you have because you haven't taken care of yourself?

- Now choose to be the best physical specimen of a human being you can possibly become?

- _____
  _____
  _____

- _____
  _____
  _____

Immediately write down the reasons you pictured specifically or heard yourself say or felt within yourself. These sensory descriptions are the pleasure-seeking or pain-avoiding reasons that are motivating you! The goals you set will require you to choose methods to gain these pleasures or to avoid these pains.

## *Motivation*

True motivation lies internally within each of us. Once you identify the pleasure you're seeking or pain you're avoiding, you can request assistance externally, from other people or your environment, to temporarily coach and support your decision. Instructors, classmates, friends, and attractive workout settings can give you the immediate information, encouragement, and gratification you need to get started on your fitness journey.

No one can be with you for all 1440 minutes available to you in your day to make the choices that reflect upon your fitness. Other people and your environment can be only temporary motivators in your lifetime fitness journey because they are all external to you. It's the "Kleenex® analogy."[1] Use them when you need to. Then discard them and carry on!

True motivation and lasting change have to be developed or happen internally. This type of motivation is not difficult to acquire. Your internal coach is there just waiting to be called upon.[2] Internal motivation

is simply a matter of understanding *how* to use your unlimited internal resources.

## What Are My Internal Resources?

Your internal resources are thoughts reflecting

— past and present life experiences

— past, present, and future needs, wants, and goals.[3]

You can use your internal resources to empower you when you need motivation, or to give you ideas on how to or how not to set your physical fitness goals.

Defining what these resources are within you will give you the key to accessing and enhancing your future and provide you with the ability to set powerful goals. These resources consist of your:

- Hereditary and environmental influences

- Positive and negative life experiences

- Wants, needs, priorities, and goals

- Strengths, talents, and interests

- Weaknesses, risk factors, and poor choices

- Beliefs/truths/rules you follow

- Attitudes (interpreting an experience as positive or negative)

- Feelings (emotions)

- Actions/behaviors/choices you have expressed (resulting from all of the above)

Take a contemplative moment and review these points. What mental pictures, self-talk, and feelings surface as thoughts reflecting your life experiences, needs, wants, and goals? In terms of your physical fitness, the resources that surface will represent pleasure-filled or painful memories—thoughts with resulting actions that you'll choose to experience again and ones you don't choose to experience ever again!

Moving toward pleasure-based results and away from painful ones are the driving forces behind motivation. The direction you've just stated (toward pleasure or away from pain) reflects *how* and *where* you've stored your internal resources.

## How Internal Resources Affect Motivation

How and where have you stored your thoughts (internal resources) sensory-wise regarding your physical fitness? Do you remember an earlier attempt at aerobics, step training, fitness walking, strength training, or stretching as a positive experience that met your goal at the time? How do you picture, hear, taste, smell, self-talk, and feel about that experience? You might say, "Great workout! The fitness facility looked clean, the music was easy to follow, I was energized, and I made lots of friends!" or, "The room smelled terrible, the people were unfriendly, and I felt awkward. I'll never go back there!"

What answers your thoughts are your *sensory representations*. Visual pictures, sounds, feelings, tastes, or smells come to mind. You can hear yourself stating them. You can see yourself in the situation. And, a feeling comes over you that is either pleasant or painful. Motivation, thus, has the following sensory components:

- Images, sounds, tastes, smells

- Internal self-talk

- Body sensations (movements, touch, emotions)

### Images, Sounds, Tastes, Smells

Individuals can take ownership of, or responsibility for, *how* they are picturing or imaging the fitness goals they're choosing to set. Images that are big, bright, up close, in color, and moving are more powerful than small, dim, far away, black-and-white, freeze-frame images.

The same applies to tastes, sounds, and smells. They are fresh or tangy, soft or loud, strong or weak. Apply this concept now and ask yourself: "How *large* are the images I'm making in my head? Are they small like a postcard or large like a poster?" (see Figure 2.1). More powerful images are more motivating. Goals established with powerful images will be accomplished much more quickly.

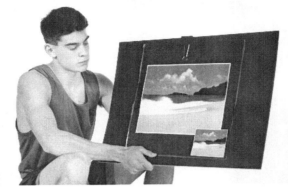

"How large are the images I'm making in my head? Are they small like a postcard or large like a poster?"

**Figure 2.1** Self-Talk

### Self-Talk

Internal dialogue, or self-talk, that is in the present tense, positive, moving (verb has "ing" on the end), and enabling is more motivating than self-talk that is in the past tense or future tense, negative, and disabling (see Figure 2.1 text). For example, stating, "I'm confident of my ability to learn new aerobics moves quickly and am enjoying my instructor's creative, improvising style" is more powerful and motivating than stating to oneself, "I will begin to feel confident of my ability in aerobics class as soon as I learn all the basic moves and get to know the instructor."

Listen to the verbs and adverbs in your sentences, and construct talk that is as if it's already accomplished, for this is how you state your goals to yourself on paper and in your head. An assessment of your self-talk is provided in Exercise 2.1 located at the end of the chapter.

### Body Sensations

Body sensations that focus on gaining pleasure instead of avoiding pain ("doing my best" instead of "not coming in last") and sensations that are quick, powerful, big, high, and the like are the most motivating. For example, if you want to get up in the morning and are lying in the comfort of bed, what will motivate you to get up? Actually, what *did* motivate you to get up at 6:30 a.m. on a Saturday morning this past winter? Did you:

- *Picture* how cold, gray, and dreary it was outside?

- *Say*, "Gosh, it's so *early*, and I'm so *tired*," and *move* slowly out of bed?

or did you:

- *Picture* a fun event you had planned for the day, complete with great smells and tastes?
- *Say* to yourself, "It's great to be alive! Today is a fresh new day with no mistakes!"
- *Spring* up quickly?

If you're not motivated to do something you must change your images, sounds, tastes, smells, self-talk, movements, touch, and feelings.

## Changing Sensory Representations

Changing your sensory representations requires you to understand how you *experience* or perceive your world, how you *store* these perceptions in your head, and how you *retrieve* the information. Immediately following retrieval of information, you respond with actions and choices. It is important to realize that you can *change* those perceptions (or experience), storage, and retrieval of information and subsequently change your actions and choices. Understanding that you have the power to change your thinking *physiologically* and, therefore, to change the results you get is exciting!

### Eye Accessing

Eye accessing is a natural and instinctive process. It is not trained eye movement (e.g., eye contact).

According to established research on eye and head positions during various modes of thought,[4–7] when you are making *visual pictures*, you hold your head at chin level or higher (Figure 2.2). Your eyes are looking forward or up, and to one side (left or right, specifically according to your "internal map" or "timeline"). If you are making *remembered* pictures, your eyes are up and to one specific side (left or right according to your map), or up and forward. If you are making *constructed* pictures (future pictures), as occurs when you are goal setting, or if you can't remember something, or if you recall incorrectly or lie, your eyes are up and to the other side (the opposite side from your remembered images), or up and forward.

When remembering or constructing *sounds and words*, the eyes turn toward the ears in a horizontal movement. The *remembered* sounds/words are accessed toward the memory side. The sounds/words a person has not experienced yet, can't recall, recalls incorrectly, or that are lies, are accessed toward the *constructed* side.

When carrying on *internal dialogue* (engaging in positive or negative self-talk), the head will

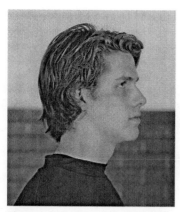

**Figure 2.2** Accessing Visual Images

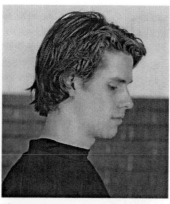

**Figure 2.3** Accessing Self-talk or Recitations; Feelings, Touch, or Movement

**Eye Access Cues**

Note: All visuals here are from the perspective of
YOU OBSERVING OTHERS,
i.e., seeing their accessing sides, from your perspective.

Step 1:

LEFTY

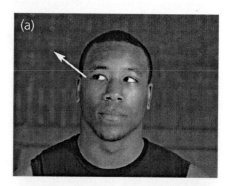

RIGHTY

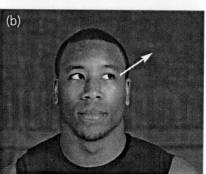

**Figure 2.4** Determining Visual Remembered Side of *Others*

lower, the chin will drop, you will be looking down and to one side (*remembered side*) and talking to yourself (Figure 2.3). When you access how you *feel*, especially painful emotions such as anger, sadness, and fear, your head and chin again will be in the lowered position, looking down and to the other side (opposite the self-talk side).

The *location* sides of visual and auditory remembered and constructed thought, self-talk and recitation, and feelings have been coded and are individual. They can be determined easily by your observing others, or by others observing you. Using Figures 2.4 and 2.5, determine your own "map" (your remembered information side and your constructed side) by asking someone to observe how you access the answer to a fact that is a remembered visual picture you've stored such as:

- What color was the first automobile you drove as a new driver?
- What color and design was your bedspread when you were a grade-school child?
- What color and shape is your current toothbrush?

- What were your high school colors?
- Describe an unforgettable toy from your childhood.

From *their perspective,* the side your eyes immediately travel to instinctively to retrieve/access the information (Figure 2.4), is your *remembered* visual side (this memory-side location never changes). Knowing a person's remembered visual side is the first step in understanding his or her eye access cues and internal map.

---

*Any change or goal setting must begin at the sensory representation, internal-thought level.*

---

Figure 2.5 represents the two basic internal processing maps possible and will help you observe others' accessing all of their stored perceptions. As you look at a person *from your perspective* does he or she look left or right to 'access remembered information? (It is easier to begin watching others before

you begin to understand your own internal map.) From others watching you, did they say that you access memory like the Lefty or the Righty (left or right from their perspective)? The answer tells you the location and map regarding how and where you can begin to change the images, sounds, feelings, tastes, or smells you've stored. Physiologically, this is where all permanent change begins.

Some people's maps tend to travel directionally more in a back-center-forward direction when describing past-present-future. They appear to look up and back, through the top of their skull, for information located in the past (behind them), look directly in front of themselves for the present, and defocus and look far in front of themselves when detailing future thought.

# Lefty

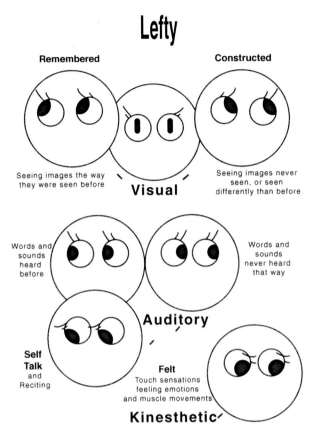

# Righty

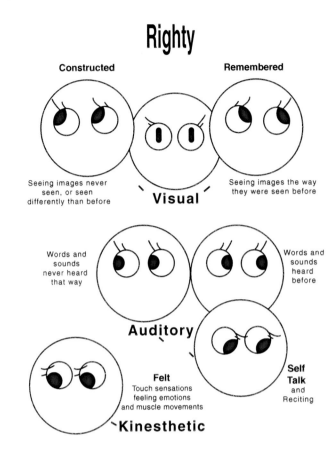

**Figure 2.5** Coding of Eye-Accessing Locations

## Hand Gesturing and Predicates

Various other physiological directional movements enable you to determine internal maps or timelines. Directional movement of your hand gestures indicating the past, the present, and the future match eye accessing. Either hand will gesture the *past* toward your *memory* side, your present in the center in front of you, and the *future* toward your *constructed* side.

In addition, among other physiologies not discussed here, you can experience accessing your information through predicates in your sentences. "I *see* what you mean" cues your eyes to travel upward. "I *hear* you" cues your eyes to travel horizontally. "I *feel* depressed" cues your eyes downward toward the side where your kinesthetics are stored.

The "eye accessing" information can be a key to understanding your internal resources and what motivates you. It can assist you with setting and achieving powerful goals that may have eluded you in the past. Once you understand how you make images, sounds, smells, taste, self-talk, and the body sensations of movement, touch, and feelings, *you*

---

*If you're not motivated to do something, you must physiologically change your images, tastes, sounds, smells, self-talk, movements, touch and feelings. It's as simple as that.*

---

*will know exactly how and where to begin the change process.*

A final example may clarify accessing and how you've stored your thoughts. Picture in your mind experiencing first "the thrill of victory" and then "the agony of defeat." When people are experiencing victory, physiologically the head and chin are level or up and pictures and sounds are being made. When they are experiencing defeat, physiologically the head and chin drop, and feelings or self-talk are tapped into. To get out of this agony-of-defeat mindset, you literally must physiologically "keep your chin up" so you no longer are accessing the disabling feelings or self-talk that is spatially located down. It's just as simple as that.

## Goal-Setting Strategies

To use your full potential to set powerful goals, you must take ownership of your internal resources. This requires you to take responsibility and *not to blame others or the environment* for your successes and failures. Retaining ownership of your total fitness program goals provides you with the ability to change, to set powerful goals that you choose, and to go about the business of systematically achieving them.

If a goal you're setting for yourself doesn't happen soon enough and any type of blame enters the internal picturing, feelings, and self-talk—stop. Take ownership and state: "*I own this situation. How can I get the results I need? How can I repicture or talk differently about this situation so it is helpful to me?*" Taking ownership of your internal resources—your thoughts—is the key to personal freedom and to achieving goals. You have a free will, and you are in charge of your life.

## Establishing Priorities

It's time to apply your new knowledge of internal motivation and plan your future by first acknowledging, and perhaps re-establishing, your time priorities. This is important so that you are providing yourself with enough time to achieve the goals you're setting.

Priorities reflect how you spend your time and are the *means* to reach your goals (the *ends* you seek). Exercise 2.2 at the conclusion of this chapter invites you to record your time by providing columns for you to identify how many hours per day and week you devote to each priority, and to record "time robbers" (any activity that *takes you away from the priority*—it may be another priority).

Can you associate an excellent role model with each priority? Record the names of your role models in the column provided. Positive role models provide us time-saving, short-cut ideas on how to do something the quickest, most efficient, and best way possible. Take advantage of their strategies by asking them how they do what they do, or by reading their biographies.

In the last column of this exercise, rank each priority by how you feel about its importance (not which takes the most time). A key to setting powerful fitness goals includes prioritizing your activities toward meeting the goals you're setting.

## Creating the Future in Advance

The foundation for successful goal setting has been established and consists of:

1. Identifying reasons you're choosing to change (pleasure seeking or pain-avoidance values)

2. Becoming aware of how you're motivated—which senses you use and how—and, consequently, how to change your actions at the sensory-thought level

3. Assessing and re-establishing your time priorities, providing the time to enable change to happen.

You now are prepared to set very powerful goals. The goal-setting procedure in Exercise 2.1 tells your brain precisely what goal you are choosing to set and provides solid (positive, pleasure) reasoning for why you're choosing this goal. It then breaks the link to old programming by stating all of your negative pain-avoidance reasons for having the goal. Heap them on big here! Make it *painful* to continue to make poor choices! Then make immediate positive action choices to create the motivational

pictures, self-talk, and movements necessary to initiate active change in your program, starting this moment.

Do you need more help with making change? Make an audiotape of yourself responding to the questions and statements for each goal you set. You'll find that listening to a tape provides the needed repetition for the blueprinting process to occur and is a unique short-cut to achieving your goals. During the entire goal-setting process, have fun during your pursuit of fitness!

## Developing a Goal Script

Exercise 2.3, Fitness Course Goals: A Sample Goal Script to Model will help you write your own goal script. After carefully reviewing this four-step procedure, begin writing one goal for both Chapter 1 (if you have not yet written this) and Chapter 2. Record all course goals in a Fitness Journal that you develop or purchase. This procedure is designed so that you can set goals for all of the chapters of this text, after you have studied the material. You will end up with all of your goals in one handy location, to review and continually update.

In sum, setting goals helps keep you focused daily on improvement and positive change. It encourages consistency in your fitness program and helps keep you on target.

When they are properly set internally and nourished continually, goals will become reality. Believe it, and you will see it. Your future resides within you as a rich resource of possibilities.

*One simple decision:*
*consciously*
*actively*
*make your choices.*

Shad Helmstetter

## Exercise 2.1  Motivation: What Do You Say When You Talk to Yourself?

### Step One:   Assessment

Have you ever listened to your intrapersonal (self) communication? We talk to ourselves all of our waking hours, and our internal dialogue is either positive and enabling or negative and disabling to us.

What do you say when you talk to yourself? Become aware and listen to yourself for an hour, a day, 2 days, or a week, and write your internal dialogue statements (both positive and negative) as shown in the examples.

Our self-talk usually takes the form of "I" statements followed by am/enjoy/hate/fear/think/feel/want/need/worry about, and so on.

Examples:
"I enjoy Peter and his attention to details."
"I've been such a klutz! I've dropped everything today."
"I need to get in shape; I can't breathe after going up a flight of stairs."
"I want to lose ten pounds before Spring Break."

_____

_____

_____

_____

_____

_____

_____

_____

_____

_____

_____

_____

_____

_____

_____

Continue listing self-talk statements on a separate paper and staple to this assessment.

### Step Two:   Evaluation

After you've recorded your self-talk for up to a week, go back and evaluate each comment as positive or negative. Place an "N" before the comment if it was negative and a "P" in front of those that are positive.

Total your entries as positive and negative below.

Totals:   Positive  =  _____

Negative  =  _____

### Step Three:   Reprogramming

The next step in the reprogramming a negative disabling attitude (expressed through self-talk) is accomplished by updating and actually rewording each negative statement you wrote so each reads positive and enabling to you. This opens a channel for you to begin to achieve your goal of an improved attitude.

1. Replace all use of past or future tense verbs and adverbs (negative language in regard to personal attitude and fitness mindset improvement): need to, want to, going to, ought to, should, could, wish, used to be, have been, was, and so forth.

2. Rewrite each of the predicate phrases using positive, present-tense language (I am, I enjoy, I can), and use verbs with "ing" as much as possible to represent movement. State these phrases as if you have already achieved the outcome of your new script.

   Example:   *Old*:  I need to quit smoking.
   *New*:  I *enjoy being* a non-smoker.

3. Add another helpful line or two, to each new script, if you wish.

   Example: *Old*: I need to cut out eating high-fat, high-salt, and highly sugared foods such as cookies for snacks when I get hungry mid-morning at work.

   *New*: I enjoy selecting a highly nutritional, low-calorie snack such as fruit or juice when I get hungry at work mid-morning. *I feel better about myself every time I make this better choice!*

4. State positives of positives. If, however, you choose to add the negative because you think it will help, place it as the second or last sentence of your new script.

   Example: *Old*: I need to exercise more than once a week, and to eat less junk food such as doughnuts.
   *New*: I am pace walking 3 miles every day and enjoy being a "fat-burner" instead of a "fat-storer." *I don't eat FAT PILLS (doughnuts) any more!*

# Exercise 2.1 Motivation: What Do You Say When You Talk to Yourself? (continued)

5. Be specific as to the outcome of each new script's goal. Tell your brain exactly what you want and are now choosing to do.

Example: *Old*: I enjoy exercising to improve my health.

*New*: I enjoy exercising *at my target heart rate for 40 continuous minutes, 4 or more days every week*, to continue achieving my goal of dropping a pound of body fat a week.

_____

_____

_____

_____

_____

_____

_____

_____

_____

_____

_____

_____

_____

_____

_____

_____

_____

_____

_____

_____

_____

### Step Four: Taping Your Own "Reprogramming-for-Improvement" Audio Tape

Developing your own "tape talk" tool can prove to be one of the most influential and rapid ways for you to achieve the changes you're choosing to make.

1. Purchase a good, blank audiotape. Give it an interesting title.

2. Review your self-talk assessment (Step 1) and take note of some of your most used negative self-talk ideas or phrases (Step 2). Select 15–18 reprogrammed scripts (Step 3) to tape.

3. You can also reword new beliefs/philosophies that you now choose to adopt that haven't "stuck" yet. Use positive, present-tense language throughout.

4. Take your transcribed new scripts, and on recording tape slowly repeat each of the suggestions three times, pausing briefly between each suggestion.

5. Repeat this procedure for each new script. (If you have 15 new scripts, you will have a total of 45 suggestions; if you use 18 new scripts, you will have 54 new suggestions).

6. End the taping session by recording each of the phrases/scripts one more time each, but this time change "I" to "You." This provides for the external validation that we all need. The total number of scripts on your entire tape now will be 60/72. Example: "I am a good listener and enjoy hearing what others have to say" becomes, "*You* are a good listener and enjoy hearing what others have to say."

7. If possible, add appropriate instrumental background music while you tape record. Soft, pulsating music seems to affect the way the brain receives and permanently stores information. To do this, you'll need an additional CD/tape player, playing the music on it separate from your taping instrument.

8. Talk your scripts onto your tape with emotion! Any programming you currently have in your head is etched more permanently if you experience it in a highly emotional state.

9. Rework your thoughts in language you will like to hear. This taping can be a lot of fun.

10. Play your tape while you are doing something else—getting ready each morning, during a break while you are relaxing, during a drive in the car to or from class or work, or as you are getting ready for bed. Play it once or twice a day the first 3 weeks, then once a day until you realize that you've mastered all of these challenges. When this occurs, it's time to make a new tape on other new challenges!

# *Exercise 2.2  Establishing Your Top 20 Time Priorities*

Time priorities are the *means* to your ends (goals). They are interests and activities that you give time to in the wellness areas (physical/social/emotional/spiritual/intellectual/talent expression) of your life, from the minute that you arise in the morning until you go to bed at night—every day, or at least once a week.

| **Top 20 Time Priorities** (listed In any order) | **Role Model** | **Hours Each Day** | **Hours Each Week** | **Time Robbers** (takes you away from the priority) | **Rank Order (1–20) of Importance** |
|---|---|---|---|---|---|
| • | | | | | # |
| • | | | | | # |
| • | | | | | # |
| • | | | | | # |
| • | | | | | # |
| • | | | | | # |
| • | | | | | # |
| • | | | | | # |
| • | | | | | # |
| • | | | | | # |
| • | | | | | # |
| • | | | | | # |
| • | | | | | # |
| • | | | | | # |
| • | | | | | # |
| • | | | | | # |
| • | | | | | # |
| • | | | | | # |
| • | | | | | # |
| • | | | | | # |

# Exercise 2.3  Fitness Course Goals

## A Sample Goal Script to Model

*Directions*: For every goal you'll set, follow the four steps presented next. Each uses one or several full sentences for each step. All of the responses to these four components of a goal collectively become one goal or goal script—the precise language you'll repeat to yourself at least twice daily until you achieve the goal. (If you make an audiotape of your goal scripts, you'll achieve your goals more quickly.)

**Step 1:** All powerful goals use the SMART formula: specific, measurable, achievable, realistic, timely. Now state one goal, using positive, present-tense verbs, as if you have already achieved it. Do not use past or future tense verbs such as: want to, need to, going to, ought to, should, wish, etc. Begin by asking yourself, "What am I choosing to experience—see, hear, taste, smell, or feel—when I achieve it?" You'll recognize these as the components of motivation.

*Example:* "I am choosing to be labeled 'physically fit' within the next 10 weeks and to continue dropping 1–2 pounds of fat per week during that time, by practicing everything I learn in this class, for two additional 40-minute sessions per week, at the 5:00 p.m. aerobics session at the student recreation center."

**Step 2:** Again using complete sentences, state your pleasure-value reasons, using positive, present-tense verbs. Ask yourself, "Why am I totally committed to achieving each goal?" This involves your positive, "moving-toward" values. Values you are choosing to feel by achieving this goal may be any of the following: adventure and change, commitment, freedom, giving pleasure to others, happiness, health, love, power, prestige, and worth, security, life purpose, success, expression of talent, trust, loyalty, and any other positive values important to you.

*Example:* "Having this goal and continually working on it proves that I am able to make and keep commitments to myself. I look and feel healthier and am able to breathe easier. I feel a new sense of self-discipline and in charge of my life."

**Step 3:** Using complete sentences, state your pain-avoidance reasons, but for this step only, use future-tense verbs. Because we do more to avoid pain than to gain pleasure, heap on the painful thoughts so you are really motivated to change! Break the link of the old programmed ways by first asking yourself, "What painful values am I choosing to avoid?"

Some pain-avoidance values that you'll feel if you don't achieve this goal, or at least immediately begin working on it, are: anger and resentment, anxiety and worry, boredom, depression, embarrassment, frustration, guilt, humiliation, jealousy, overwhelmed, physical pain, prejudice, rejection, sadness.

*Example:* "If I don't continually work on this goal I've set, I will feel angry, guilty, and depressed at myself that I can't follow through on something that is extremely important to me at this time in my life. Why would I choose to continually feel this way?!"

**Step 4:** Finally, reestablish the pleasure link by picturing, hearing, feeling, "what actions do I choose to take or do immediately to master this goal? What is something I can start doing right now and within the next 24 hours?" Use full sentences, present-tense verbs, and specific, measurable, achievable, realistic, and timely wording.

*Example:* "I am choosing to practice all of the physical fitness moves I am learning in class this term at least every other day, for 40 continuous minutes per session, at my target heart rate. In addition, I choose to be aware continually of all the mental training aspects I am learning and incorporate them into my daily total fitness program, too. Following each workout session, I am journaling my progress in this text. I am starting this program at 5:00 p.m. today."

This is your entire goal, stated in the form of a script of motivational language that you alone have chosen. This is the format used by individuals in the professional world and private sector alike who daily achieve excellence, success, and their goals!

## Writing My Personal Goals

Write one goal script for each chapter of this book after you have studied it. Directly relate the goal to the information covered in that chapter. Keep all of your goals in a Fitness Journal by developing your own (or purchasing a blank) journal book for recording. As goals are accomplished remember to establish new goals to work on, so that your growth and change continue.

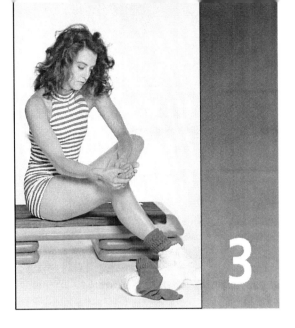

# Safety First

**3**

All physical activities have an element of risk. By taking proper preventive measures, however, problems and injuries can be minimized. The following discussion will alert you to some of the more common concerns.

Self-discipline is required to become and stay physically fit. The dividends of wellness and vitality are well worth it.

## Signs of Overexertion

Monitoring your pulse helps to determine how hard to exercise your body, but you also need to be aware of your own bodily signs of overexertion. Signs are:

- Severe breathlessness.

- Poor heart rate response (continually monitoring too high an exercising heart rate that does not drop significantly after 1 minute of recovery, or final heart rate not below 120 beats per minute after 5 minutes of cool-down.

- Undue fatigue during exercise and inability to recover from a workout later in the day.

- Insomnia.

- Persistent, severe muscle soreness. (The type of muscle soreness to guard against is not immediate but instead, becomes apparent 24–48 hours after exercise.)

- Nausea, feeling faint, dizziness.

- Tightness or pains in the chest.

These symptoms do not indicate that you shouldn't exercise. Rather, they suggest a reduced level of activity until you develop the capacity to handle more intense workouts. You should undertake an exercise program cautiously, and increase the frequency, intensity, and duration of each session gradually.

If you have any of the following symptoms, ease gradually to a slow walk, sit with your head between your knees, or lie down on your back and elevate your feet. The latter will help the blood move to your head more readily and carry the needed oxygen to your brain. If any of these symptoms persist, contact your doctor.

1. Abnormal heart action

   - Irregular pulse

   - Fluttering, jumping, or palpitations in chest or throat

   - Sudden burst of rapid heartbeats

   - Sudden, very slow pulse when a moment before it had been on target (immediate or delayed)

---

Some general tips for sensible training are:

1. Progress gradually in your sessions.
2. Be sure to both warm up and cool down.
3. Progress from easy to advanced in the stretches, aerobic options, and strength-training exercises.
4. Learn to read your body signs. You're going to perspire, and you're going to tire a little. With an effective fitness program, you may encounter some initial, slight, temporary discomfort, but do not perform to the point of exhaustion.
5. Pace yourself. For example, after engaging in numerous aerobics moves, a complete step-training routine, or one lap in your fitness walking, you may be short of breath. This should subside within minutes. If it doesn't, you've worked too hard.
6. If you are unsure about a specific discomfort or pain, ask a reliable person (such as your physician) about it before continuing with exercise.

---

*Undertake an exercise program cautiously, and increase the frequency, intensity, and duration of each session gradually.*

---

2. Pain or pressure in the center of the chest or the arm or throat precipitated by exercise or after exercise (immediate or delayed)

3. Dizziness, lightheadedness, sudden incoordination, confusion, cold sweat, glassy stare, pallor, blue skin tone, or fainting (immediate)

Do not try to cool down. Stop exercise and lie down with your feet elevated, or put your head down between your legs until the symptoms pass.[1]

## Safety Variables

Numerous variables can affect a fitness program. These include illness, infection, or injury, lack of exercise for a while, location and environment, and shoe selection, among others.

### Illness, Infection, or Injury

Illness, infection, or injury will show up in your "thermometer of fitness," your pulse. The pulse will be higher at rest and will escalate to the training zone with less than your usual effort. In that event, take it easy and decide whether to "walk through" your program mentally to maintain your discipline of exercising or to curtail exercise until you're completely well again.

### Lapse in Exercising

If you have missed aerobic exercise for a time, return to it slowly. When you miss activity several times, you will need to start more cautiously, as if beginning a new program. For example, you may have a bout of flu, which renders you unable to exercise for a week. When you are able to

exercise again, do not plan to start where you left off. Return cautiously to the fitness level where you were before the illness.

A leading cardiologist in the United States has stated that you will lose approximately half of your fitness program gains after just 5 weeks if you discontinue your program totally. After 10 weeks of no aerobic activity, you will have lost most of your fitness gains.[2] Whenever a circumstance curtails your program, return to it slowly and systematically.

## Location and Environment

Select a convenient and physiologically safe location for your workouts. Choose a *wood*-based floor or an area carpeted with flat nap and thick padding. (Carpeted surfaces tend to make lateral moves and turns risky, however.) Try not to exercise on concrete, as it has no "give" or buoyancy. Concrete surfaces impose unnecessary stress on your legs and feet.

> A resilient floor should be selected for exercise that involves repeated foot impacts. If such a surface is not available, the exercise routines should be modified to ensure that the feet remain close to the floor throughout the program (low-impact exercises).[3]

If relative humidity is high and the temperature is 85° (room or outside), curtail your aerobics, step training, or fitness walking program. Seek another option, such as aerobic swimming in a cool-air environment.

For aerobic exercise a cold environment is fine as long as you protect yourself thoroughly, especially your air passages. (At 40°F and below, cover your air passages.)

Heat, however, *does* matter. You can incur heat stress injuries if you abandon caution.

## The Proper Shoes

The shoes you wear constitute one of your major requirements. When you jump or run, you place three to six times more force on your feet than when you are stationary. If you weigh 125 pounds, you are placing 375 to 750 pounds of pressure on your feet with each jump. Your body can withstand the stress of exercise better if you wear shoes that shock-absorb this pressure or exercise on a surface with a giving quality. Select a shoe that totally supports your foot for your exercise modality. The following criteria[4] give specific guidelines for personalizing your shoe selection.

- Inquire about midsole composition. For durability and performance, select shoes made from either compression-molded ethyl vinyl acetate (EVA) or polyurethane.

- Stay with the same brand and model of shoe you are replacing if it has been satisfactory.

- Do not allow yourself to be forced or pressured into buying a shoe that does not feel comfortable.

- About every 4 months replace a single pair of shoes worn at least 4 days per week for any fitness-related activity. If the shoes have a polyurethane midsole, the wear may be extended up to 6 months. If they have a standard, open-cell EVA midsole, they might last only 3 months.

- Examine the inside of the shoe as well as the insole. Shoes with removable insoles are preferable because they tend to be better cushioned and allow the fit of a custom foot orthotic, if needed.[5]

- Get nylon uppers rather than leather uppers if you want a cooler shoe. If you prefer an

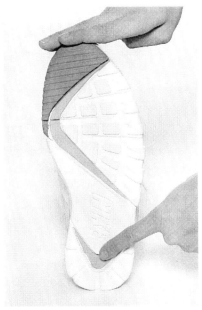

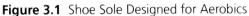

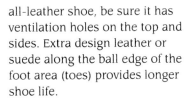

This sole, with the rubber designed for sideward movement, and the heel unflaired, is suitable for aerobics.

**Figure 3.1** Shoe Sole Designed for Aerobics

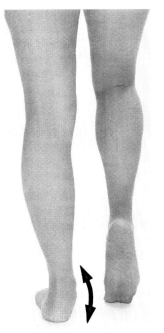

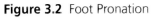

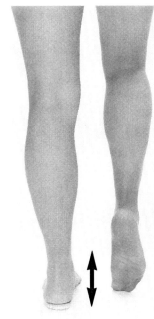

**Figure 3.2** Foot Pronation

**Figure 3.3** Foot Pronation Corrected with a Sports Orthotic

all-leather shoe, be sure it has ventilation holes on the top and sides. Extra design leather or suede along the ball edge of the foot area (toes) provides longer shoe life.

- Choose a shoe that has a sole with a relatively smooth tread[6] and of white rubber, designed for aerobics or court use (Figure 3.1). Jogging shoes with black rubber soles, designed for road and track running and with rubber triangles, squares, circles, or thick waves provide excellent forward movement, but because aerobics consists of forward, backward, and lateral movement, this is not the best choice of shoe sole.

   The rough treads of most running shoes can be hazardous during aerobic exercise dance as they can cause the feet to come to an abrupt halt each time they strike the floor. Thus, most shoes designed for running are unsuitable for aerobic dance.[7]

- If you have a tendency toward *pronated ankles* (the lower leg bones do not sit directly on the ankle, as shown in Figure 3.2),

do not select a wide heel flair of rubber. This heel flair will limit, to some extent, your lateral (sideward) movement and also will not provide the appropriate correction to avoid possible future injury to naturally weak ankles, as it does in jogging, which is all forward movement. Pronation of the ankles can be corrected inside the shoe by means of:

- an extra firm heel box
- raising the arch with a specifically designed wedge
- controlling the floor contact of various portions of the foot by a specially designed orthotic (prescribed corrective device) for the foot, as shown in Figure 3.3

*Sports orthotics* are devices that are custom-made to control the function of your specific foot. They are not arch supports. They are shaped to control your foot closely the entire time it is on the floor or ground. The bones in your foot are moved so the muscles can function and adapt normally, decreasing or eliminating foot problems. The orthotics are made of an unbreakable, reinforced

material and are worn inside your athletic shoe.[8]

A person doesn't have to live with the pain that structural imbalances cause, such as the entire bottom of the foot aching from the forward movement of running or shin splints from the lateral movement of aerobics. Sports orthotics can be prescribed by a qualified specialist, such as a podiatrist.

## Comfort While on the Move!

Consider taking a therapeutic foot massage using Hydropedes™ to relieve the discomfort and fatigue your feet feel daily. Whether participating in your high or low impact aerobic workouts, standing on your feet all day at work (especially if you're on cement), or even during the time in between when you're just moving about, Hydropedes™ glycerin-filled insoles with Cambrelle® (see Figure 3.4) can provide the comfort you need for your active lifestyle.

## Features and Benefits[9]

**CUSHION** — Hydropedes™ provide a cushion to the entire bottom of

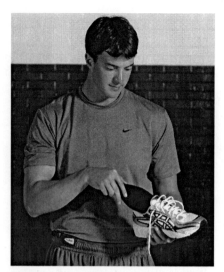

**Figure 3.4** Hydropedes™ glycerin-filled insoles provide an all-day therapeutic foot massage.

the feet. Some people begin to lose this padding at an earlier age than others, and some never lose it. When this erosion begins to occur, certain bones in the bottom of the foot become closer to the skin. Hydropedes™ help considerably in the reduction of pain due to heel spurs, stone bruises, and pain suffered by individuals who spend long hours standing and/or walking on hard surfaces.

**MASSAGE** — Hydropedes™ offer a constant massage to the bottom of the feet. With each step, the glycerin gel is moved forward, and as the ball of the foot descends, the gel moves back to the heel of the foot. By creating this action, there is a constant massage on the bottom of the feet, as long as the Hydropedes™ are in place. There are thousands of nerve endings located at the bottom of the feet. These nerve endings lead to various parts of the body (refer to a Reflexology Chart on the packaging). The nerve areas are set in small clusters and have a tendency to accumulate deposits. Massaging these little nodes, over a period of time, can actually break up the deposits that have formed on the nerve clusters. By massaging the bottom of the feet, Hydropedes™ work constantly to

break up these deposits. The glycerin gel is of a dense consistency, which makes it slower in movement than many other liquids. The slower movement creates a deeper massage action and therefore is very therapeutic.

**ABSORBS SHOCK** — Hydropedes™ can dramatically reduce shock on the lower skeletal system. The glycerin gel actually "floats the foot," therefore the shock is absorbed by the insole and not the ankles, knees, and lower back.

**EVEN DISTRIBUTION OF WEIGHT** — It is a known fact that liquid seeks its own level. The glycerin gel in Hydropedes™ will, therefore, float the foot, allowing an even distribution of weight. A foam rubber or plastic insole is not able to do this. The even distribution of weight also reduces the amount of friction on the feet, which can lead to relief from painful calluses, plantar warts, and excessive perspiration.

The brochure accompanying Hydropedes™ provides complete instructions and answers to all of your questions.[10] Insert the insoles with the black side up and the gray side down.

## Proper Clothing

Choosing what to wear for the environment in which you are exercising is important. Safety, comfort, and ease of movement are the variables for aerobics apparel. Dressing in layers is best. A warm-up sweatsuit or jogging suit will help to increase the temperature of your arm and leg muscles during warm-up. On very warm or highly humid and warm days this, of course, is unnecessary. Cotton material is best, as it absorbs perspiration better than other fabrics. When cotton clothing becomes damp, the surrounding air causes the moisture to evaporate, and this cools the body.

During laps or routines you'll need to be free to move in all directions and sweat freely. Therefore, choose to wear as little as possible, especially when the temperature and

relative humidity are high. Avoid long, loose slacks, as they can catch under the feet. The same is true for tight-fitting garments, as they restrict flexibility. The best advice for someone who exercises vigorously is to keep clothing to a comfortable minimum. This allows unrestricted motion and facilitates loss of excessive body heat.[11]

Exercise apparel kept to a comfortable minimum is a solid guideline for all participants, to avoid heat stress injuries. Individuals who are overweight or obese are prime targets for overheating because they have a thick layer of fat tissue between the internal organs and the outer layer of skin. It works like insulation, retaining internal heat.

The internal body systems may overheat and cause heat exhaustion or heat stroke. Therefore, don't try to "sweat" off water pounds by wearing lots of clothing or rubber-lined sweatsuits. Sweat and water loss are body cooling mechanisms and are not to be used in measuring weight loss. Water is *not* fat!

To prevent friction in your shoes, wear cotton socks, and smooth out any wrinkles. Cotton absorbs sweat. This will help keep your feet drier and free from blisters.

Finally, do not wear a towel around the neck during exercise. The major artery from the heart to the brain is located in the neck area, and it has to be free for cooling by exposure to air of the skin surface in that area.

## Fluid Intake

Water is the principal means of transporting heat (and substances) within the body. In warm inside and outside environments, it is the *only* means of dispersing body heat. This is accomplished by the evaporation of released perspiration on the surface of the skin. When the room air contacts the sweat, the skin surface is cooled, and the cooling then is conducted internally. Production of body heat increases greatly during physical exercise.

Unless water for perspiration is available, the body temperature increases beyond normal, causing overheating. When fluid loss exceeds supply, dehydration follows. When dehydration sets in, even modest physical activity causes the heart rate and body temperature to increase. When the water loss is approximately 5% of the total body water, evidence of heat exhaustion may become apparent. When losses are 10%, the condition could lead to heat stroke soon. This is fatal unless the person receives immediate attention (through submersion in an ice bath).

As the work level and environmental temperature increase, fluid intake must be increased to maintain fluid balance.[12] You should replace water loss by continuous daily fluid intake. A few guidelines to facilitate water balance are as follows. (Additional information is provided in Chapter 13, Figure 13.4.)

1. Drink plenty of liquids at least 20 minutes before beginning an aerobic exercise session. Frequent, small intake of fluid throughout the day is best.

2. If you have been drinking plenty of water prior to aerobic sessions, you probably will not need to drink water during the session (room temperature and humidity usually are the determining variables). If you get thirsty, however, drink water. Your thirst mechanism is a late sign that you need water, so don't ignore it.

3. After aerobic exercise, relax and sit with a tall glass of ice water or a homemade electrolyte ("sports drink") solution:[13]

   > 1 quart frozen reconstituted orange juice
   > 3 quarts water
   > ½ teaspoon salt

This will provide immediate rehydration and is a pleasant way to conclude your session.

4. If you use any of the sports beverages or commercial preparations, dilute them with water to decrease the concentration of sugar and thereby decrease the time the fluid stays in the stomach. Recommended dilutions are given in Table 3.1.[14] Many "sports beverages" are promoted as sources of available sodium, potassium, and sugar. Replacement needs for sodium and potassium can be met much better through a diet that contains a variety of foods and supplies these and other nutrients, including proper amounts of water.

Deliberate dehydration (by loading on the clothes and promoting profuse sweating), of course, is not an acceptable method of weight management. This will cause a temporary loss of weight, which is regained rapidly by rehydration. Loss of weight should be body fat, not water or protein.

## *Table 3.1  Dilution of Replacement Fluids*

| Fluid | Concentration |
|---|---|
| Fruit juices | 1 part juice; 3 parts water |
| Soft drinks | 1 part soda; 3 parts water |
| Vegetable juices | 1 part juice; 1 part water |
| Gatorade® | 1 part drink; 1 part water |

# *Common Injuries and Conditions*

Common injuries include, among others, blisters; bunions, muscle cramps and soreness; injuries to muscles, tendons, and joints; and ventricular fibrillation.

## Blisters

A blister arises in seconds but takes days to heal. Even a small blister that goes untreated will affect your workout. The best advice is to do everything you can to prevent blisters from forming in the first place.

Blisters are caused by friction as the surface of the shoe rubs against the skin of the foot. The best preventive measure is to wear shoes that fit well, not too loose or too tight.

Also, to help prevent blisters, lubricate any trouble spots with petroleum jelly before you put on your shoes for a fitness session. If you sweat a lot, powder your feet as well. Before purchasing shoes, do a few exertive moves in your local shoe store to size up comfort *in motion*.

If you get a water blister, care for it as follows:

1. Scrub the area gently with soap and water to clean it thoroughly.

2. Gently swab with alcohol or a surgical preparation.

3. Make two incisions at the outer edges of the blister. Slowly press out the superficial fluid.

4. Apply ointment or first-aid cream.

5. Bandage until healed completely.

If you get a blood blister, care for it as follows:

1. Ice the area.

2. Do not puncture. This increases the chance of infection as blood circulates throughout the body.

3. Place a "doughnut"-type compress around the blister until it is reabsorbed and healed completely.

## Bunions

A bunion is a large, bony protuberance on the outside of the big toe. It indicates inflammation of the joint. The main causes of bunions are overpronation and faulty foot structure. Podiatrists treat foot problems, including bunions.

## Muscle Cramps

A cramp is a painful muscle spasm that sometimes occurs during or after a vigorous exercise session. Cramps result from two different phenomena. Muscle cramping *during* an exercise session usually reflects an electrolyte and fluid imbalance in your system.[15] Electrolytes are sodium, calcium, chloride, potassium, and magnesium. Cramping usually occurs because you have not properly replaced your water loss while conditioning and training.

If a person has lost a lot of water through perspiration (8 or more pounds of water), those elements have to be replaced. With moderate sweating and water loss, regular, daily water intake and proper diet will replace the needed fluids and electrolytes and do much to eliminate this type of cramping.

The second, and most common, type of cramps associated with exercise are those occurring in the 24 hours *after* exercise, especially after having gone to bed or after a sudden movement. These post-exercise cramps are not associated with electrolyte imbalance.[16] They are believed to be caused by swelling of muscle fiber, agitating the peripheral nerves that service the muscle tissue. If these cramps are frequent and severe, the treatment prescribed may be .2 grams of quinine sulfate.

---

*Immediate relief from cramping is to do a static stretch in the exact opposite direction for a few moments.*

---

## Muscle Soreness

Two types of muscle pain are associated with exercise:

1. Pain during and immediately after exercise, which may persist for several hours
2. Localized soreness that usually does not appear for 24–48 hours

The first is associated with metabolic wastes deposited on pain receptors, and the second with torn muscle fibers or connective tissue.[17] The first type need not cause great concern because it has no lasting effects. The delayed type requires attention in the form of a more adequate warm-up and cool-down stretching program and incorporating a strength segment into your program. Gradual, sensible use of muscles during exercise is the best preventive measure.

## Muscle, Tendon, and Joint Injuries

"I've found that most injuries are caused not by poor form, but by previously undiagnosed joint problems and overuse. The main way to prevent these injuries is to always *listen to the body.* I've found that most people either over-train or under-train. Very few people are exercising at an optimal intensity and frequency to elicit fitness progress and minimize risk. . . People need to work hard to overload their muscles during the exercise session, but should not normally leave the session completely exhausted."[18]

For *muscle strains or sprains*, the treatment is to ICE (ice, compress, and elevate). Injuries are iced (or cold whirlpools are administered) to inhibit swelling and promote healing by making the body internally (rather than at the surface) supply more blood to the affected deep area. When cold applications are applied, the body forces more blood to come to the area by making the body work harder pumping away the old cells and pumping in fresh oxygen and nutrients to begin the repair process at the deep site rather than the surface skin area.

Ice applications are administered twice daily, about 20 minutes each time. When the affected area no longer is warm to the touch (using the back of your hand) but seems to be the same temperature as the surrounding area, ice compresses can be stopped.

When heat is applied, it brings more blood to the skin surface, but it doesn't make the body work hard on its own to pump in a fresh supply of oxygen and nutrients to the deep affected area. The less comfortable application of ice will hasten the repair process.

*Achilles tendonitis* is an inflammation of the thick tendon that connects the heel to the calf muscle. This injury results from wearing shoes with soles that do not provide a proper cushion for the foot. Aggravating the problem are biomechanical problems such as bowed legs, tight hamstrings and calves, high-arched feet, overpronation, and excessive toe-running.

Adequate heel-cord stretching helps to prevent Achilles tendonitis. Any aggravation of this problem can cause a serious and permanent condition. Therefore, anyone with this problem should not continue to exercise with the pain.

## Shin Splints

The most common injury to new participants in aerobics is shin splints, characterized by pain on the front and inside of the lower leg (Figure 3.5). Although it is common in runners, this malady can affect anyone who engages in physical activity that uses the legs. Most cases of shin splints occur at the beginning of an exercise program because the lower leg muscles are weak.

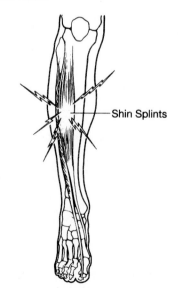

**Figure 3.5** Shin Splints

Jumping and running activities cause the leg muscles in the back of the leg to develop and become stronger while the leg muscles in front develop only slightly. This muscle imbalance can cause shin splints if it is not treated correctly.[19] When the strength of one muscle or muscle group is disproportionate to that of the antagonist(s) for that muscle or group, the weaker muscle should be strengthened to restore balance around the joint.[20]

Preventive measures for shin splints include light, flexible shoes with good arch support. Track running should be avoided, as the repeated turns put great stress on the lower leg. Stretching before and after physical activity helps the muscles absorb shock.

Performing a stretch using three repetitions of straight-leg and bent-knee wall leans for 20 seconds may alleviate the problem (Figure 3.6). Another preventive measure is to develop the strength of the anterior lower leg area. This can be accomplished by performing an exercise such as the lower-leg flexor, using a towel rolled lengthwise or resistance/rubber tubing. Sit tall with your legs together in front of you and place the center of the towel or tubing securely under the toes of your shoes. Place your hands comfortably in front of the abdomen and don't move them during the exercise. Slowly point your toes down and toward the wall in front of you (Figure 3.7), and hold 15 seconds. Relax a few seconds, then flex your feet at the ankle and draw your toes up tightly toward your knees (Figure 3.8), and hold 15 seconds. Repeat the entire exercise for several minutes. This can be done one leg at a time or both feet working together simultaneously.

Of utmost importance in caring for shin splints are *rest and immediate icing* in the tender area. The icing should be for 8–10 continuous

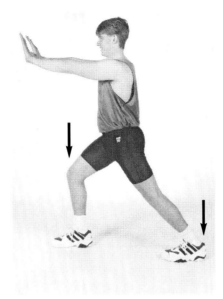

**Figure 3.6** Exercise for Relief of Shin Splints

minutes while gently massaging the problem area. A second gentle ice massage later in the day for the same time duration will give the desired relief. Follow this routine for several days. You'll be amazed at how quickly you will heal within a week.

If icing, rest, aspirin (4–6 per day), strengthening, and stretching do not create relief within 10 days, see a physician to rule out more serious conditions such as stress fractures, structural imbalances that might require orthotics, or anterior compartment syndrome.[21]

## *Ventricular Fibrillation*

As many as half of all deaths from heart attack possibly occur because of *ventricular fibrillation*. This rhythm disturbance of the heart muscles is deadly if it cannot be reversed within minutes.[22] Some drugs can trigger this condition. In recent years the drug-related deaths of superstar athletes have been attributed to ventricular fibrillation induced by cocaine intoxication.

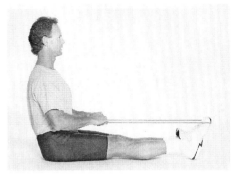

**Figure 3.7** Strength Exercise to Develop Anterior Lower Leg Muscles, Down Position

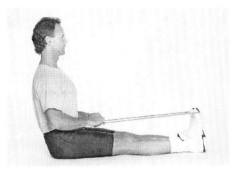

**Figure 3.8** Strength Exercise to Develop Anterior Lower Leg Muscles, Up Position

## Professional Help

Understanding cause and effect will help prevent problems or injuries during the quest for fitness. Whenever problems or injuries do arise, you should seek answers from qualified professionals—medical doctors, sports medicine specialists, physiologists, athletic trainers.

Follow the diet, exercise, and mental training programs promoted by scientific professionals. Read and believe authors whose credentials are impressive in the various fields of total fitness and who publish their researched findings in professional journals. In this way, you will have access to the most accurate, up-to-date knowledge available—and a safer, more fun way to good health.

## Goal-Setting Challenge

Correct any safety concern or fear you may have that you have let slide without proper attention. Write one Safety Goal for Chapter 3 following the four steps presented in Chapter 2, Exercise 2.3, then recording it in your Fitness Journal.

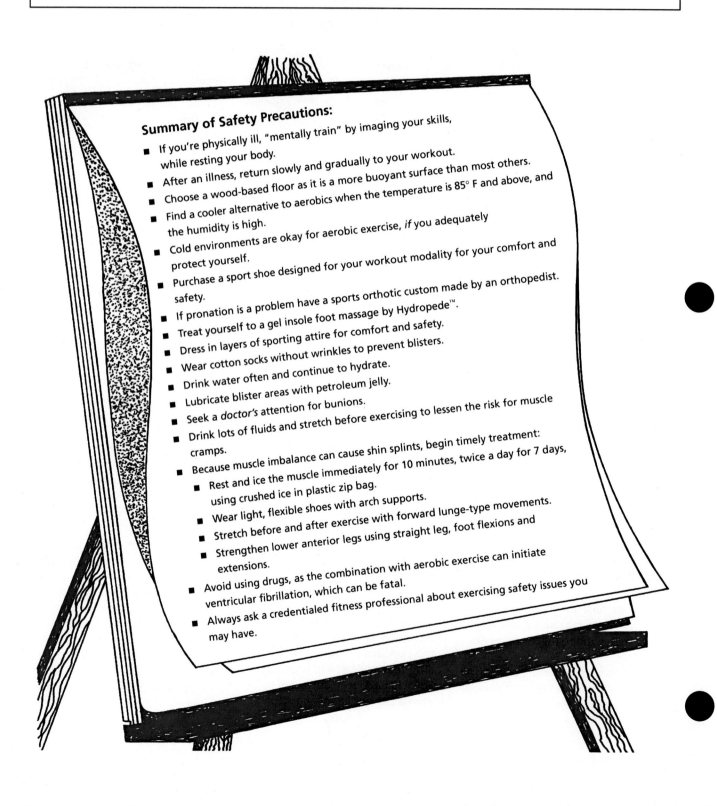

### Summary of Safety Precautions:

- If you're physically ill, "mentally train" by imaging your skills, while resting your body.
- After an illness, return slowly and gradually to your workout.
- Choose a wood-based floor as it is a more buoyant surface than most others.
- Find a cooler alternative to aerobics when the temperature is 85° F and above, and the humidity is high.
- Cold environments are okay for aerobic exercise, *if* you adequately protect yourself.
- Purchase a sport shoe designed for your workout modality for your comfort and safety.
- If pronation is a problem have a sports orthotic custom made by an orthopedist.
- Treat yourself to a gel insole foot massage by Hydropede™.
- Dress in layers of sporting attire for comfort and safety.
- Wear cotton socks without wrinkles to prevent blisters.
- Drink water often and continue to hydrate.
- Lubricate blister areas with petroleum jelly.
- Seek a *doctor's* attention for bunions.
- Drink lots of fluids and stretch before exercising to lessen the risk for muscle cramps.
- Because muscle imbalance can cause shin splints, begin timely treatment:
    - Rest and ice the muscle immediately for 10 minutes, twice a day for 7 days, using crushed ice in plastic zip bag.
    - Wear light, flexible shoes with arch supports.
    - Stretch before and after exercise with forward lunge-type movements.
    - Strengthen lower anterior legs using straight leg, foot flexions and extensions.
- Avoid using drugs, as the combination with aerobic exercise can initiate ventricular fibrillation, which can be fatal.
- Always ask a credentialed fitness professional about exercising safety issues you may have.

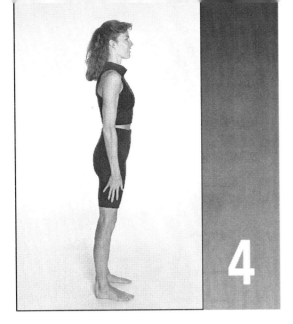

# Posture and Positioning

4

The best reason to include posture information in a fitness course is to *save your back!* To ensure that you are exercising in the safest possible fashion, you must understand good postural techniques, regardless of the activity. Poor posture is illustrated in Figure 4.1. Correct posture is shown in Figure 4.2.

## Getting a Picture of Yourself

Have someone photograph a set of "before" and "after" pictures of you: (1) from the *side* (Figure 4.3a) (2) from the *back* (Figure 4.3b), both with arms at your sides and standing with your weight evenly distributed on both feet. You will be able to use these for a specific purpose: to note your postural habits, from both a side view and a back view.

Attach the side and back views onto Exercise 4.1 Posture: Detecting and Correcting Problems at the end of this chapter. You will use these for a postural analysis that will be discussed shortly.

## The Mechanics

The downward pressure of gravity applied to the bones of the upright, balanced skeleton tends to cause it to buckle at three main points: hip, knee, and ankle. Because the body weight is largely in front of the spinal column, the body tends to fall forward.

To counteract these tendencies toward buckling and falling forward, five muscles or muscle groups are antigravity in nature, allowing for an upright, balanced skeleton. The antigravity muscle groups responsible for holding us erect are located in the:

- back (along with the spinal column)
- abdomen
- buttocks
- front of the thighs
- calves

To develop good posture, the position of the spine, pelvic girdle, and hip joints (which act as the main hinges of the body) have to be controlled. This is done primarily by the five muscle groups. *How* you control them determines posture.

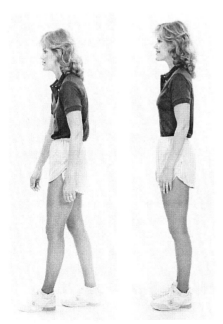

**Figure 4.1**
Poor Posture

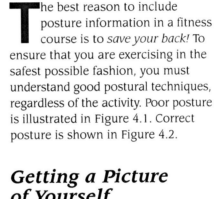

**Figure 4.2**
Good Posture

## (a) Side View

Line of gravity passes:

1. Through tip of ear
2. Through center of shoulders
3. Slightly behind center of hip
4. Behind kneecap

5. In front of ankle joint
6. Perpendicular vertically through weight center

Head is up.

Chin is parallel to floor.

Ear is above middle of shoulder.

Tip of shoulder is over hip joint.

Shoulders are relaxed and down.

Chest and rib cage are lifted.

Abdomen is flat.

Pelvis is balanced; front of pelvis and thigh are in a continuous line.

Knees are unlocked or slightly flexed.

Feet are parallel; body weight is centered between heel and toe and carried on outer half of feet.

## (b) Back View

Line of gravity passes through:

1. Mid-head
2. Mid-trunk
3. Mid-waist
4. Mid-ankle

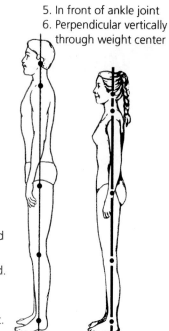

Head is erect.

Body is symmetrical.

Shoulders are level.

Spine is straight.

Hips are level.

Legs are straight.

Feet are parallel; toes are pointing forward.

Weight is distributed equally on both feet and toward outer half of each foot.

**Figure 4.3** Characteristics of Good Posture

## Balanced Static Posture

A balanced standing posture (Figure 4.3) is established when:

- The head and stretched neck are balanced on top of the spine and centered above the shoulders, while keeping the chin parallel to the floor.
- The shoulders are pulled back and down in a relaxed position.
- The chest and rib cage are raised up.
- The abdominal muscles are pulled in and up, under the rib cage.

- The pelvic girdle is pulled down and under, tightening the buttocks. The pelvis rests on the two thigh bones balanced over the two arched feet.
- The knees are relaxed. Locking the knees in a hyperextended position causes imbalance and increases susceptibility to knee injury.
- The weight is distributed equally on both feet while standing with the feet parallel and toes pointing forward, taking the weight on the outer half of the feet.
- The arms are relaxed.

## Dynamic Posture

Performing aerobics or step training gesture and step patterns or fitness walking will require you to take a body position or posture, different from the posture when you are standing stationary and poised. You are preparing dynamically to move in some direction through space (forward, backward, laterally, up, down).

While preparing to move through space, the broader your base of support, the lower your center of gravity (weight center) becomes.

---

### *Goal Setting Challenge*

 Set a goal to start looking good throughout your entire day by becoming aware of, and improving, your position in every type of physical activity you do. Write one Good Posture/Positioning Goal for Chapter 4 that you would like to achieve, following the four steps presented in Chapter 2, Exercise 2.3, then recording it in your Fitness Journal.

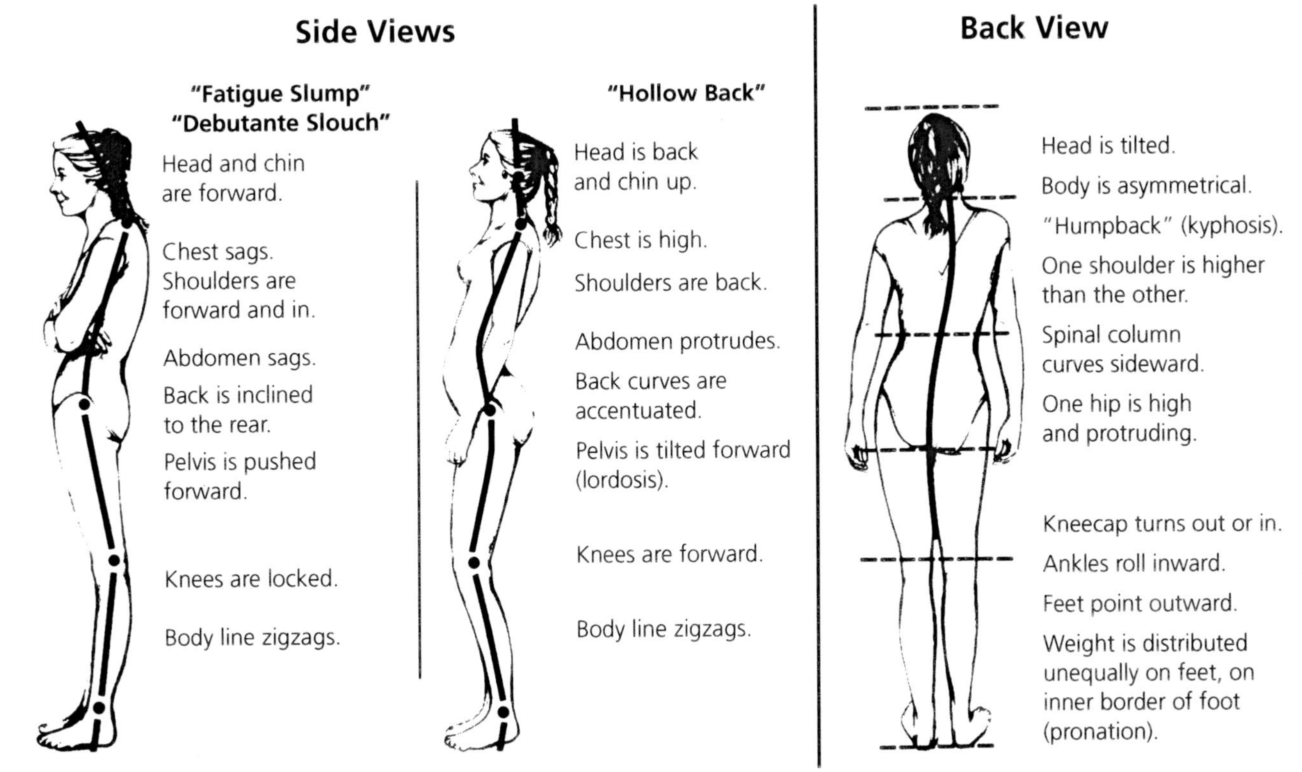

**Side Views**                                    **Back View**

**"Fatigue Slump"**          **"Hollow Back"**
**"Debutante Slouch"**

Head and chin              Head is back              Head is tilted.
are forward.               and chin up.
                                                     Body is asymmetrical.
                           Chest is high.
Chest sags.                                          "Humpback" (kyphosis).
Shoulders are              Shoulders are back.
forward and in.                                      One shoulder is higher
                           Abdomen protrudes.        than the other.
Abdomen sags.
                           Back curves are           Spinal column
Back is inclined           accentuated.              curves sideward.
to the rear.
                           Pelvis is tilted forward  One hip is high
Pelvis is pushed           (lordosis).               and protruding.
forward.

                           Knees are forward.        Kneecap turns out or in.

Knees are locked.                                    Ankles roll inward.

                           Body line zigzags.        Feet point outward.
Body line zigzags.
                                                     Weight is distributed
                                                     unequally on feet, on
                                                     inner border of foot
                                                     (pronation).

**Figure 4.4** Characteristics of Poor Posture

## Poor Posture

If any part of the body is out of alignment, weight distribution will be uneven over the base of support and will put unnecessary strain on muscles, bones, and joints. This soon causes fatigue. Figure 4.4 shows the characteristics of poor posture.

Poor posture is a habit that can be changed. It takes time, though, for it has been a part of a person for a long time.

Most muscles are in pairs. If a muscle is shortened constantly, its opposing muscle lengthens and becomes weak from disuse. Therefore, stretching (lengthening) one set of muscles while simultaneously contracting (shortening) the opposing set of muscles, and then repeating vice versa, will strengthen both, especially if additional weight resistance is used.

With this information, you can understand why stretching and strengthening the muscles will lead to better posture. If your body is to move freely, every muscle has to be able to shorten or lengthen in either a strong, quick manner or a slow, relaxed manner. Fully understanding the principles of stretching and strength training will assist you further in understanding and obtaining good posture goals.

## *Postural Analysis and Change*

Now that you understand the benefits of good posture and the mechanics involved, turn to Exercise 4.1, Posture: Detecting and Correcting Problems at the end of the chapter. Take a look at the two photos of you taken earlier. Compare the criteria for balanced postures and those for the more common postural problems (as shown in Figures 4.3 and 4.4) with your photos, or by looking into a three-way mirror.

Fill in Exercise 4.1. The only item that may require further explanation is "body line." To check if your body line is perpendicular through the center of your weight (the center of gravity), determine if a line goes from the tip of your ear through the center of your shoulder joint, slightly behind the center of your hip joint, behind your kneecap, and in front of your ankle joint.

Do this by placing a straightedge on your sideview photo and carefully drawing a vertical line from one point of reference to the next. If most of your body *weight* falls in *front* of the line, your body line will be *backward* (from a balanced, perpendicular line perspective). If most of your *weight* falls *behind* the line, your body line will be *forward*. You also will be able to tell immediately if your body

This allows for better balance so you can move quickly and more efficiently in any direction.

line is straight (perpendicular) or a combination of zigzags.

After you have completed your evaluation, have your instructor review your impressions and make her or his own additions and corrections. At the conclusion of the course, evaluate your change and progress toward good posture.

This can best be achieved by again being photographed in your new, current standing posture, from both side and back views. Attach the new photos to Exercise 4.1, and do a post-assessment. Your instructor may want to go over your final posture evaluation and give you suggestions for continual improvement.

## Efficient Positions

If you now have poor posture during aerobic movement activities, you will have to reeducate your neuromuscular system. This takes patience, persistence, and a sincere desire to want to improve your appearance and the efficiency of your body.

If you were born free of hereditary or congenital deformities, you can obtain good posture (Figure 4.3). It's all a matter of:

■ understanding balanced postures
■ developing a kinesthetic (sensory) awareness of your body positions during all movements
■ developing strong, yet relaxed, muscles and flexible joints
■ desiring to obtain good posture
■ having the discipline to continue what you have learned

As you understand correct techniques, you can challenge yourself to try to use these positions in every total fitness component of your program (stretching, aerobics, step training, fitness walking, and strength training exercises). At first you'll be thinking through the activity, but with persistent practice and desire you can exchange former faulty habits for safe, more

complementary ones. If you can attain a balanced standing posture, you've mastered this task already.

## Practice

For your total daily well-being, good posture must become important enough to you to make it a lifelong endeavor. Are you sitting correctly while reading how to improve your posture?

Daily practice is required for good posture to become an integral part of you. Good posture is established through discipline. Setting aside time to do exercises such as those that follow to encourage good posture and develop strength and flexibility, accompanied by constant attention to posture throughout your daily living tasks, will turn this into reality. You can improve as you move—all day, every day.

## *Exercises to Promote Postural Awareness*

Exercising the antigravity muscles is a fundamental part of any total physical fitness conditioning program. To develop and then maintain a good posture, these muscles have to be:

■ *strong* enough to perform their functions
■ *flexible* enough to allow a variety of movements
■ *relaxed* enough to perform with ease

Therefore, establishing a program of *strength* exercises for the abdomen, lower back, hip, thigh, and calf areas (see Chapter 10, Figures 10.20–10.25) will help you to obtain a balanced pelvic alignment and provide the means for efficient and painless movement. Each joint involved has to be flexible enough to permit the full range of movement possible from these groups of antigravity muscles so that any new position can be maintained properly.

The following exercises will help you develop joint *flexibility* of the

antigravity muscle groups needed to maintain correct postures. Establishing a *program of relaxation* will assist with ease of performance while moving or while motionless.

The best exercise you can do for yourself is both a physical and mental one: *Become aware of correct postural technique with every move you make.* Then practice this physical and mental conditioning constantly until it becomes a habit.

## Finding Correct Standing Posture

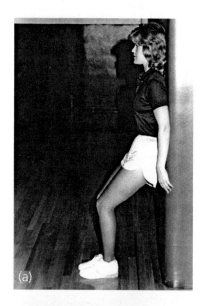

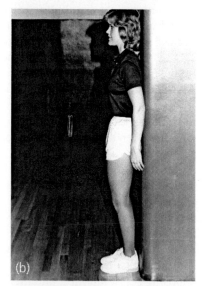

**Figure 4.5** Finding Correct Standing Posture

To find your correct posture, follow these steps:

1. Stand one foot away from the wall, facing out. Now "sit" against the wall, bending your knees slightly (Figure 4.5a). Tighten your abdominal and buttock muscles. This will tilt the pelvis back and flatten the lower spine.
2. Holding this position, inch up the wall to a standing position by straightening your legs (Figure 4.5b).
3. Now walk around the room, maintaining the same posture.
4. Place your back against the wall again to see if you have held the correct posture.

---

*** Posture is where a total program for physical fitness begins.***

---

## Elbows Wide and Close

To become aware of the space between the shoulder blades *contracted* and then *widely stretched* (see Figure 4.6):

1. Clasp your hands loosely behind your head (a). Do not lace fingers tightly behind the neck. Pulling on the cervical spine is not a good body position. Keep your *elbows out and high*, shoulders down, and your chin parallel to the floor. (4 counts)
2. Exhale, and widen the space between your shoulder blades by bringing your elbows *together* in front of your nose (b). (Hold for 4 counts)
3. Inhale, and return *elbows wide to* the sides (a). (4 counts)
4. Exhale and pull your elbows *up and back* (not shown), tightly contracting the space between your shoulder blades. (Hold 4 counts)
5. Inhale and return *elbows wide* (a) to the sides. (4 counts)

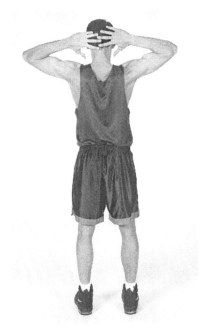

(a) Elbows Wide

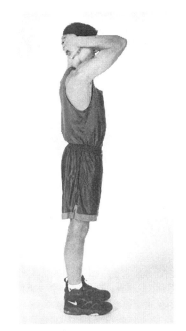

(b) Elbows Close

**Figure 4.6** Elbows Wide and Close

6. For variety, again attempt to touch your elbows together, first *in front of forehead* and *below the chin*, maintaining the good posture position.

*Cues*: "Elbows out and high, together, wide, up and back, wide."

## Rib Lifter

To establish awareness of the all-important position of "chest high" (and not sagging), the rib lifter (Figure 4.7) will help to isolate and stretch the intercostal (rib) muscles:

1. Stand in correct alignment, with your *arms forward* and *parallel* to the floor. Place your thumbs and index fingers of each hand together, hands forward, palms down (a). (4 counts)
2. Bend your elbows, bring your arms back, and place your palms parallel to the ground above your breast, with your *thumbs* snugly *under the armpits* and elbows held wide and parallel to the floor (b). (4 counts)
3. Without lifting your shoulders or bending forward, *lift your entire rib section as high as you can.* Breathe deeply, inhale, and exhale. (8 counts)
4. Now *lift* one elbow high and *stretch* your rib cage on that side (c). (4 counts)
5. *Lower* the raised elbow to shoulder level. (4 counts)
6. Repeat with lifting and lowering of the other elbow. (8 counts)
7. Repeat *raising both* elbows together (d). Lower. (8 counts)

*Cues*: "Stand; thumbs under armpits; lift ribs, breathe and stretch; lower; repeat other side; repeat both; lower."

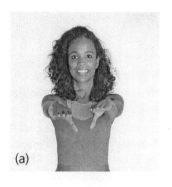

(a)

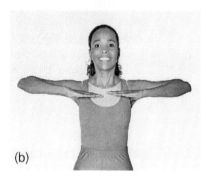

(b)

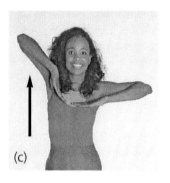

(c)

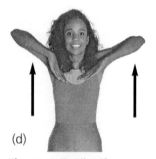

(d)

**Figure 4.7** Rib Lifter

## Posture Improvement and Coordination Exercise Routine

The Bounce 'n Tap Series (Figure 4.8) pattern can be performed rhythmically to any 4/4 time music, as follows, or in another improvised way. There are

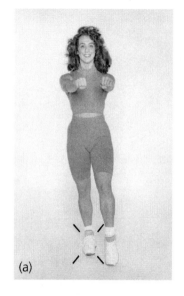

(a)

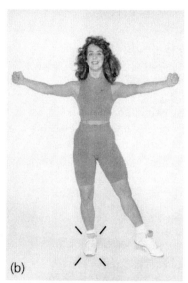

(b)

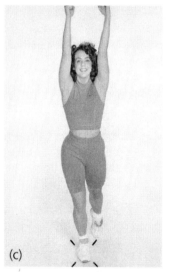

(c)

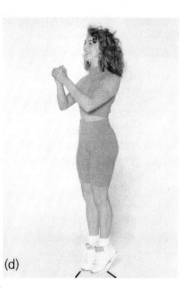

(d)

**Figure 4.8** Bounce 'n Tap Series

three basic directional positions and one "hold" position. The *weight-bearing foot*, or important movement, *is accented with slash marks* and the exercises are photographed and described by the mirroring technique (described in the Introduction).

*1. Forward* (Figure 4.8a):

**Feet:** Hop on left foot, with right foot *forward*—toe pointed and tapping.

**Arms:** Stretched *forward*, parallel thumbs down.

*2. Sideward* (Figure 4.8b):

**Feet:** Hop on left foot, with right foot out to right side (toe pointed and tapping).

**Arms:** Shoulder high, *out* from sides, fists.

*3. Back 'n Up* (Figure 4.8c):

**Feet:** Hop on left foot, with right foot *back* behind you (toe pointed and tapping).

**Arms:** Stretched *skyward*, arms close to ears, thumbs in.

*4. "Hold" and Bounce* (Figure 4.8d):

**Feet:** Hop or bounce on *both* feet together.

**Arms:** Close to body, elbows down at sides, hands in either a jogging position or hands clasped.

## Suggested Sequence of These Movements

1. Repeat four times, right foot pointing and tapping *each* direction (*forward* 4-*side* 4-*back* 4-*hold* 4). Repeat four times, left foot pointing and tapping (hopping on right).

2. Repeat three times, right foot pointing but before each directional change, hop on both feet together, with arms close to body, one time (a *hold and bounce* once would be the fourth count for a 4/4 time rhythm).

   *Forward* 3/*hold* 1-*side* 3/*hold* 1-*back* 3/*hold* 1-*hold and bounce*.) Repeat three times, left foot pointing.

3. Repeat two times, right foot pointing. Repeat two times, left foot pointing.

4. Repeat one time, right foot pointing (each direction; the fourth count is hop 'n hold, two feet in place). Repeat one time, left foot pointing.

5. Repeat 1s; 2s; 3s; 4s!

6. Repeat 4s; 3s; 2s; 1s! And continue to do 1s for the remainder of the music.

*Note:* For *high intensity,* do the previous steps (hopping while pointing and tapping). To lower your workload and thus your heart rate:

- Don't hop, but do both arms and legs.
- Don't hop, and lower or eliminate the arm moves.
- Don't do the leg movements, just the arm movements.

This posture/coordination rhythmic exercise thus can be as much, or as little, exercise as the participant can (aerobically) do. For variety, the entire group can form a large circle, facing in, and perform the exercise as a group!

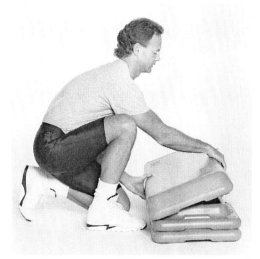

**Figure 4.9** Correct Lifting Position

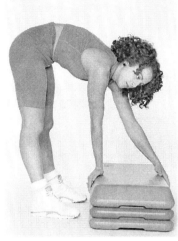

**Figure 4.10** Incorrect Lifting Position

## Correct Lifting and Lowering

To protect your muscles and joints (especially the lower back) from undue strain or fatigue, proper technique in these areas must become second nature. Disciplined practice of correct techniques now will establish good habits for the rest of your life. The leg muscles are strong, whereas the back muscles are relatively weak. All heavy lifting should be done by stabilizing the back in an erect position and making the legs provide the necessary power.

1. Get as close as possible to the object, using a forward-stride position. The object should be in front of you if you are using two hands (such as step-bench), or beside you if you are using one hand (such as luggage). Keeping your back straight and your pelvis tucked, bend at the hips, knees, and ankles to lower your body. Lower directly downward, only as much as necessary (keeping your head high and buttocks low).

2. Place both arms well under or around the weight center of the load. Lift vertically upward in a slow, steady movement by *extending your leg muscles.* Keep the object close to your weight center (Figure 4.9). Reverse the procedure to lower the object.

*Do not* bend over from your hips (head low, buttocks high) and force your back muscles to lift the load (Figure 4.10).

## Correct Carrying

1. Keep the object close to your weight center.

2. Separate the load when feasible, carrying half in each hand/arm (Figure 4.11).

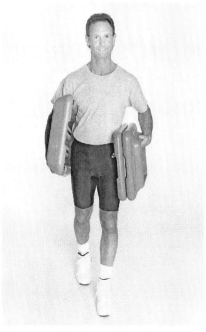

**Figure 4.11** Correct Carrying Position

# Exercise 4.1 Posture: Detecting and Correcting Problems

**Directions:** Evaluate your own posture by analyzing your photos, using both the side and back views.
Draw horizontal lines connecting both inside photo edges to "Body Segments".

ATTACH OWN **SIDE** VIEW PHOTO HERE

ATTACH OWN **BACK** VIEW PHOTO HERE

**Body Segments:**

Head/Neck
Shoulders
Chest/Upper Back
Abdomen Lower Back
Pelvis-Hips/Thighs
Knees/Ankles/Feet

| | Side View | | Back View | |
|---|---|---|---|---|
| **Body Line:** | Perpendicular through weight center ___ | | | |
| **Therefore Is:** | Balanced ___ | Forward ___ | Symmetrical ___ | Asymmetrical ___ |
| **Head:** | Up ___ | Back, with chin up ___ | Erect ___ | Tilted ___ | Zigzags ___ Backward ___ Forward with chin forward ___ |
| **Shoulders:** | Directly over hip joint ___ | Back ___ | Relaxed, down and level ___ | One shoulder high ___ (R/L) | Rounded, in and forward ___ |
| **Chest:** | Balanced with rib cage lifted ___ | High ___ | | | Sags ___ |
| **Upper Back:** | Normal curve ___ | Concave and accentuated ___ | Straight spine ___ | Curves sideward; scoliosis ___ | Convex—humpback; kyphosis ___ |
| **Abdomen:** | Contracted and flat ___ | Protrudes ___ | | | Sags ___ |
| **Lower Back, Lumbar Curve:** | Balanced and easy ___ | Hollow swayback ___ | | | Flat; inclined to the rear ___ |
| **Pelvis:** | Balanced ___ | Tilted forward; lordosis ___ | Hips level ___ | One hip (R/L) high and protruding ___ | Pushed forward ___ |
| **Knees:** | Flexed and balanced ___ | Forward; too flexed ___ | Legs straight ___ | Kneecaps turn out or in ___ | Locked; hyperextended ___ |
| **Ankles and Body Weight:** | Weight balanced on outer half ___ | Roll inward (R/L); pronated ___ | | | |
| **Feet:** | Parallel with toes forward ___ | Toe in ___ | | Toe out ___ | |

*Note:* When entire evaluation is completed, star (*) your checked body segments that are unbalanced and require correction. It also may help to study your posture using a three-way mirror, with the aid of a partner.

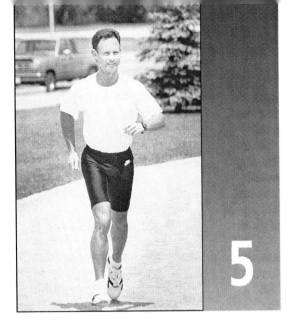

# *Fitness Testing*

**5**

The next step in the journey toward achieving and then maintaining physical fitness for a lifetime involves establishing your current fitness starting point, using scientific test and assessment procedures. Knowing yourself clearly in terms of your past history, risk factors, and present physical status will assist you in developing a lifetime fitness plan. It will enable you to set, realistically and safely, achievable short-term fitness goals. It also will provide the basis for motivating you continually to adhere to the program you do establish to achieve your long-range and lifetime fitness goals.

Initially you may find it painful to realize that you are out of shape and test poorly on a laboratory or field stress test. No one wants to see or hear scientific results that are inferior or below the norm. But having the courage and determination to find out just where you are at the outset and then, with time and dedication, progressing to the point at which your post-assessment test numbers represent an excellent state of fitness and well-being is motivating.

In most instances, specific fitness testing is appropriate only after obtaining a medical history.

Screening may uncover potential problems and determine if you should be considered for a specific exercise prescription. Most course settings require prescreening, or, if you have any limitations or known risk factors, a thorough medical exam.

## *Purpose of Testing*

The purpose of an initial pre-course fitness assessment is to establish a baseline of information, against which later changes can be compared. This starting point information lets you know if you are physically fit (compared to the test's accepted research standards) and can endure a *continual aerobic program* for 20 or more minutes working at your target heart rate. Or, if you are not classified as physically fit (using the same research standards), for safety reasons you must begin an *interval aerobic training program*, which entails working aerobically for a short time and then slowing down, to recover your breathing (a starting-and-stopping aerobic format).

At the onset, an interval training program will consist of a minute or two (or a lap or two) of aerobic exercise, followed by slowing down

(but not stopping) exercise movement to accomplish a lower heart rate so breathing becomes easy again. The intervals continue, using longer aerobic intervals, followed by recovery breathing work intervals.

In several weeks you will be working continuously in your safe training zone for 20 or more minutes (and for hours, when you become well trained, as marathon participants are). When this process of progressively overloading the heart muscle with longer and longer periods of efficient pumping is well under way, you will have experienced the training effect, and when retested, will experience the new fitness classification label of *physically fit*!

## *Understanding Fitness Assessments*

Three basic assessment principles are:

1. Nearly all assessment protocols result in *estimated* values for the fitness component being measured. Therefore, the testing is best used as a way to measure improvement in your performance over time, not as an absolute physiologic measurement.

2. By following consistent procedures of testing (using the same test, the same person administering it, the same instrument, the same time of day), you will have more accurate measurements in subsequent testing over time.

3. Results are recorded for comparison purposes. The person being tested should understand these values and ask questions as needed to ensure understanding.

## Measuring Aerobic Capacity

Preassessment of your current status via a thorough physical fitness exam will include measurement of your heart's response to increasing amounts of exercise by measuring your ability to use oxygen. Physical fitness can and should be measured in one of two ways at least every 3 years:

1. A laboratory physical fitness test
2. A field test administered by you and a friend

## Laboratory Physical Fitness Test

A properly conducted treadmill stress test is done to check the precise condition of your heart.[1] Physical fitness and health are different, and the treadmill stress electrocardiogram (ECG) helps to make that distinction.[2]

Prior to a treadmill stress test, you will be screened thoroughly. The screening will consist of: (a) a brief history-taking and physical exam, during which the technician will listen to your heart and lungs; (b) a check for the use of various heart and hypertensive medications known to affect the ECG; (c) a check for history of any congenital or acquired heart disorders; and (d) an evaluation of the resting ECG.

This screening and background check will help determine your risk factors—feature in heredity, background, or present lifestyle that increase the likelihood of developing coronary heart disease. If no risk factors are present, an exercise test usually is not necessary below age 35 if the person is following the guidelines mentioned in Chapter 1. If the person has symptoms of heart, lung, or metabolic disease, a maximum stress test is recommended for individuals of any age prior to beginning a vigorous exercise program, followed by another test every 2 years.[3]

### Submaximal Testing

Submaximal testing is accomplished by means of a physical fitness test (stress test) on a treadmill. Electrocardiogram leads transmit and record electrical (heart) impulses that a machine reads and records on a strip of paper. You are tested to only approximately 150 beats per minute, not to exhaustion.

The ECG electrodes with leads are circular rubber discs with wires attached to them. The discs are glued onto the chest and back at key sites in preparation for taking various "pictures" of your heart from different angles and sides. Usually between 7 and 10 electrodes are applied, depending on the laboratory's procedures or the individual's specific needs.

You probably will be asked to walk at a pace of 3.3 miles per hour (90 meters per minute) on the treadmill. The grade will begin flat and will increase slowly in gradation, as if you were walking up a hill. Every minute the "hill" will become steeper and more difficult to climb. When your heart rate reaches 150 beats per minute, a record is made of the amount of time you took to arrive at that reading. Then, through an indirect method of extrapolation (projecting maximum results by comparison with many others who have been tested the same way in

> If you are older than 35, you should start an aerobic exercise program by first seeing your doctor and then taking a monitored laboratory fitness test. Individuals with known cardio-vascular, pulmonary, or metabolic disease should have a maximum stress test prior to beginning vigorous exercise at any age. These people and those whose exercise tests are abnormal should get a stress test annually.

the past), your fitness ability is estimated.

Basically, the longer your heart rate takes to reach 150 beats per minute, the more fit you are; the shorter it takes, the less fit you are. Submaximal fitness testing usually is used with individuals who know of no outstanding limitations and who are interested in starting a total fitness program.

### Maximal Testing

If an individual's need is more specific, such as for diagnostic or research purposes, maximal testing procedures are administered. Maximum testing reveals directly how much oxygen you use, because you are tested to exhaustion. The exhaustion point is when you start to get markedly fatigued. Some researchers believe that maximum laboratory testing is the only conclusive form to use.

## Field Tests of Fitness

You may not have immediate access to a laboratory and qualified physiologists to monitor the results recorded through the treadmill method. Therefore, field tests have been developed to help you assess your own physical fitness by determining your current aerobic capacity (see Figure 5.1). This testing is conducted easily in a fitness class setting.

The following information and Exercises 5.1a, 5.2a, and 5.3a were developed from Dr. Kenneth Cooper's book, *The Aerobics Program for Total Well-Being*.[4] You can administer Cooper's 3-Mile Walking Test, the 12-Minute Test, and 1.5-Mile Test by yourself or with the help of a friend. You should assess your cardiovascular and respiratory endurance using one of these tests before you begin your aerobic exercise program, then reassess your cardiovascular and respiratory efficiency 8 weeks later.

As aerobic exercise becomes a lifetime activity for you, an ongoing assessment should be done every 2 months, and your results compared with those from your first assessment. This also will help you set continual, lifelong, specific physical fitness goals.

As guidelines for field-testing:

1. If you have been physically inactive previously, participate in 1–2 weeks of walking or slow jogging before undertaking any of Cooper's tests.

2. Wear loose clothing in which you can sweat freely, and a sport shoe that conforms to the guidelines suggested in Chapter 3.

3. Determine first which field test you plan to take. You can choose fitness **walking** with your *distance covered* as the stopping point, or **running** with *time* or *distance* as the stopping point.

   - If *distance* is the stopping point, take the 3-Mile Walking Test, or the 1.5-Mile Test.

   - If *time* is the stopping point, take the 12-Minute Test.

   - If you believe rather strongly that you are really out of shape, take the 12-Minute Test, because you run for this amount of time only. (You might take 20 minutes to complete 1.5 miles or 60 minutes to complete 3 miles.)

4. Have a stopwatch or a second hand on your watch, be close to a timer, or use the testing or timing capabilities of your Polar® F11™ Heart Rate Monitor or your Walk4Life™ Duo® Pedometer.

5. Immediately before performing the test, spend 5–10 minutes warming up your muscles (see Chapter 6).

6. Have a partner record your data (as the time it takes, or laps, or distance) using Exercise 5.1b, 5.2b, or 5.3b. For administering the 3-Mile Walking Test, to avoid one partner sitting for a long time counting laps, devise a method for the student performing the walking test to determine his or her own laps (with a lap counter for example), if the test is being performed around a track.

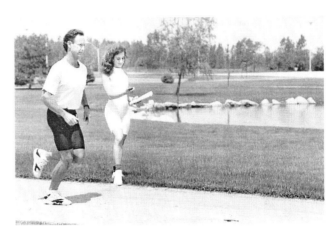

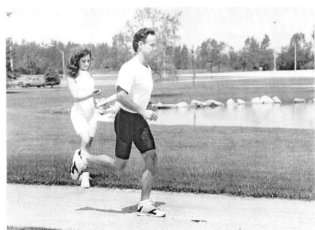

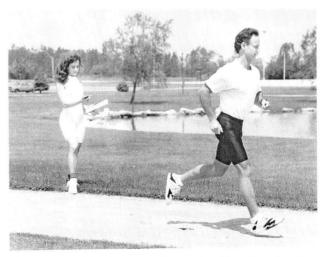

**Figure 5.1** Field-Testing to Determine Your Starting Point

7. Perform the Walking Test by covering 3 miles in the fastest time possible *without running*. Run or walk (or a combination) as quickly as you can for the 12-Minute Test or the 1.5-Mile Test. These are all-out tests of endurance.

8. When you stop, identify precisely the distance you covered in miles and tenths of miles, or the time you took, and have your partner record it, using Exercises 5.1b, 5.2b or 5.3b (the appropriate one).

9. Cool down by first walking slowly for several minutes, and then finish by doing cool-down stretching.

10. Interpret your results for the specific test you took, using Exercises 5.1a, 5.2a, or 5.3a. Results that reflect physical fitness labeled "good," "excellent," or "superior" means that you are considered *physically fit* to engage in continuous aerobic exercise for 20+ minutes.

Results that reflect a "fair," "poor," or "very poor" fitness level means that you are *not physically fit* and for safety reasons must begin with an interval aerobics program, described earlier in this chapter.

At the conclusion of your course, reassess your fitness. What changes did you experience from the pretest to the posttest?

Some beginners will not be happy with their test results. Do not be discouraged. You will be pleased with your improvement as you participate in a regular aerobics program.

---

*The quest for personal fitness must result in a complete change in lifestyle for most people.*

---

## Fitness for Life

Attaining a good or high level of physical fitness does not mean you have achieved a finished product or goal. Instead, you have found a method of getting or staying in shape that you must continue for the rest of your life. If you discontinue your program completely, all your aerobic gains will be lost in 10 weeks.[5]

The quest for personal fitness must result in a complete change in lifestyle for most people. You must prioritize and program exercise into your busy weekly schedule for the rest of your life. A "yo-yo" concept of a 10-week class now and maybe another one a year later just doesn't maintain fitness and a healthy heart.

You have just completed assessing your aerobic capacity. With this information, you can establish your cardiovascular fitness goal for the course, or for time intervals after the course is over.

---

### Goal-Setting Challenge

 Write one physical fitness goal that can be post-tested by the end of this course. Truly stretch yourself and your potential in regard to what you are actually capable of achieving. Record this Fitness Testing Goal for Chapter 5 following the four steps presented in Chapter 2 Exercise 2.3, then recording it in your Fitness Journal. Be *very specific* with this goal (regarding distance achieved, time it takes, what level you're desiring to achieve and so on).

 Immediately after each exercise session, take time to begin recording your progress and gains in your Fitness Journal, using entry ideas like these suggested in Exercise 5.4. Record any setbacks also. This will give you a visual blueprint on how successfully you are accomplishing a variety of short-term goals, and how you can do so again in the future. Include in your journaling: today's date, exercise varieties, time you spend, short-term goal set, new achievement today, and your thoughts and feelings. Enjoy the process of monitoring and changing.

## *Exercise 5.1a*   *Cooper's 3-Mile Walking Test (No Running)*

| Age (Years) | | 13–19 | 20–29 | 30–39 | 40–49 | 50–59 | 60 + |
|---|---|---|---|---|---|---|---|
| **Fitness Category** | | Time (Minutes) | | | | | |
| I. Very Poor | (men) | >45:00 | >46:00 | >49:00 | >52:00 | >55:00 | >60:00 |
| | (women) | >47:00 | >48:00 | >51:00 | >54:00 | >57:00 | >63:00 |
| II. Poor | (men) | 41:01–45:00 | 42:01–46:00 | 44:31–49:00 | 47:01–52:00 | 50:01–55:00 | 54:01–60:00 |
| | (women) | 43:01–47:00 | 44:01–48:00 | 46:31–51:00 | 49:01–54:00 | 52:01–57:00 | 57:01–63:00 |
| III. Fair | men) | 37:31–41:00 | 38:31–42:00 | 40:01–44:30 | 42:01–47:00 | 45:01–50:00 | 48:01–54:00 |
| | (women) | 39:31–43:00 | 40:31–44:00 | 42:01–46:30 | 44:01–49:00 | 47:01–52:00 | 51:01–57:00 |
| IV. Good | (men) | 33:00–37:30 | 34:00–38:30 | 35:00–40:00 | 36:30–42:00 | 39:00–45:00 | 41:00–48:00 |
| | (women) | 35:00–39:30 | 36:00–40:30 | 37:30–42:00 | 39:00–44:00 | 42:00–47:00 | 45:00–51:00 |
| V. Excellent | (men) | <33:00 | <34:00 | <35:00 | <36:30 | <39:00 | <41:00 |
| | (women) | <35:00 | <36:00 | <37:30 | <39:00 | <42:00 | <45:00 |

## *Exercise 5.2a*   *Cooper's 12-Minute Walking/Running Test*

| Age (Years) | | 13–19 | 20–29 | 30–39 | 40–49 | 50–59 | 60 + |
|---|---|---|---|---|---|---|---|
| **Fitness Category** | | Distance (Miles) Covered in 12 Minutes | | | | | |
| I. Very Poor | (men) | <1.30 | <1.22 | <1.18 | <1.14 | <1.03 | <.87 |
| | (women) | <1.0 | <.96 | <.94 | <.88 | <.84 | <.78 |
| II. Poor | (men) | 1.30–1.37 | 1.22–1.31 | 1.18–1.30 | 1.14–1.24 | 1.03–1.16 | .87–1.02 |
| | (women) | 1.00–1.18 | .96–1.11 | .95–1.05 | .88–.98 | .84–.93 | .78–.86 |
| III. Fair | (men) | 1.38–1.56 | 1.32–1.49 | 1.31–1.45 | 1.25–1.39 | 1.17–1.30 | 1.03–1.20 |
| | (women) | 1.19–1.29 | 1.12–1.22 | 1.06–1.18 | .99–1.11 | .94–1.05 | .87–.98 |
| IV. Good | (men) | 1.57–1.72 | 1.50–1.64 | 1.46–1.56 | 1.40–1.53 | 1.31–1.44 | 1.21–1.32 |
| | (women) | 1.30–1.43 | 1.23–1.34 | 1.19–1.29 | 1.12–1.24 | 1.06–1.18 | .99–1.09 |
| V. Excellent | (men) | 1.73–1.86 | 1.65–1.76 | 1.57–1.69 | 1.54–1.65 | 1.45–1.58 | 1.33–1.55 |
| | (women) | 1.44–1.51 | 1.35–1.45 | 1.30–1.39 | 1.25–1.34 | 1.19–1.30 | 1.10–1.18 |
| VI. Superior | (men) | >1.87 | >1.77 | >1.70 | >1.66 | >1.59 | >1.56 |
| | (women) | >1.52 | >1.46 | >1.40 | >1.35 | >1.31 | >1.19 |

## *Exercise 5.3a*   *Cooper's 1.5-Mile Run/Walk Test*

| Age (Years) | | 13–19 | 20–29 | 30–39 | 40–49 | 50–59 | 60 + |
|---|---|---|---|---|---|---|---|
| **Fitness Category** | | Time (Minutes) | | | | | |
| I. Very Poor | (men) | >15:31 | >16:01 | >16:31 | >17:31 | >19:01 | >20:01 |
| | (women) | >18:31 | >19:01 | >19:31 | >20:01 | >20:31 | >21:01 |
| II. Poor | (men) | 12:11–15:30 | 14:01–16:00 | 14:44–16:30 | 15:36–17:30 | 17:01–19:00 | 19:01–20:00 |
| | (women) | 16:55–18:30 | 18:31–19:00 | 19:01–19:30 | 19:31–20:00 | 20:01–20:30 | 21:00–21:31 |
| III. Fair | (men) | 10:49–12:10 | 12:01–14:00 | 12:31–14:45 | 13:01–15:35 | 14:31–17:00 | 16:16–19:00 |
| | (women) | 14:31–16:54 | 15:55–18:30 | 16:31–19:00 | 17:31–19:30 | 19:01–20:00 | 19:31–20:30 |
| IV. Good | (men) | 9:41–10:48 | 10:46–12:00 | 11:01–12:30 | 11:31–13:00 | 12:31–14:30 | 14:00–16:15 |
| | (women) | 12:30–14:30 | 13:31–15:54 | 14:31–16:30 | 15:56–17:30 | 16:31–19:00 | 17:31–19:30 |
| V. Excellent | (men) | 8:37–9:40 | 9:45–10:45 | 10:00–11:00 | 10:30–11:30 | 11:00–12:30 | 11:15–13:59 |
| | (women) | 11:50–12:29 | 12:30–13:30 | 13:00–14:30 | 13:45–15:55 | 14:30–16:30 | 16:30–17:30 |
| VI. Superior | (men) | <8:37 | <9:45 | <10:00 | <10:30 | <11:00 | <11:15 |
| | (women) | <11:50 | <12:30 | <13:00 | <13:45 | <14:30 | <16:30 |

< = less than; > = more than.

## Exercise 5.1b     Cooper's 3-Mile Walking Test (No Running)

Check off laps (for example, 28 for 190-yard track; 42 for 126-yard track):

1 - 2 - 3 - 4 - 5 - 6 - 7 - 8 - 9 - 10 - 11 - 12 - 13 - 14 - 15 - 16 - 17 - 18 - 19 - 20 - 21 - 22 - 23 - 24 - 25
26 - 27 - 28 - 29 - 30 - 31 - 32 - 33 - 34 - 35 - 36 - 37 - 38 - 39 - 40 - 41 - 42

Time: _____

Or, record below if using an open roadway.

      Stop Time: _____

   minus Start Time: _____

        Time: _____

**Circle Fitness Category:**

Very Poor     Poor     Fair

Good     Excellent

**Course Goal:** _____

**2-Month Goal:** _____

---

## Exercise 5.2b     Cooper's 12-Minute Walking/Running Test

Start Time: _____    Stop Time: _____    Distance Covered: _____

**Circle Fitness Category:**     Very Poor    Poor    Fair    Good    Excellent    Superior

**Course Goal:** _____

**2-Month Goal:** _____

---

## Exercise 5.3b     Cooper's 1.5-Mile Run/Walk Test

Check off laps (for example, 14 for 190-yard track; 21 for 126-yard track):

1 - 2 - 3 - 4 - 5 - 6 - 7 - 8 - 9 - 10 - 11 - 12 - 13 - 14 - 15 - 16 - 17 - 18 - 19 - 20 - 21

Time: _____

Or, record below if using an open roadway.

      Stop Time: _____

   minus Start Time: _____

        Time: _____

**Circle Fitness Category:**

Very Poor     Poor     Fair

Good     Excellent     Superior

**Course Goal:** _____

**2-Month Goal:** _____

---

## Exercise 5.4 Fitness Journal

**The Goal-Setting Challenge mentions the importance of recording your progress and gains in a Fitness Journal. Record these types of entries after each exercise session:**

Date/ Exercise Mode/ Time Duration/ Short-Term Goal/ Today's Achievement/ Thoughts and Feelings/ Additional Entries

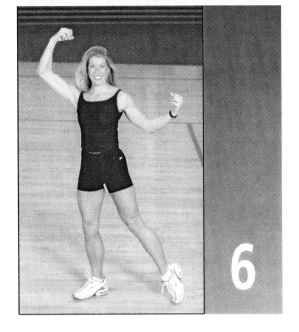

# Warm Up

**6**

The foundation for understanding physical fitness has been set. The terminology and criteria have been defined. The sensory-based components of motivation have been explored. You've become aware of the key questions to ask so you can set powerful, life-changing goals for every phase of your program. Strong encouragement has been (and will continue to be) given constantly to facilitate setting SMART goals—short-, medium-, or long-term—whatever works best for you. You've been informed about the risk and safety factors involved and good positioning that must be incorporated into all parts of your program to see results that last! And you've been given several fitness testing procedures for estimating your cardiovascular starting point.

Now we can build upon this base with principles and techniques that represent a safe, beneficial, and fun total fitness workout session.[1-10] The first of these program segments is the warm-up.

## Limbering Exercises

The warm-up begins with activities that are active, medium-to-low-level, rhythmic, limbering, standing, range-of-motion types of exercises that raise the body's core temperature slightly, initiate muscular movements, and prepare you for more strenuous moves to come. Examples such as step-touch with arm-curl swings (shown in the chapter opening photo),

wide stride squats with side-claps, sweeping punches, and other smooth, sweeping motions of low intensity (Figure 6.1) are good to initiate the warm-up. The timeframe is approximately 3 to 5 minutes.

> *Note:* All techniques are photographed and described by the "mirroring technique," in which the words and movement are to be done exactly as shown.

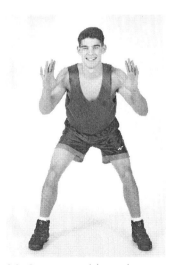

(a) Step-out wide and squat. Hold.

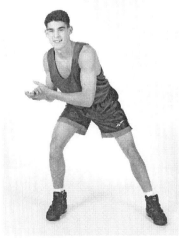

(b) Side-clap left, side clap right. (4 counts)

**Figure 6.1** Step-Out Wide and Squat

## Static Stretching

Slow-sustained, static stretching follows the initial warm-up exercises when the muscles, tendons, ligaments, and joints now are loose and pliable. Static stretching is done from head to toe (Figures 6.2–6.14).

Static stretching is probably the most popular, easiest, and safest form of stretching. It involves stretching a muscle or muscle group gradually to the point of limitation, then holding that position for approxi-

mately 15 seconds. The stretch is repeated to the opposite side. Each stretch is repeated several times. Static stretching is recommended when the muscles are warm—after the initial active phase of the warm-up, and later after intense physical activity.

## Breathing Techniques

Breathing should be continuous. Your entire system, especially your working muscles, constantly needs oxygen. Holding your breath and turning

red is not acceptable! While doing the warm-up or cool-down stretching (or any strengthening exercise), *exhale when you stretch*, by puckering your lips and breathing out, and *inhale deeply through your nose, filling your lungs completely (engage the use of your diaphragm) when you relax your muscles*. Cue yourself: "Breathe out and stretch; breathe in and relax." The timeframe suggested for the warm-up stretching segment is approximately 5 minutes.

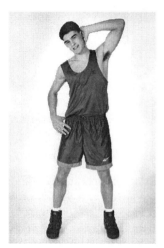

Drop head to *L* side and press with *R* palm, keeping elbow high. Stabilize with *L* hand on hip. Hold. (8 counts)

Reverse *R* side. (8 counts)

**Figure 6.2** Lateral Neck Stretch

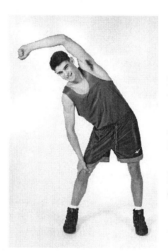

Sliding *L* hand down to *L* thigh, lean *L*; *R* hand and arm reach and stretch, close over head. Hold. (8 counts)

Reverse *R* side. (8 counts)

**Figure 6.3** Trunk Sideward Lean

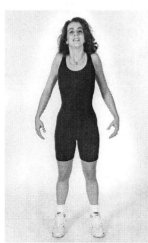

Up, back, down, forward; or alternate, one at a time. (4 counts in each direction)

**Figure 6.4** Shoulder Circles

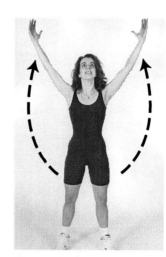

Arms low and center; wide and palms up; raise, reach high. (8 counts)

Reverse. (8 counts)

**Figure 6.5** Arm Sweeps

## *Static Stretching Moves*

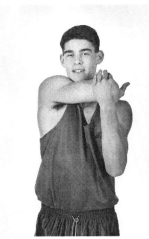

(a) Bring *L* upper arm under chin, keeping *L* elbow shoulder high; gently *press L* elbow toward you with *R* palm. Hold. (8 counts)

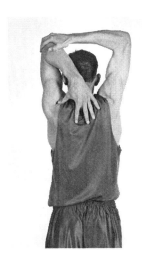

(b) Raise *L* arm/ elbow above head, placing *L* palm on center back; raise *R* arm, framing head, *R* elbow kept high; *R* palm gently *presses* *L* elbow backward. Hold. (8 counts)

Reverse (a), then (b). (16 counts)

**Figure 6.6** Shoulder/Upper Back Stretch

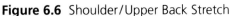

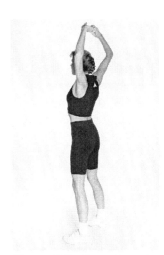

(a) Grasp hands very high, elbows bent, press back, and hold. (8 counts)

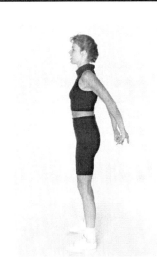

(b) Grasp hands low, behind back, lift and hold. (8 counts)

**Figure 6.7** Chest Stretch

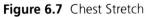

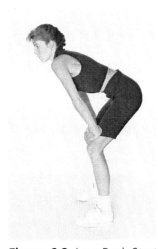

(a) Feet apart, hands on thighs, flatten back. Hold. (8 counts)

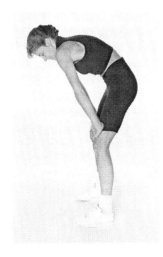

(b) Now round lower back upward, contract abdominals, tuck buttocks under hips. Hold. (8 counts)

**Figure 6.8** Low Back Stretch

## Static Stretching Moves

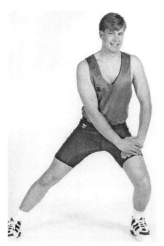

Feet apart/toes forward, shift weight/hips *R*; flex *R* knee over *R* toe. Hold. (8/16 counts)

Reverse.

**Figure 6.9**  Inner Thigh Stretch

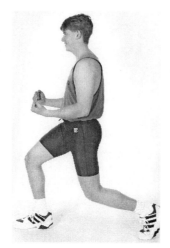

Forward/back stride, feet forward, fists at waist; firmly tuck buttocks under hips, flex and lower front knee. Contract hip flexors by bringing the back knee forward, with weight on ball of back foot and forward foot. Hold. (8/16 counts)

Reverse. (8/16 counts)

**Figure 6.10**  Hip Flexor Stretch

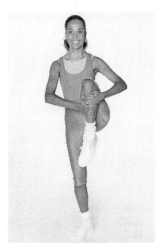

Weight *L* and turned out; encircle *R* knee and bring to chest, keeping spine upright. Hold. (8 counts)

Reverse. (8 counts)

**Figure 6.11**  Hamstring Stretch

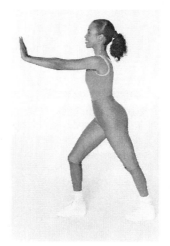

Immediately step backward with same leg held, feet in forward/backward stride; bend front knee just over toes, *keeping back foot flat on floor*. Straight arm forward press. Hold. (8 counts) Walk through and reverse. (8 counts)

**Figure 6.12**  Calf and Achilles Tendon Stretch

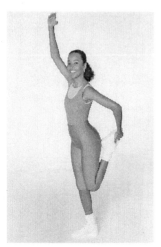

*L* foot turned outward carrying weight, bend *R* knee/leg backward, grasping shoestring area with *R* hand; *L* hand high and back for balance. Keeping knee pointing down and legs together, bring heel close to buttocks. Hold. (8 counts)

Reverse. (8 counts)

**Figure 6.13**  Quadriceps and Iliopsoas Stretch

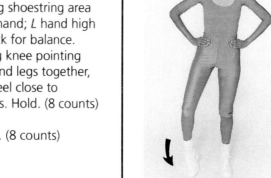

Weight on *R* foot and ball of *L* foot. Circle *L* ankle, stretching out, back, in, forward. (8 counts)

Reverse. (8 counts)

Repeat, weight *L* stretching *R* ankle. (16 counts)

**Figure 6.14**  Ankle Stretch

## Monitoring Progress

At the conclusion of the warm-up and stretching from head to toe, determine how hard you are working (intensity) by taking your pulse. The pulse tends to be in the range of 90 to 120 beats per minute (bpm), and the accompanying number of how you feel on the Borg Scale Ratings of Perceived Exertion should be approximately a "2" (see Chapter 1, Figure 1.6). Determine at this point in each class the ratings of perceived exertion "number" *you* are feeling, remember this number, and at the conclusion of class record it on Exercise 1.3, Part III, as your specific RPE warm-up reading for that day.

Immediately after each exercise session, take time to record your progress and gains (or setbacks) in your Fitness Journal.

---

*Static stretching is probably the most popular, easiest, and safest form of stretching.*

---

### Goal-Setting Challenge

✓ Write one Warm-Up Goal for Chapter 6 that you would like to achieve, following the four steps presented in Chapter 2, Exercise 2.3, then recording it in your Fitness Journal.

✓ Set an additional goal to stretch for *5–10 minutes every day* of your life. This provides you with mobility and comfort for a lifetime.

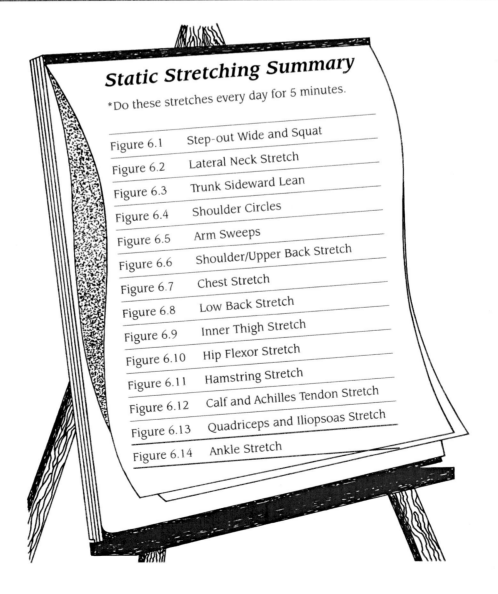

### Static Stretching Summary

*Do these stretches every day for 5 minutes.

| | |
|---|---|
| Figure 6.1 | Step-out Wide and Squat |
| Figure 6.2 | Lateral Neck Stretch |
| Figure 6.3 | Trunk Sideward Lean |
| Figure 6.4 | Shoulder Circles |
| Figure 6.5 | Arm Sweeps |
| Figure 6.6 | Shoulder/Upper Back Stretch |
| Figure 6.7 | Chest Stretch |
| Figure 6.8 | Low Back Stretch |
| Figure 6.9 | Inner Thigh Stretch |
| Figure 6.10 | Hip Flexor Stretch |
| Figure 6.11 | Hamstring Stretch |
| Figure 6.12 | Calf and Achilles Tendon Stretch |
| Figure 6.13 | Quadriceps and Iliopsoas Stretch |
| Figure 6.14 | Ankle Stretch |

# Exercise 6.1  Fitness Course Self-Assessment Checksheet

## Techniques / Skills / Knowledge

DIRECTIONS: Here is a listing of all physical fitness skills you'll be learning in this text. As you master each one, ✓ check it off. This can prepare you for the practical testing, at the end of the course.

**KEY:**

| | |
|---|---|
| 4 / A = always | |
| 3 / U = usually | |
| 2 / O = occasionally | |
| 1 / S = seldom | |
| 0 / N = never | |

### Aerobics / Step Training (column headings)

- Know how to determine resting heart rate.
- Know how to determine target heart rate.
- Use warm-up exercises—active, medium-to-low level, rhythmic, limbering, standing, full range of motion.
- Perform slow sustained static stretching (no bounce).
- Engage in continuous breathing.
- Exhale during stretch; inhale as release from stretch.
- During low-impact: keep legs low, arms below heart.
- During power low-impact: follow hip, knee, ankle extending moves by a knee flexion, ankle-springing action; one foot always in contact with the floor; space is well used.
- During high/low-impact: perform higher knees and arms overhead more frequently; use both airborne and grounded moves.
- During low-impact cool-down: use active, rhythmic, slower, half-tempo moves.
- Post-aerobic stretching: perform standing stretches for hamstrings, quadriceps, and calves.
- Know how to vary intensity and impacts.
- Know how to select proper bench height.
- Use proper posture: keep back straight, head and chest up, shoulders back, abdomen tight and buttocks tucked under hips.
- Lean forward slightly with the whole body. Don't bend at hips.
- Step up lightly, making sure the whole foot lands on platform.
- Do not lock knees when stepping up.
- Step down close to platform, not back.
- Bring heel down to floor before taking next step.
- Avoid excess arm movements over head.
- Maintain appropriate speed for safe movement.
- Do not pivot or twist on weight-bearing leg.
- Maintain muscular balance by working opposing muscle groups.
- Know bench/step directional approaches / orientations.
- Can perform single lead basic step.
- Can perform alternating lead basic step.
- Can perform touch step (w/bench tap, floor tap, lunge).
- Can perform v-step.
- Can perform straddle down.

## Techniques / Skills / Knowledge

**KEY:**

| | |
|---|---|
| 4 / A | |
| 3 / U | |
| 2 / O | |
| 1 / S | |
| 0 / N | |

### Step Training (cont.) / Fitness Walking / Strength / Flexibility / Relaxation (column headings)

- Can perform straddle up.
- Can perform single and alternating bypass moves (knee, kick back, side leg lift).
- Can perform lunge (from side and end).
- Can perform turn step.
- Can perform over the top.
- Can perform repeaters.
- Limit propulsions and power moves.
- Can perform propulsion steps.
- Can perform single-skill sequence (change one element at a time).
- Can perform double-skill sequence.
- Can perform multiple-skill sequence.
- Can pace-walk with proper heel-first mechanics.
- Use arms (short-lever or long-lever) efficiently.
- Keep body in a good alignment while pace-walking.
- Can keep pace to the beat of 120–128 bpm music for 1 song.
- Can keep pace to the beat of 120–128 bpm music for 20–40+ mins.
- Precede strength training with static stretching.
- Stabilize joints and spine before each exercise.
- Perform smooth, continuous, full range of motion movements.
- Maintain slow timing, and not jerky.
- Take 2 seconds to overcome resistance.
- Take 2 to 4 seconds during release/lowering phase.
- Exhale during lifting phase; inhale during lowering phase.
- Engage in visualization and self-talk.
- 1–3 sets, 8–12 reps format.
- Can add 1–4 lbs. resistance.
- Take brief rest periods between bouts.
- Can lift and lower whole body against gravity
- Can properly add weight resistance to body part used.
- Can control use of hand-held weights.
- Can use rubber resistance bands efficiently and effectively.
- Can use rubber resistance tubing efficiently and effectively.
- Can combine tubing with bench workout.
- Can combine step with strength using tubing and the bench in intervals of 3 min. step, to 1 min. strength-with-tubing.
- Can actively stretch slowly with position held at joint extreme.
- Can gently press slowly beyond this point without motion.
- Can mentally relax, visualize, self-talk, and hold for 15 seconds
- Can withdraw slowly from stretch.
- Perform to opposite side of body for each stretch.
- Can perform at least one PNF stretch.
- Can construct powerful images to relax.
- Can construct positive self-talk affirmations.
- Can deep-breathe and effectively lower after-workout heart rate.

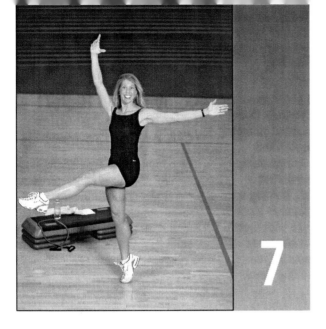

# Aerobic Exercise: #1 Aerobics

**7**

**T**he aerobic segment of your fitness program can consist of any activity that promotes the supply and use of oxygen, provided that it adheres to the aerobic exercise criteria established in Chapter 1. The aerobic exercise modalities presented in this book are *aerobics* (in this chapter), *step training* (Chapter 8), *fitness walking* and Elliptical Trainer use (Chapter 9).

## Principles of Aerobics

In addition to how often (frequency), how much work (heartbeats per minute/intensity), and how long to work out (duration of time per session), the concept of *impact* has to be considered when determining your fitness program.

Basic step movements in aerobics have changed considerably since the origin of the activity. These changes have centered on reducing and preventing injury, with the primary focus on amount of vertical force exerted on the feet as they contact the floor surface and how this stress subsequently affects the musculoskeletal system.

Early programs included many steps and gestures with great bodily elevation and corresponding great compression upon foot contact with the floor. Research has given the aerobics enthusiast a variety of safe alternatives regarding impact and movement possibilities.

## High-Impact Aerobics (HIA)

High-impact aerobics (HIA) involves steps and gestures in which both feet are off the floor at the same time briefly. This step movement results in great force exerted when the foot meets the floor surface. The force is absorbed by the landing, floor surface, shoes, orthotics (if worn), and musculoskeletal system (muscles, tendons, ligaments, joints, and bones).

Several examples of basic movements that are considered high-impact are jogging, hopping, and jumping. A few characteristics of high-impact aerobics are:

- Music between 130 and 160 beats per minute (bpm).
  - Faster music—smaller moves.
  - Slower music—greater range of motion.
- Landing through toe/ball/heel.
- Avoiding more than eight repetitions (reps) on one limb.
- Strengthening anterior tibialis (shin area).
- Strengthening hamstrings.
- Limited to every other day.
- Higher intensity = $>VO_2$ max.
- Moderate intensity > fat utilization.[1]

High-impact aerobics is generally *not recommended* for:

- Individuals who obviously are in poor condition or out of shape, especially obese people.
- Anyone who is susceptible to specific injuries (such as shin splints) caused by, or likely to be aggravated by, upward impacts on the feet.
- Women in the latter stages of pregnancy, who usually have loosened joints.
- Individuals who are incontinent (unable to control urination).
- Individuals who are uncomfortable with high-impact steps.[2]

## Low-Impact Aerobics (LIA)

Low-impact aerobics (LIA) involves steps and gestures that produce less force than those in high-impact movements when the feet strike the floor. LIA controls the landing and force of foot impact because one foot is in contact with the floor at all times.

*Low-impact does not mean low-intensity!* Cardiovascular and respiratory conditioning still can be achieved as long as you are working within the target heart rate training zone you've established. To help elevate your heart rate if it is not in

---

*LIA controls the landing and force of foot impact because one foot is in contact with the floor at all times.*

---

your zone, place more emphasis on weight-bearing moves that lower your center of gravity. Suggested ways to accomplish this include deepening knee flexion (bending motions) that uses the large leg and buttocks muscles (quadriceps and hamstrings, and gluteals) and gesture actions of the upper body. Examples of low-impact moves are step-touch, lunge, grapevine, marching, and vigorous walking in place. Characteristics of low-impact aerobics are:

- Heart rate is kept in the target heart rate (THR) training zone.
- Moves can be modified if the THR is not maintained.
- Any music tempo can be utilized.
  - With faster tempos, less space is covered.
  - With slower tempos, more space is covered.
- Feet are kept closer to the ground to decrease impact.
- Moves require traveling from side-to-side and forward-and-back so large muscles of legs and trunk are engaged continuously.
- Controlled, vigorous arm movements compensate for reduction in activity of the leg and back muscles when the height of hops and jumps is reduced. Research has shown that up to 25% more work can be performed with the arms and legs combined, compared to work performed by the legs alone.[3]

- Arms are not used above shoulder level for extended periods. Doing so necessitates extended isometric contractions of the arm and shoulder muscles and probably causes more soreness after exercise. In addition, holding the arms over the head raises blood pressure, and anyone with high blood pressure or a history of angina pectoralis should be discouraged from doing these movements.[4]

- Toes/knees are turned out, with wide legs.
- Center of gravity is raised and lowered.
- In lateral moves, legs are turned out.
- Angle of knee flexion is 90°.
- Vastus medialis (front, inner thigh) and hamstrings are strengthened.
- Adductor muscles are used for correct mechanics.[5]

Low-impact aerobics (LIA) is generally *not recommended* for:

- Anyone who complains of knee discomfort during prolonged knee flexion.
- Individuals who have severely flattened or pronated feet. (Knee flexion, and some side-to-side movements in which one foot crosses in front of the other, tends to cause the kneecap to shift toward the outer side of the knee joint, which increases stress.)
- Well-conditioned, injury-free individuals who are unable to achieve their target heart rate, even in the most intense LIA program. (Although many instructors use LIA exclusively in the interest of safety, conventional high-impact choreography may be acceptable for these participants as long as they remain injury-free.[6]

## Combination High-/ Low-Impact Aerobics (CIA or Combo-Impact)

The combination style of choreography, which utilizes characteristics of both high- and low-impact movements can be a safe and exciting blend. Combination high-/low-impact choreography can be defined in two ways.[7]

1. *Routines that offer both a high-impact and a low-impact version of a movement.* Programs that offer both of these versions work best in classes with mixed fitness levels so individual participants can select the amount of impact appropriate for them. A beginner in the program, therefore, might choose to do the low-impact version, whereas an experienced dance-exerciser might feel more challenged by the high-impact movements.

2. *Routines combining a series of varied high-impact and a series of varied low-impact movements.* This style lends itself well to classes of experienced aerobics exercisers whose primary concern is to improve cardiovascular and respiratory fitness while minimizing the risk of injury.

Combo-impact aerobics offers a wide range of choices and possibilities. It allows you to individualize how much physical stress you choose to experience safely at various times and stages of your life according to your fitness level, personal goals, and special interests. Especially if you are a beginner, or coming off an illness or injury, obese, older, or pregnant, you will want to choose the less biomechanically stressful, low-impact movements. Athletes in training and well-conditioned, injury-free individuals may choose the high-impact movements and series more frequently, or even exclusively. As another option, they might wish to blend their HIA and LIA techniques into

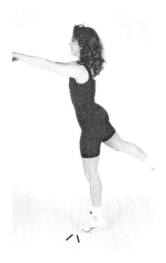

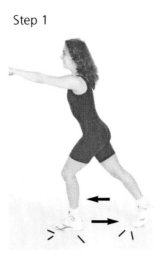

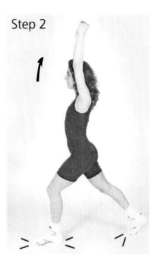

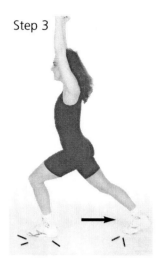

Step 1                   Step 2                   Step 3

**Figure 7.1** High-Impact Version of a Lunge (Momentarily Airborne)

**Figure 7.2** Lower Impact by Stepping Backward or Forward Instead of Jumping

**Figure 7.3** Increased Intensity by Raising Arms

**Figure 7.4** Increased Use of Space by Reaching Farther

the *moderate-impact aerobic* (MIA) style explained in the next section.

The unique feature of a combination approach is that participants can choose from the various possibilities the impact that best fits their current lifestyle needs. Some people, of course, can never participate in the high-impact movements because of permanent physical limitations.

As illustrated by Figures 7.1–7.4, a three-step process for interpreting any high-impact steps into acceptable low-impact movement can be accomplished by:

1. Lowering the foot impact.
2. Increasing the arm movement.
3. Increasing the use of space.

Step 1 of this process minimizes the impact, and steps 2 and 3 increase the intensity of the movement. The idea is to change one element at a time. Combining a series of varied high-impact and a series of varied low-impact movements will produce fewer of the large upward impacts typical of a HIA program and fewer of the large side-to-side impacts typical of many LIA programs.

Keen attention to the beat of the music becomes important when converting high-impact movement to

low-impact movement, to ensure an injury-free workout. The sum of all the stresses on the vulnerable parts of the body is what determines whether injury occurs.

## Moderate-Impact Aerobics (MIA)

The fourth alternative style of impact aerobics is called moderate-impact aerobics (MIA). It was designed as the result of laboratory and dance-exercise class research done at San Diego State University.[8] By adapting the gesture style (non-weight-bearing body parts) and foot impact, this choreographic style combines the best elements of both HIA and LIA, for movements that keep the intensity needed to maintain target heart rate while reducing foot-impact forces.

This key technique is called *plyometric*.[9] At least one foot remains in contact with the floor most of the time to reduce potentially injurious stresses on the body. The center of gravity of the body, however, rises and falls almost as much as it does during HIA, thereby avoiding prolonged knee flexion.[10] This raising and lowering of the center of gravity, by extending the hip, knee, and ankle joints without

actually leaving the floor, requires *work*, the expenditure of energy. This provides for a relatively high exercise intensity.

Athletes have used the plyometric technique for many years, in sports such as track and skiing, to increase power in a workout. These athletes have used plyometric techniques to increase their springing or bounding abilities. For example, picture yourself engaged in either sport and landing and recovering after a forceful jump. The lifting and springing action is plyometric. You are forcefully loading the weight as you jump and then undergoing a powerful unloading, or springing out of this move.[11]

Although this is an effective method to increase power, it can be stressful to the musculoskeletal system of the average person. In moderate-impact aerobics the plyometric principle of power in movement is used, but you will load the weight with much less force by simply bending or flexing the knees and the hips, then springing out of this position. This will allow you to increase the intensity safely and also safely increase power in your leg and hip muscles.

In many LIA routines the emphasis is placed on flexing the knees, lowering and then raising the body to an erect position. This can be stressful to the knees of some participants. In addition, many beginners have found that this *down-up* movement is unnatural and requires a great deal of concentration. If the amount of knee flexion is decreased and *emphasis is placed on extending the knees and ankle joints without the feet actually leaving the floor*—as in moderate-impact aerobics—the center of gravity can be raised and lowered effectively. The physiological cost is high, but the bouncy motions are comfortable and stimulating for many participants.[12]

To clarify the differences between the three distinct methods of impact, an example of *stepping-in-place* is:

- *High-impact aerobics:* jogging—both feet off the ground briefly.

- *Low-impact aerobics:* marching—one foot always in contact with the floor.

- *Moderate-impact aerobics:* plyometric techniques using the lift-and-spring action depicted in Figure 7.5.

The main difference between high-impact jogging and the moderate-impact version is the *rate at which the force on the foot is increased*. Even though the final load on the foot for the MIA step is close in magnitude to that for the HIA step, the load increases much more gradually during the MIA step.

Researchers believe that when high levels of force are exerted on the feet suddenly, the human body is vulnerable to injury. The body is equipped with reflex mechanisms that can control muscle contractions to protect it from mechanical stress. Damage can result, however, if the forces reach high levels before the reflex mechanisms can provide protection. In practical terms, the spring-like motions of MIA are less jarring than the high-impact versions because the body is raised and lowered with control. In HIA, the body is

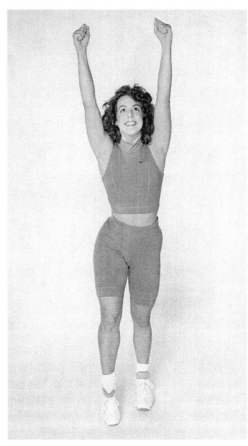

Keeping your *R* foot flat on the floor, raise your *L* foot until the tip of your *L* toe is just barely in contact with the floor. Now alternate the position of the feet to the same tempo that you used for the two previous movements. Lift your body as high as possible as you shift your weight from foot to foot by using the full range of motion of your ankle joints and moderate amounts of knee flexion and extension. Make certain that the heel of the supporting foot is pressed to the floor to maintain a good range of motion of the ankle joint.

**Figure 7.5** Lift-and-Spring Plyometric Technique

under less control as it falls freely, colliding suddenly with the floor.[13]

---

***The sum of all the stresses on the various vulnerable parts of the body is what determines whether injury occurs.***

---

Guidelines for using moderate-impact aerobics are as follows:

1. Begin movements by lifting your body upward, rising onto the balls of your feet. Complete each step, whenever possible, by lowering your heels and pressing them gently against the floor. This action produces the spring-like motion characteristic of MIA steps. The lifting and lowering of the center of gravity is what increases exercise intensity.

2. Concentrate on leaving at least one foot on the floor most of the time. The purpose of MIA is to reduce the magnitude of impact. Steps such as MIA jogs, jumps, and twists are performed with both feet on the floor, either bearing the weight on both feet, as in a jump, or bearing it on one foot with the second foot touching the floor lightly, as in a twisting step.

MIA steps that require lifting one foot off the floor, such as kicks and knee-lifts, must be timed carefully so the airborne foot is back on the floor before the opposite foot leaves the floor.

3. Exercise intensity can be increased by traveling directionally across the floor and using the arms through a wide range of movement.

4. To adapt your present LIA or HIA moves to MIA, concentrate on taking the movement up and down while keeping one foot on the floor most of the time. (Not all LIA and HIA steps can be modified to suit MIA. Practice and common sense will help you determine which steps can be adjusted best.) Examples of steps that adapt well to MIA are heel-jacks, jogs, jumps, kicks, knee-lifts, ponies, step-touches, and twists.

5. For variety, mix MIA with LIA and HIA steps.

6. Because the ankle joint is used through a wider range of motion with MIA than with HIA and LIA, it is particularly important to strengthen the tibialis anterior (shin area) and stretch the gastroc-nemius and soleus (back lower leg area) muscles during warm-up and cool-down. These precautions will help prevent tightness of the calf, as well as muscle imbalance.[14]

## *Caloric Expenditure From Aerobics*

If all of the variables are attended to and duplicated carefully, aerobics can cause substantial energy expenditure of more than *12 calories per minute, with no significant difference in caloric expenditure between low- and high-impact routines* (if these routines are duplicated in style, content, and energy level).[15] Certified instructors (IDEA Foundation and AFAA) conducted the research, which involved two 11-minute sequences of high-impact and low-impact aerobics at a tempo of 148 bpm. For those concerned with weight management, it is exciting to realize that one can engage in high- or low-impact moves and still expend significant energy and burn calories.

Because the average peak force of LIA can result in impact forces of approximately 1½ times your weight and HIA can result in foot impact approximately 3 times your weight,[16] the impact you choose can be important—especially if you have

physical limitations (for example, obesity, pregnancy, susceptibility to joint injury). Choice of *impact,* therefore, does not have to be made in regard to caloric expenditure.

## Intensity Matters

*Intensity*, or how fast your heart beats, however, matters. If you are exercising far too intensely, it makes your aerobic training very uncomfortable. If you *stay in your individualized training zone*, your comfort level and enjoyment is greatly enhanced. When you exceed your appropriate training zone, your body shifts from burning fat into burning blood sugar (glucose). When you are burning mostly glucose, cardiovascular exercise tends to become very uncomfortable to sustain, both during a single exercise session, and even more so, with repeated bouts of too intense exercise.[17]

## Decide, What Is Your Primary Goal?

When initiating your fitness program, decide the following.

- Is my goal primarily to train my heart to become more fit? If so, your program design is to:
  1. warm up
  2. **aerobically train**
  3. **strength train,** especially your upper body (since most aerobic activity includes impact activity that trains the lower body)
  4. cool down
  5. relax

- Is my goal to primarily train my heart *plus* lose unwanted body fat? If so, your program design is to:
  1. warm up
  2. **strength train** (especially the upper body)
  3. **aerobically train**
  4. cool down
  5. relax

The difference in the sequence of these two program designs is simple and it deals with the kind of fuel you are using...glucose (blood sugar) or body fat.

"Always resistance train (weight training or strength training) first, followed by cardiovascular training (aerobics) *especially if the goal includes losing body fat.* Here's why: Our bodies use two primary sources of energy to fuel most of our activity, blood glucose and body fat. The body will always use glucose first before using body fat; it's just an easier source of fuel to access.[18] So, when we perform cardiovascular exercise, our body uses either glucose, or stored body fat as its fuel to perform the work. *Strength training, on the other hand, uses primarily a glucose energy system (blood sugar) and very little fat as its fuel source.* If someone was to start their exercise session with cardio, during the training session glucose will be utilized as the primary fuel source until the point that blood sugar is depleted. Only then will the body begin to use its fat reserve to fuel the cardio session. And, chances are, if cardio is performed first, the exercise session may not completely deplete glucose and tap into body fat. Now, once a person is finished with cardio and moves into the strength training, they may have very little energy left in reserve to get through resistance training, since much of the body's glucose was used during the cardio training. (Remember, glucose is the primary energy source for weight training.")[19]

"Opposite scenario... Starting with resistance training and finishing with cardio, the exerciser uses most and in some cases all, of their available glucose during the strength training session. As they progress into their cardio activity, they will quickly begin using stored body fat as fuel. Remember strength training uses glucose for fuel, cardiovascular training uses either glucose or body fat, but prefers glucose if it's available. Doing the strength training first, followed by cardio training, allows the body to utilize excess body fat most effectively."[20]

Here is a sample effective cardio program where your goal is also to lose body fat:

**Session 1:** Perform strength training first, followed by a long (45–60 minute) but *lower intensity* cardiovascular session. Lower intensity specifically means elevating your heart rate 60–70% of your maximum heart rate, as determined by the formula in Exercise 1.3 How To Figure Your Target Heart Rate Training Zone.

**Session 2:** Strength training followed by 25–35 minutes of a *moderate intensity* cardiovascular session (70-80% range of your maximum heart rate).

**Session 3:** (To be followed only by healthy people with no signs of heart disease) Strength training followed by a short (20 minutes) *intense* bout of cardio-training. In this session, an exerciser would incorporate 3–4 very intense, but short (60–90 seconds) sprints of up to 95–100% of your maximum heart rate. Specifically the 20 minutes breaks down as follows: maintain heart rate between 60–70% of maximum for first 5 minutes, then begin the first sprint lasting for 60–90 seconds shooting for up to 95% maximum heart rate. After sprinting, allow heart rate to come back down to 60–70%. Repeat this sequence two more times, first at the 10 minute mark and

then again at the 15-minute mark. Once you hit 20 minutes, you're finished with the session and your energy will feel amazingly elevated throughout the day!

*Note:* If you're new to participating in an exercise program, give yourself plenty of time (2–3 months) for your body to work up to this type of cardio training (used by personal trainers in private sessions with clients). Check with both your doctor and a well-qualified fitness professional for direction and advice on your specific readiness for the Session 3 workout.[21]

**Time of Day/Nutrition:** Regarding best time of day for a workout session...this is specific to when you feel at your best. There is a slight metabolic advantage to working out first thing in the morning on an empty stomach, provided you have enough fuel from the previous day's nutrition to complete the session. If you feel like you need some additional nutrients to make it through a training session first thing in the morning, eat a little protein and very few carbs or fat. The protein will feed your working muscles while allowing you to burn fat throughout the exercise session. Try having a shake made of 30 grams of protein (no carbs or fat) just before your morning workout.[22]

## *Aerobics Techniques*

The aerobics segment of your fitness hour can be subdivided into six parts, each focusing on the impact in relation to the heart rate intensity you are building, sustaining, or lowering and according to which phase of the hour you are in.

These six parts are:

1. Low-impact aerobics warm-up
2. Power low-impact aerobics
3. High-/low-impact aerobics
4. Power low-impact aerobics
5. Low-impact aerobics cool-down
6. Post-aerobics stretching.

### Low-Impact Aerobics Warm-Up

The LIA warm-up consists of simple, low-intensity moves that increase the heart rate gradually. They start with the legs down low and arms below heart level. To increase the intensity

gradually, the range of motion of each movement is first increased, and then the use of air and floor space is widened. For example: Step-touch in place with hand claps, punching, or arms shoulder high (Figure 7.6) with hands pointing in

(a), and then both hands and toe-touch extending far out, to the side (b). Progress to a grapevine (Figure 7.7), using large arm reaches, then the other low-impact moves (Figures 7.8–7.16). The timeframe is 5 minutes.

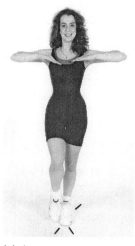
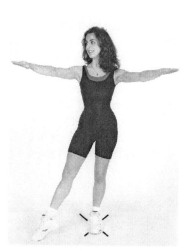

(a) In         (b) Out

**Figure 7.6** Step Touch

## Low-Impact Aerobics Warm-Up

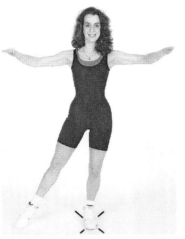 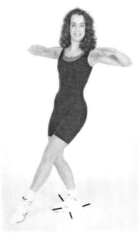 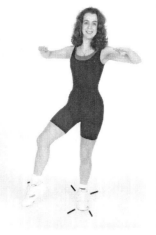 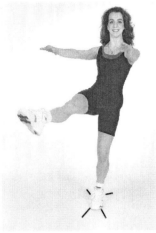

(a) Step to *R* side, arms out shoulder high.

(b) Step back *L*, and bring arms in, still shoulder high.

(c) Step *R* side.

(d) Weight still *R*, kick *L*, arms forward and parallel.

**Figure 7.7** Grapevine

**Options:** Instead of kick: ▪ touch ▪ knee-lift ▪ lift-touch forward or backward.

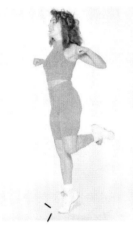

(a) One-foot bounce while bending other knee, with lower leg pointing back. (1 count)

> **Low-impact aerobics require that one foot is always in contact with the floor.**

**Figure 7.9** Bounce 'n Tap Series

(Shown and completely described in Chapter 4.8a-d.)

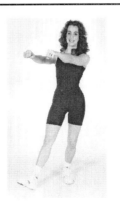

(a) Bounce *R* foot while *L* heel extends forward. Arms forward. (1 count)

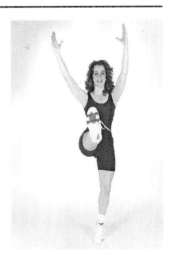

**Figure 7.11** Kicks

Weight on one foot, kick other leg to only a 90° waist-high level (or lower). Forward or sideward. (1 count)

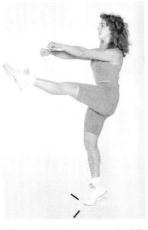

(b) One-foot bounce and kick same leg forward, waist-high or lower. (1 count)

(b) Bounce *R* foot while *L* toe taps in close. Draw arms in to chest. (1 count)

Repeat heel out, followed by feet back in together in a transitional move. (2 counts)

**Figure 7.8** Bounce 'n Hitch-Kick

**Figure 7.10** Heel-Toe Bounce Series

**Options:** Add bounce. (2 counts)

## Low-Impact Aerobics Warm-Up

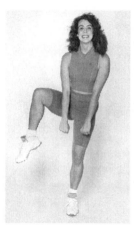

(a) Bounce *R* foot, lifting *L* knee to *L* side. Arms parallel, punch down. (1–2 counts)

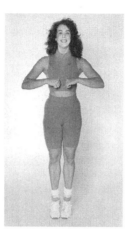

(b) Feet together bouncing, lift arms chest-high in a half upright-row position (transitional move). (1 count)

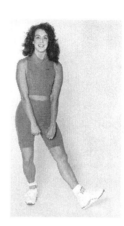

(c) Bounce *L* foot, extending *R* heel forward. Arms parallel, punch down. (1–2 counts)

Last, repeat (b) transitional move. (1 count)

**Figure 7.12** Hoe-Down

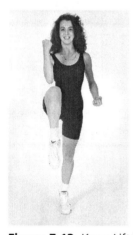

(a) Step *R*, knee-lift *L* knee forward, touch same elbow. (2 counts)

Reverse.

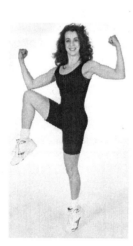

(b) Step *R*, knee-lift *L* knee sideward, same elbow out wide and touch. (2 counts)

Reverse.

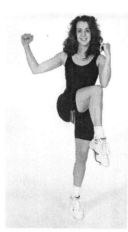

(c) Step *R*, knee-lift *L* knee across body center forward, *R* (opposite) elbow across chest and touching the lifted knee. (2 counts)

Reverse.

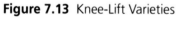

**Figure 7.13** Knee-Lift Varieties

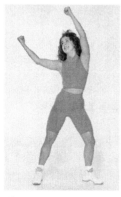

Step and bounce-lunge *R*, arms overhead, parallel and diagonally high *L*, head following direction of arms. (2 counts)

Reverse, shifting weight. (2 counts)

**Figure 7.14** Lunge Side and Bounce

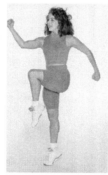

Step-lift, one count each step pattern. Swing arms opposite and big. (1 count)

**Figure 7.15** Marching

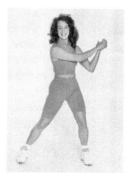

Step out wide stride to *R* side, bending knees. (1 count)

Clap hands *R*. (1 count)

Reverse. (2 counts)

**Figure 7.16** Side Step-Out

## Power Low-Impact Aerobics

The moves illustrated here increase the load on the large muscles of the legs by bending and extending more, with the accent on lifting or raising the center of gravity while keeping at least one foot firmly on the floor and recovering with an ankle-flexion springing movement. Traveling through space is characteristic with these movements, which really challenge the leg muscles. The examples in Figures 7.17 to 7.23 are strong low-impact with plyometrics. The time-frame is approximately 10 minutes.

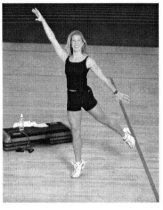

**Figure 7.17** Bouncing and Reaching—Side

Reach *L*, extend *L* arm high, weight on *L* foot. (1 count)

Bring feet together, arms into center and two-foot bounce. (1 count)

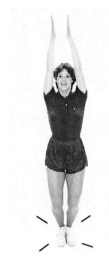

Two-foot bounce and reach high above you. (2 counts)

**Figure 7.18** Bouncing and Reaching—Center

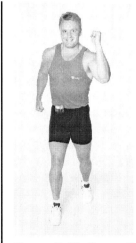
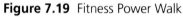

Walk with force, using short-lever or long-lever arms.

**Figure 7.19** Fitness Power Walk

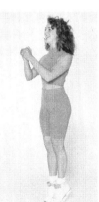

(a) Lift high on balls of feet, without leaving floor. (1 count)

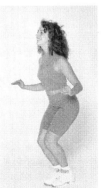
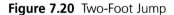

(b) Land and gently press the heels into the floor. (1 count)

**Figure 7.20** Two-Foot Jump

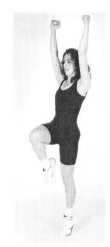
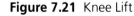

Lift knee while rising to ball of foot. (1 count)

Lower heel of support foot as lifted foot returns to floor. (1 count)

Arms forcefully assist in raising entire body, reaching above shoulder level.

**Figure 7.21** Knee Lift

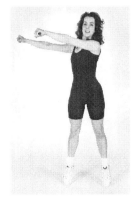

Shift weight from ball of foot to ball of other foot as you lift your body and twist from side to side. (2 counts)

**Figure 7.23** Twist

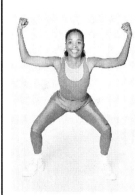

With feet in a wide base of support, toes out, bend knees and hips, and "sit"; curl arms wide and shoulder high, and in. (1 count)

**Figure 7.22** Squats

Extend arms out, legs upward to full extension. (1 count)

*Note:* **You also can easily use these moves as moderate-impact plyometric moves: lunges, jumps, kicks, step-touches, jogs, heel-jacks, ponies.**

## High-/Low-Impact Aerobics

Here you'll intersperse high-impact moves, in which both feet may leave the floor momentarily, with low-impact moves, in which one foot always remains on the floor. You'll raise your arms overhead more frequently, and raise the knees and feet up higher.

A key point in this segment is that the intensity of the moves you choose must remain high so the heart rate maintains the high, but safe, training zone you've established for cardiovascular and respiratory improvement. *Not more than four high-impact repetitions are performed on the same leg at one time.* Examples are: two high-impact jacks in the wide-stride-and-together leg and arm positions (Figure 7.33), followed by four low-impact power-walking moves with forceful arms (Figure 7.19).

Most *high-impact* moves can be converted easily to *low-impact* moves simply by removing the five basic high-impact movements outlined in Table 7.1. Instead of a take-off and landing, those moves are changed to the following moves:

- One foot remains on the floor as the free foot uses floor and air space.
- Both feet remain on the floor, incorporating the lifting and lowering plyometric principles described earlier.

To change *low-impact* moves to *high-impact* moves, you simply replace the stationary-foot move and incorporate the high-impact locomotor moves of take-offs and landings (hops, hitch-kicks, leaps, rocks, hop astride, two-foot jumps, or hopscotch-type moves replace a low-impact step move). The time-frame is approximately 15 minutes.

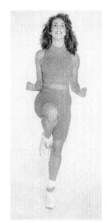

**Single Hops:**
Hop *R*, forward lifting *L* knee.
(1 count)

**Double Hops:**
Repeat *R* hop.
(2 counts)

**Figure 7.24** Hops—Single and Double

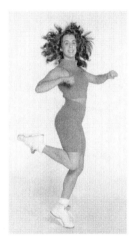

(a) Hop on *L* as *R* foot lifts back, knee bent.

**Options:**
Pull arms back forcefully.
(1 count)

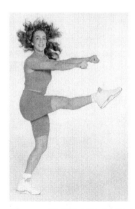

(b) Hop *L* again, kicking *R* forward, waist-high or lower.

**Options:**
Arms forcefully parallel, punching forward.
(1 count)

**Figure 7.25** Hitch-Kick    Reverse.
(2 counts)

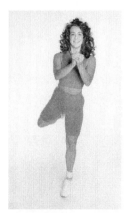

With weight *L* (not shown) take off, propelling body forward and upward, *R* foot.
(4 counts)

**Figure 7.26** Leap

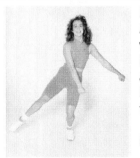

Hop on *R* foot to *R* side, placing weight over *R* leg (knee and ankle flexed), lifting *L* leg out to side. (1 count)

Reverse.

**Figure 7.27** Rock Side-to-Side

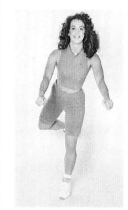

Rock (hop) *R* into forward lean, lifting *L* leg back and up for balance.
(1 count)

**Figure 7.28** Rock Forward

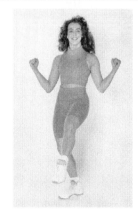

Rock (hop) *L* backward into backward lean, lifting *R* leg forward and up for balance.
(1 count)

**Figure 7.29** Rock Backward

## Two-Foot Jump

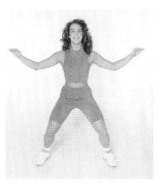

**Figure 7.30** Astride

With weight *R* or *L* (not shown), hop to astride or straddle position, loading weight onto both feet by bending knees. (1 count)

(Usually preceded by or followed with another move.)

*Table 7.1 Basic High-Impact Locomotor Movements*[23]

| Take-Off | Landing | Example | Figure |
|----------|---------|---------|--------|
| One foot | same foot | hop; hitch-kick | 7.24; 7.25 |
| One foot | opposite foot | leap; rock | 7.26; 7.27–7.29 |
| One foot | two feet | astride | 7.30 |
| Two feet | two feet | jump (widestride or together) | 7.31–7.33 |
| Two feet | one foot | hopscotch; polka | 7.34–7.35 |

Source: *Aerobic Dance—A Way to Fitness*, 2d ed., by Karen S. Mazzeo et al. (Englewood, CO: Morton Publishing, 1987), p. 112.

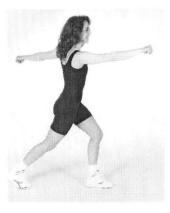

**Figure 7.31** Lunge

Two-foot scissors jump forward on *R* foot, bending *R* while keeping *L* leg extended back (still bearing weight on *L*) in wide forward/backward lunge position, *L* arm forward, *R* arm back. (1 count)

**Options:**

- Jump back to two feet together and center (1 count), then reverse the forward and backward legs and arms, lunging and jumping back to center. (2 counts)
- Reverse directly from forward/backward lunge (1 count), to opposite forward/backward lunge position. (1 count)

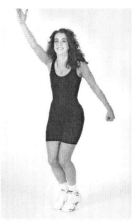

(a) Jump sideward, forward, or back. Hold. (2 counts)

Reverse.

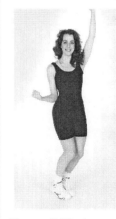

(b)

**Options:** Use skiing arms position with *L* elbow close, *R* elbow high and wide, when jumping *R*. Reverse arms when you reverse feet.

**Figure 7.32** Jumps—Feet Together

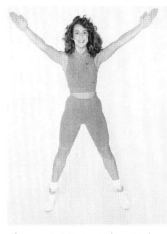

**Figure 7.33** Jumping Jacks

(a) When executing two-foot jump to side in *wide-stride position*, followed by two-foot jump *together*, (b) this becomes a jumping jack. Arms can work wide and together with legs, or in opposition (not shown).

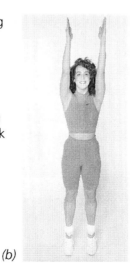

(b)

**Options:**
Coordination Pattern: Jump wide (a); together with high arms (b); jump wide (a); together with low arms (not shown). (4 counts)

*Many popular social dances, or dance steps and gestures, are aerobics possibilities.*[24]

## High/Low-Impact Aerobics

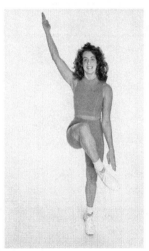

**Figure 7.34** Hopscotch

**Forward** (a) Hop to astride position (Figure 7.30) and with weight on *R* foot, hop and touch *L* foot raised forward to lowered *R* hand (a knee-open position). (2 counts)

For balance, reach *L* hand diagonally skyward, thumb back.

Reverse.

**Back** (b) Hop to stride position (Figure 7.30), and with weight on *L* foot, hop and touch *R* foot raised backward to lowered *L* hand. (2 counts)

For balance, reach *R* hand diagonally skyward, thumb back.

Reverse.

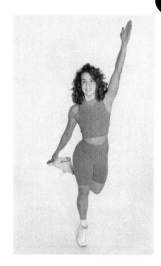

**Note:** If you have sensitive (injury-prone or recent surgery) knees, avoid this exercise.

---

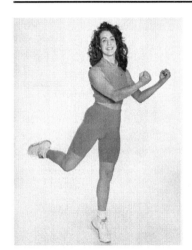

**Figure 7.35** Polka

(a) Hop *R*, lifting *L* leg backward. (1 count)

(b) Step *L*, in close quickly. (1/2 count)
Step *R*, in close quickly. (1/2 count)
Step *L*, in close quickly. (1/2 count)

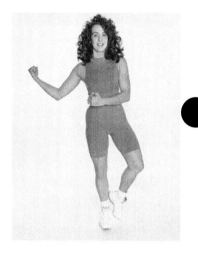

---

## Aerobics Variety: Funk Moves

Funk aerobics are exercise moves developed from the culturally rich areas of jazz dance, ballet, street dance, gymnastics floor-exercise competition, and other rhythmical forms of aesthetic, emotionally expressive movement.

Funk aerobics include numerous expressive trunk, elbow and knee moves (Figure 7.36), funk walking (Figure 7.37) that mimics movie and television characters, and animation moves such as the funky chicken.

Creative expression and attitude prevail in funk exercise movement. Body gestures include the extremely big and wide-open positions (Figure 7.38), followed quickly by closed, tight, head gesture or hair-tossing moves (Figure 7.39). The only limitation for funk aerobics lies in your own resources, experience, and individual creativity—which for all of us are unlimited!

For yet another creative option, combine your favorite aerobics moves with the step bench (Chapter 8). "Step Training the Funky Cha-Cha" and other dance moves open up the possibilities of unlimited program variety.

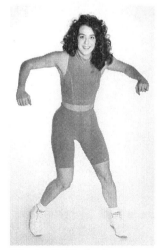

**Figure 7.36** Funky Elbows and Knees

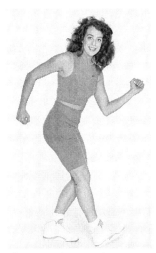

**Figure 7.37** Funky Walks/Animation

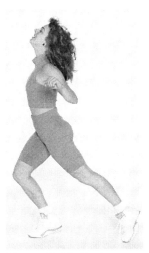

**Figure 7.38** Funky Open Position

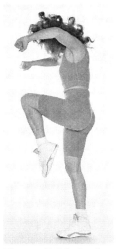

**Figure 7.39** Funky Closed Position

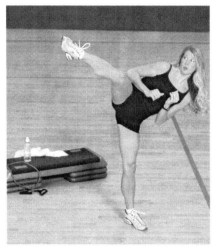

**Figure 7.40** Box Aerobics—Kicks

## Sports Conditioning

An aerobic sports conditioning workout uses movements that simulate sports, such as box aerobics.[25] Movement patterns are basic and simple to follow, emphasizing coordination, speed, agility, and quickness. These fun movements can be a great way to energize your workout.

*Box aerobics* utilizes the upper body during the aerobic segment of the workout.[26] Researchers have found that an hour of noncontact boxing uses as much energy as running 5⅝ miles in an hour.[27]

A box aerobic class incorporates the *boxer shuffle* (shifting your weight in little bounces from left to right) while throwing punches and kicking. Before throwing a punch, you must have the proper *stance*: feet a comfortable distance apart in a forward-backward position with both knees slightly bent. Arms are kept close to the side and slightly to the front of the body.

Punching movements used in boxing include *jabs* that extend the arm without locking the elbow, thumb tucked and down, and leading with the first two knuckles. *Upper cuts* entail forcefully swinging the bent arm up and following with the elbow. *Hooks* are punches that use

the back muscles to propel the arm,[28] extending it across the chest. *Kicks* (in any direction) may be added to a box aerobics workout (Figure 7.40).

## Aerobics Gesture, Step, and Pattern Cues

Here is a list of gesture, step, and pattern cues to assist you with designing an individualized program for yourself, according to your favorite moves and combinations.

- **Arm Circle:** Circle-back; forward; big; small.

- **Bounce, Hitch-Kick:** One-foot bounce, kick; other-foot bounce, kick. (Figure 7.8)

- **Bounce 'n Tap Pattern:** Forward, side, back, together (or hold); forward, side, back, together (or hold). (Figures 7.9, 7.12b)

- **Bounce 'n Tap Sequences:** Right forward 4, side 4, back 4, hold 4; repeat left forward 4, etc. Right forward 3 and hold 1, side 3 and hold 1, back 3 and hold 1, hold 4; repeat left forward 3 and hold 1, etc. Right forward 2, side 2, back 2, hold 2; repeat left forward 2, etc. Right forward, side,

back, hold; left forward, side, back, hold. (Figures 4.8a–d)

- **Bounce, Two Feet:** Bounce. Or: Lift, bounce. (Figure 7.12b)

- **Bounce, Two Feet Variation:** Punch, bounce.

- **Bounce-Step, Bounce-Touch:** Two-foot bounce-step, one foot bounce and touch; two-foot bounce-step, one foot bounce and touch. (Figures 7.12b, 4.8b)

- **Bounce Steps, with Side Touch:** One foot bounce, touch, one foot bounce, touch.

- **Box Aerobics:**

  **Hooks:** Cross and punch; return.

  **Jabs:** Extend knuckles and punch; return.

  **Upper Cuts:** Cut up and punch; return.

  **Boxer Stance:** Forward-backward comfortably wide-stance; slight bend of knees; arms side-close-front.

  **Boxer Shuffle:** Shift-little bounce left, right; repeat. Add arms or kicks.

  **Boxer Kicks:** Face forward, weight left, kick right side right; Alternate: weight right, kick left side left. (Figure 7.40).

- **Cha-Cha:** Cross (right forward), (left step) back, step-step, step;

cross (left forward), (right step) back, step-step, step.

■ **Cha-Cha, with Kick Pattern:** Cross, back, step, kick, step, step, step-step, step.

■ **Charleston Flapper Walk:** Step and swing forward, step and swing back.

■ **Cross-Step Forward, Touch to Side:** Cross, touch; cross, touch.

■ **Cross-Step, Hop:** Cross, hop; cross, hop.

■ **"Doubles" Knees and Kicks:** Knee-lift, down, up, down; kick, down, up, down. (Figures 7.13, 7.11)

■ **Double Hops:** Hop, hop and punch; hop, hop and punch.

■ **Double Hop, Hitch Kick:** Hop, hop-kick; hop, hop-kick.

■ **Fall Back 'n Jump Forward Pattern:** Hop, step-step, rock-back, rock-forward. (Figures 7.35, 7.29, 7.28)

■ **Funk:**

**Elbows and Knees:** Bend/extend/wide/out, relax; repeat left. (Figure 7.36)

**Walks and Animation:** Attitude walkin', walkin'. (Figure 7.37)

**Open and Closed:** Strut wide, in, wide, in (Figures 7.38, 7.39), and reverse.

■ **Gallop:** Step, slide and lift.

■ **Grapevine:** Side, back, side, touch; side, back, side, touch. (Figure 7.7)

■ **Grapevine Varieties:**

**'n Kick:** Side, back, side, kick. (Figure 7.7)

**'n Hop:** Side, back, side, hop-clap (or hop-click, or hop-punch).

**'n Jump-Clap:** Side, back, side, jump-clap.

■ **Heel-Out, Toe-in Bounce Pattern:** Out, in, out, bounce; out, in, out, bounce. (Figures 7.10, 7.12)

■ **Hip Thrust:** Astride, thrust; astride, thrust.

■ **Hoe-down:** Bounce/lift, punch down; two-foot bounce;

bounce/heel touch; two-foot bounce. (Figure 7.12)

■ **Hops, Single:** Hop/lift; repeat left.
**Double:** Hop, hop (same foot). (Figure 7.24)

■ **Hop, Hitch-Kick:** Hop, hop-kick (or kick-back, forward). (Figure 7.25)

■ **Hop, Kick:** Hop, kick; hop, kick. (Figures 7.24, 7.11); reverse.

■ **Hopscotch:** Astride, hop, astride, hop. (Figures 7.30, 7.24)

■ **Hopscotch, Variety:** Astride, hop-touch; astride, hop-touch. (Figures 7.30, 7.34)

■ **Hustle:** Jog, jog, jog, lift-clap; jog-back, jog, jog, lift-clap.

**Cross-Elbow Touch:** Jog, jog, jog, elbow-touch; jog, jog, jog, elbow-touch.

**High Impact:** Hop, hop, hop, lift; hop, hop, hop, lift.

**Low Impact:** Pace-walk, walk, walk, lift; pace-walk-back, walk, walk, lift.

■ **Jazz Touch—Out 'n In pattern:** Out, in, out, shift-your-weight; out, in, out, weight-right. (Figure 7.6)

■ **Jazz Touch—Forward 'n Backward Pattern:** Forward, back, forward, shift-your-weight; forward, back, forward, weight-right.

■ **Jog:** Jog—heel first.
**Circling:** Jog, 2, 3, 4, 5, 6, 7, 8. Jog—left, 2, 3, 4, 5, 6, 7, 8.

■ **Jumps:**

**Big/Little:** Big, turn-clap, little and clap; turn-clap, little-clap; turn-clap, little-clap; turn-front-clap, little-clap.

**One-Foot Jump:** Jump-right; jump-left.

**Two-Foot Jump:** Jump and clap! (Figure 7.20)

**Circling:** 3 o'clock, 6 o'clock, 9 o'clock, noon; reverse-and-9 o'clock, 6 o'clock, 3 o'clock, 12 o'clock.

**Forward 'n Backward:** Jump-forward, jump-back.

**'n Land, Widestride:** Jump and land-wide, hold. (Figure 7.33)

**Side Jump, Clap:** Jump-side, clap; side, clap. (Figure 7.32a)

**Ski Jump:** Jump-side, hold; jump-side, hold. (Figure 7.32b)

■ **Jumping Jacks:**

**Regular:** Stride-clap, together-slap.

**Coordinated:** Astride-wide, together-clap. (Figure 7.33)

**Crazy:** Stride, cross; stride, cross.

**Double Pattern:** X, high I, X, low I. (Figure 7.33)

■ **Kicks:** Kick right; repeat left. Or, kick, bounce, kick, bounce. (Figure 7.11)

■ **Knee-Lift:** Power lift, power lower; repeat left. (Figure 7.21)

■ **Knee-Lift Elbow-Touch, Varieties:**

**Same Side:** Step-lift, elbow-touch-same; repeat left. (Figure 7.13a)

**Open to Side:** Step-lift, elbow-touch-open; repeat left. (Figure 7.13b)

**Crossed:** Step-lift, cross-elbow-touch; repeat left. (Figure 7.13c)

**High Intensity:** Hop-lift, elbow-touch-(same/open/crossed).

■ **Leap:** Push-off, leap forward, and clap; repeat left. (Figure 7.26)

■ **Lunges:**

**Forward:** Forward lunge, 2, 3, 4, 5, 6, 7, 8; walk-through-and-lunge, 2, 3, 4, 5, 6, 7, 8.

**Scissor:** Jump-forward, scissor-jump. (Figure 7.31)

**Side:** Lunge-side and bounce (the holding counts). (Figure 7.14)

**Side, with Arm Circling:** Lunge-3 o'clock, hold; 6 o'clock, hold; 9 o'clock, hold; noon, hold; reverse counterclockwise.

**Side-Bounce 'n Sway:** Lunge-side and bounce; sway-lunge and bounce. (Figure 7.14)

- **March:** Left, right; forward, to-the-rear, side. (Figure 7.15)
- **Polka:** Hop-step, step-step; hop-step, step-step. (Figure 7.35)

  **Circling:** To-the-right, back, side, forward.

  **Low-Impact:** Step, step, step, hold; step, step, step, hold.

  **Side-to-Side:** To-the-left; to-the-right.
- **Prance:** March, hop-lift march, hop-lift march. (Figure 7.15 with a hop)
- **Quads 'n Hams Coordination Pattern:** Step, lift-front, step, lift-back. (Figure 7.34)

  **Variety:** Step, lift-front left, step, lift-front right; step, lift-back left, step, lift-back right. (Figures 7.30, 7.34)
- **Reach:** Bounce-step, reach; bounce-step, reach. (Figures 7.17 and 7.18)
- **Rock:**

  **Big, Forward 'n Backward:** Rock-forward and back. (Figures 7.28 and 7.29)

  **Side-to-Side:** Rock-side; side. (Figure 7.27)

  **Side-to-Side Variety:** Rock-side and punch; side and punch.
- **Shake Up, Shake Down:** Shake, two, three, four; shake-down, six, seven, eight.
- **Side Coordination Pattern:** Side (right), together (left), side (right), touch (left); side (left), together (right), side (left), touch (right).
- **Side Step-Out:** Side, clap; side clap. (Figure 7.16)
- **Skip:** Step, hop; step, hop. (Figure 7.24)
- **Slides:** Step, together-step.
- **Slide, Bend, Jump, Clap Pattern:** Slide, bend, jump, clap; slide, bend, jump, clap.
- **Squats:** Sit, extend. (Figure 7.22)
- **Step, Hop:** Step, hop. (Figure 7.24)

**Circling:** Step, hop to the side; step, hop to the back; step, hop to the side; step, hop front.
- **Step, Hop, Step, Kick Pattern:** Step (right), hop (right), step (left), kick (right).
- **Step, Kick:** Step, kick; step, kick.

  **Circling:** Step, kick; two; three; four; five; six; seven; eight.

  **'n Punch-Down:** Step, kick-side and punch down, step, kick-front, and punch down.

  **Sidekick:** Step, side-kick and click; step, side-kick and click.
- **Step, Lift, Touch, Lift Pattern:** Step (right), lift (left), touch (left), lift (left); step (left), lift (right), touch (right), lift (right).
- **Stride 'n Twist Pattern:** Stride, cross, turn, hold, lift, touch, kick, touch.
- **The Twist:** Step forward and twist-down, 2, 3, 4; twist-up, 2, 3, 4; walk-through-forward (or back) and twist, 2, 3, 4; twist-up, 2, 3, 4.

  **Power Twist:** Lift and twist, down; lift and twist, down. (Figure 7.23)
- **Walk:** Power-walk-forward and (count each pace walk). (Figure 7.19)
- **Walk Varieties, with Creative Arm Gestures:**

  **Backward:** Pace-walk back and (count).

  **Diagonally:** Pace-walk diagonally-right, and (count).

  **Sideward:** Pace-walk-side, and (count).
- **Widestrides:**

  **Arm Crossover:** Stride-bend and cross, up, raise, out and down.

## Chair-Aerobics

Chair-bound and love aerobics? Not a problem! Practically every move and gesture in this listing can be performed *seated in a chair!* Position: Move to a position on your chair that is *forward of the center,* sit tall, hold

onto the arm of the chair (if necessary) and turn on your favorite upbeat music. You can get a great cardio workout in this seated position, as well as on your feet.

Don't stop there! Turn to Chapter 10 on Strength Training, get out your resistance tubing or handheld weights, and try as many moves as you can (using good form) from all of those shown. To use your tube with appropriate resistance, you'll need to roll it up in your hands or at your wrists.

## Power Low-Impact Aerobics

Again, power LIA consists of the center-of-gravity lifting, hip-knee-ankle extending moves, followed by the knee-flexion, ankle springing-action moves in which one foot is always in contact with the floor, to keep the force of impact low (Figures 7.17–7.24). The timeframe is approximately 5 minutes.

## Low-Impact Aerobics Cool-Down

These are the lower intensity moves needed to lower your heart rate gradually. The moves are still active and rhythmic, using a full range of motion, but now are low-level and slower, half-the-tempo moves. They are the same as those used in the warm-up, Figures 7.6 to 7.16. The timeframe is approximately 10 minutes.

## Post-Aerobics Stretching

Stretching the lower-body muscles to aid blood returning to the heart and preventing blood pooling in the legs is performed by standing static stretches for the hamstrings (Figure 6.11), quadriceps/iliopsoas (Figure 6.13), and calf muscles (Figure 6.12). The timeframe can be approximately 3 to 5 minutes.

## Goal-Setting Challenge

 Set a goal that challenges your ability to master the moves, and develop sequences and then entire routines. Write this Aerobics Goal for Chapter 7 following the four steps presented in Chapter 2 Exercise 2.3, then recording it in your Fitness Journal.

 Then, using Exercise 7.1, Creating Aerobics Exercise Routines, create a routine, using the variables for steps and gestures, and a variety of movement.

## Exercise 7.1  Creating Aerobics Exercise Routines

| Impact | Low-Impact | | | | | | | | | | | | High-Impact | | | | | | | | | | | | | | |
|---|---|---|---|---|---|---|---|---|---|---|---|---|---|---|---|---|---|---|---|---|---|---|---|---|---|---|---|
| **Aerobic Moves:** | Bouncing | ■2Ft/HK/'n Tap | 1/2 Galloping | Hoe-Down | Heel-Toe | Kicks | Knee-Lifts | Lunging | Marching | Pace Walking | Side Step-Out | Step-Touches | Galloping | Hitch-Kick | Hopping | ■Single/Double | ■W Kick | ■W Knee Lift | Jogging/Run | Jumping 2 ft. | ■Stride/Closed | ■Hopscotch | Leaping | Polka | Prancing | Rocking | Skipping | Sliding |
| **Gesture Basics:**<br>■ Bending-Twisting | | | | | | | | | | | | | | | | | | | | | | | | | | | | |
| **Gesture Style:**<br>■ Athletic-Western | | | | | | | | | | | | | | | | | | | | | | | | | | | | |
| **Added Sounds:**<br>■ Claps/Snaps/Audibles | | | | | | | | | | | | | | | | | | | | | | | | | | | | |
| **Levers:**<br>■ Arms short/long<br>■ Legs short/long | | | | | | | | | | | | | | | | | | | | | | | | | | | | |
| **Planes:**<br>■ Horiz./Vert./Diag. | | | | | | | | | | | | | | | | | | | | | | | | | | | | |
| **Levels:**<br>■ Low/Medium/High | | | | | | | | | | | | | | | | | | | | | | | | | | | | |
| **Direction:**<br>■ Up/Down<br>■ Right/Left<br>■ Forward/Back<br>■ Diagonal | | | | | | | | | | | | | | | | | | | | | | | | | | | | |
| **Pathway:**<br>■ Straight<br>■ Curved<br>■ Zigzag | | | | | | | | | | | | | | | | | | | | | | | | | | | | |
| **Rhythm/Beat**<br>Accented 1–2–3–4 | | | | | | | | | | | | | | | | | | | | | | | | | | | | |
| **Symmetry:**<br>■ Symmetrical<br>■ Asymmetrical | | | | | | | | | | | | | | | | | | | | | | | | | | | | |
| **Force of:**<br>■ Foot Impact<br>■ Gestures | | | | | | | | | | | | | | | | | | | | | | | | | | | | |

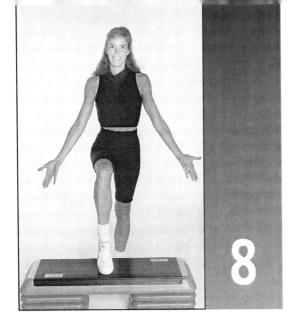

# Aerobic Exercise:
## #2 Step Training

**M**otivation to stay with any fitness program will be enhanced by adding variety to your program when you need a change. Two unique possibilities to add to the aerobic segment of your program are (a) bench/step training and (b) aerobic intervals of bench/step training with strength training, involving the bench/step and resistance tubing.

## Principles of Bench/Step Training

Because bench/step training continues to be a popular mode of aerobic fitness training, much research has been conducted to determine the physiological and biomechanical effects of bench/step exercise. The following information and guidelines are derived from various researchers promoting the activity and companies promoting products to use with the activity.[1-5]

Step training involves stepping up and down on a platform or bench, adding a variety of upper-torso movements for further challenge. This form of exercise is known by many names, including bench or step aerobics, bench or step training, bench stepping, and stepping.

The key advantage to a step training program over other aerobics is that it is primarily a *high-intensity activity* used to promote

cardiovascular and respiratory fitness but *with low impact* to satisfy safety concerns. A vast majority of the moves involve one foot supporting the weight, either on the bench platform or on the floor. Other benefits include the following:

- It's a terrific conditioning workout for every major muscle group in the lower body, specifically the hamstrings, quadriceps, gluteals, and calves.

- Upper-torso movements provide conditioning work for muscles of the arms, shoulders, chest, and back, and therefore a balanced and complete workout that strengthens and tones the entire body. This becomes especially apparent later if you combine training modes within one class format or perform step and strength intervals.

- This workout allows versatility in the class using basic moves that are very simple. The variety can

> An effective cardiovascular workout has aerobic benefits equal to running 7 miles per hour (mph), yet has the potentially low-impact equivalence of walking at a 3-mph pace, minimizing the chance of injury.[6]

encompass step patterns with fewer (or more) arm gestures, adjusting the height of the bench, increasing or decreasing the range of motion, incorporating long or short levers, and incorporating propulsion or low-impact moves, and including participants of all ages, skill and fitness levels, and both genders.

Step training is similar to all other forms of physical activity because it has an element of risk. The concerns and subsequent research associated with this exciting and challenging modality of exercise have focused on evaluating:

- Energy cost of aerobic bench/step techniques
- Physiological benefits
- Musculoskeletal safety of step training exercise.[7-12]

Research to date has produced the following highlights:

- Step training provides the sufficient cardiovascular and respiratory demands needed to attain cardiovascular and respiratory fitness in accordance with American College of Sports Medicine (ACSM) guidelines.[13]
- Determining exact energy costs depends upon various factors including height of the step bench, rate of stepping, and step pattern/technique.[14]

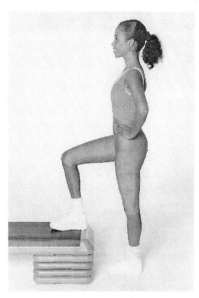

**Figure 8.1** Knee Position Indicating Correct Height for Bench

- Bench step height and rate of stepping significantly affect metabolic cost. This varies among participants because of differences in muscle mass rather than height of participants.[15]

- Specific step moves used within a workout all have specific effects on energy cost (that is, different movement patterns result in different intensities). For example, moves such as the basic step, step touch, and bypass moves expend less energy than lunging, traveling, and repeater moves.[16]

- Propulsion or power movements significantly increase heart rate and exercise intensity.[17]

- Stepping at accelerated speeds (33–35 cycles per minute) results in an increase in lactic acid levels, indicating anaeobic metabolism.[18]

- Step training injuries vary with the ground force impact and are related to step height, speed of music, and movements performed.[19]

In summary, and in keeping with research data, step training performed according to ACSM guidelines can improve cardiovascular fitness significantly. And because several variables can affect heart rate intensity, programs can be designed to meet the needs of each individual participant, to facilitate both optimum safety and effectiveness.

## Choosing Your Bench Height

When choosing a bench height, the following factors should be considered:

- Beginners who have not exercised regularly, have limited coordination, or have no experience in step training should select a 4"–6" bench initially. For the bench pictured in the chapter opening photo, this represents the basic 4" platform, and at most one 2" support block on each end.

- Intermediate or regular step trainers with a "physically fit" level of cardiovascular and respiratory fitness should choose an 8" bench. An 8" bench equals a 4" platform plus two 2" support blocks.

- Taller individuals and those with longer legs than most people should consider using a bench of 8".

- An advanced or a regular and skilled step exerciser can choose up to 10".

- Regardless of level of fitness or experience, the bench height should not allow the knee to flex less than 90° (Figure 8.1) when the knee is weight-bearing. *If the knees advance beyond the toes while stepping up, the platform is too high.*

- Choosing a platform that is too high for your energy or fitness level may affect your body alignment and result in injury. For example, if you are leaning too far forward, the platform may be too high and can cause undesirable pressure on the lower back.[20]

An optional test for bench height is shown in Figure 8.2. Place one foot flat on top of the bench; allow a 3" drop from hip to knee for safe movement up to the top of the bench.

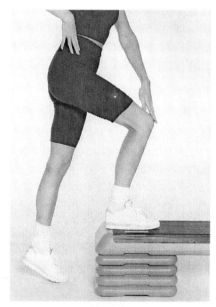

**Figure 8.2** Optional Test for Bench Height, Allowing 3" Drop from Hip to Knee

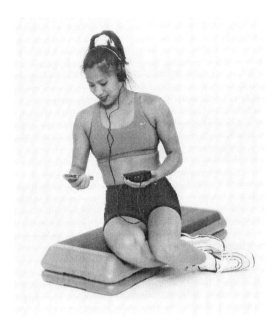

**Figure 8.3** Music at Appropriate Tempo Accompanying Step Training

## Table 8.1  Suggested Times and Tempos

| Duration (mins.) | Segment | Beats per Minute |
|---|---|---|
| 10–12 | ■ Warm-Up | 130–140 |
| | ■ Step Training: | |
| 4–5 | Pre-Aerobic | 118–124 |
| 20–30 | Aerobic Stepping | 118–122 Novice |
| | | *NTE 124 Beginner |
| | | NTE 126 Intermediate |
| | | NTE 128 Advanced[21] |
| 4–5 | Post-Aerobic | 120–124 |
| 10–15 | ■ Muscle Conditioning | 110–130 |
| 5–6 | ■ Slow Stretch | <100 |

*Not to Exceed

## Stepping to Music

Music plays a significant role, providing the underlying structure of a step training program. Fun, exciting music can motivate and challenge participants. The tempo of the music (measured as beats per minute, or bpm) determines the speed and directs the progression of the movement performed.

Using music with a bpm of 118 to 128 is best.[21] This will keep the movements controlled.

Stepping at speeds above the recommended guidelines can be unsafe and can result in the following:[22]

■ Poor postural alignment because of the tendency to bend forward at the waist in order to step onto the platform more quickly.

■ Improper foot placement and inability to make full foot contact with the bench when stepping up, and with the floor when stepping back.

■ Limited range of motion, particularly for long-limbed individuals.

■ Increase in ground force impact, which has the potential to cause overuse injuries.

The music should have a clear beat that is easy to follow (Figure 8.3).

Table 8.1 lists the suggested time duration for each class segment, followed by the tempo of music (bpm) suggested for each segment.

A listing of top companies that offer a selection of appropriate music for various exercise modalities[23] is listed on the page entitled 'Websites' at the end of the text.

## Body Alignment and Stepping Technique

Good posture is required for a safe, injury-free workout. Proper alignment and stepping technique include the following:

■ Keep your back straight, head and chest up, shoulders back, abdomen tight, and buttocks tucked under the hips, with eyes on the platform (Figure 8.4).

■ As much as possible, keep your shoulders aligned over your hips. Lean forward with the whole body. Don't bend from the hips or round the shoulders and lean forward or backward.

■ Step up lightly, making sure that the whole foot lands on the platform, with the heel bearing your weight. Placing your foot only partially on the bench (with the heel off the bench) increases your chance of slipping off, tripping, or even flipping the bench.

■ Keep your knees aligned over your feet when they're pulling your body weight onto the platform.

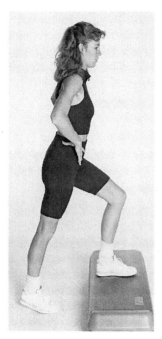

**Figure 8.4** Proper Technique for Stepping Up

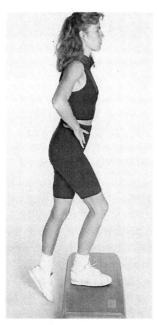

**Figure 8.5** Proper Technique for Stepping Down

- At the top, straighten your legs but don't lock your knees. Keep them "soft."
- As you step down, stay close to the platform. Step down, not back. Land on the ball of the foot (Figure 8.5), then bring the heel down onto the floor, before taking the next step. Stepping too far back with the leading leg causes the body to lean slightly forward, placing extra stress on the foot, achilles, and calf.

## Stepping Safely[24]

The following tips will decrease your risk for injury and promote safety:

- Avoid excessive arm movements over your head as this places a great deal of stress on the shoulder joint.
- Maintain appropriate speed for safe and effective movement.
- Change the lead leg after 1 minute maximum. The lead leg (leg that steps up first) experiences the most muscular skeletal stress.
- Limit propulsions and power moves. Power movements are considered advanced and can result in greater impact. Power or propulsion steps should be performed only *onto* the step and not down.
- Do not perform more than 8 counts (4 repeaters) on one leg at a time. Repeated foot impact without variation is potentially harmful.
- Do not pivot or twist the knee on the weight-bearing leg.
- Do not step up with your back toward the platform.
- Limit propulsions and power moves.
- Maintain muscular balance, working opposing muscle groups equally (quadriceps/hamstrings; calves/tibialis anterior; pectorals/upper back).
- If you feel faint or dizzy, or if any exercise causes pain or severe

discomfort, stop the exercise immediately but continue to move around.

- Limit one person to a bench at a time. Do not allow anyone to perform on the bench with you.
- If you are pregnant, check with your doctor before starting a step program. If your doctor clears you, make certain to keep your heart rate at 23 beats or below for a 10-second count (138 bpm). A step height of no more than 6" is recommended during pregnancy.

## Adjusting Your Intensity

To decrease or increase your heart rate, try the following measures:
   To decrease intensity:

1. Keep hands on hips
2. Lower bench height
3. Perform movements only on floor
4. Decrease music tempo

   To increase intensity:

1. Make larger range-of-motion arm movements
2. Add 2" support blocks to bench height
3. Increase music tempo

## Step Bench Using Tubing

Chapter 10 presents a variety of exercises using tubing in combination with the step bench for either weight training alone or for an *interval step training/strength training workout*. The key to the latter workout is incorporating 1-minute intervals of tubing exercises using the bench, with the body pressed into a bent-knees position on the action of the exercise. This position helps keep the heart rate in the training zone during strength training and provides another safe, unique variety for the aerobic exercise segment of your fitness program.

## Correct Step Training Posture

Three common step training errors and their corrections are illustrated in Figures 8.6, 8.8, and 8.10. The man is demonstrating incorrect postural techniques for each exercise. In Figures 8.7, 8.9, and 8.11, the woman is performing correctly. Additional performance suggestions are included with each position.[25]

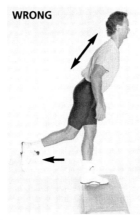

Undesirable curve of lower back with excessive rear leg lift and forward body lean.

**Figure 8.6** Incorrect Hip-Leg Extension

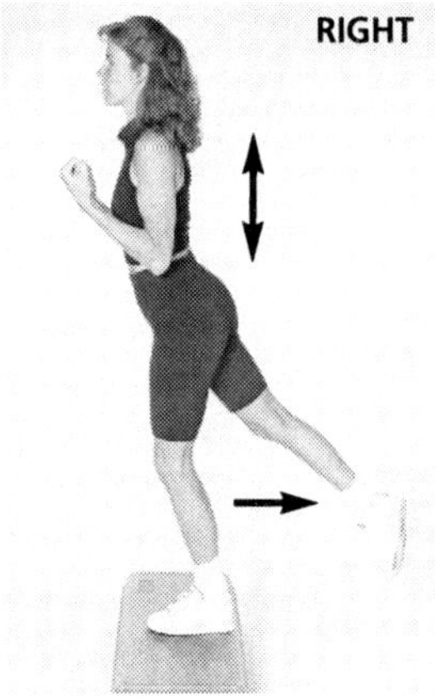

Stand tall on the platform and extend the rear lifting leg *back*, not up. This move is important to include for muscle balance.

**Figure 8.7** Correct Position for Hip-Leg Extension

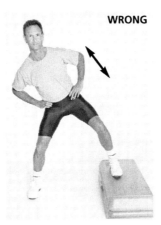

Tendency to lean too far out to the side, which places too much stress on the knee.

**Figure 8.8** Incorrect Side Step-Out Squats

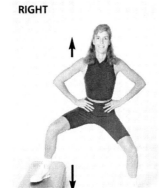

Balance your weight evenly, keeping center of gravity squarely within your legs. This move is a great exercise for the thighs and buttocks.

**Figure 8.9** Correct Position for Side Step-Out Squats

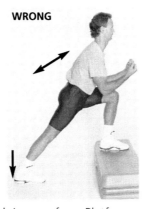

Bending too far forward at hip or having the leg reaching back in locked-knee position. Heel should not be forced to floor, as it may be too much dorsiflexion of the foot.

**Figure 8.10** Incorrect Step-Back Lunges from Platform

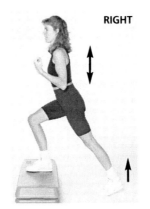

Keep body weight mainly over platform leg, and knee over toes. Leg reaching back should make floor contact, with knee slightly flexed. This reduces chance for joint trauma from ground impact. Back heel is raised off the floor.

**Figure 8.11** Correct Position for Step-Back Lunges from Platform

## Summary Step-Bench Principles

A bench/step training program has many advantages and benefits. It is a high-intensity exercise that sustains the training zone heart rate needed to produce the cardiovascular and respiratory training effect. Yet, it is low impact and safe, as one foot remains on the bench or the floor. Maintaining the safety precautions—selecting the correct bench height, having good body positioning and alignment, introducing variety in technique to prevent overuse, and following the guidelines for accompanying arm gestures—is the key to enjoying this modality of aerobic training.

At this point you have an understanding of an important step: *personal safety*. It is now time to begin your step training program, and this is initiated by considering the following goal challenge:

## *Step Techniques*

The step training techniques that follow represent movement depicting:

- the warm-up and step aerobics (the strength training and cooling down with the step/bench are presented in Chapters 10 and 11)

- directional approaches and orientations (your body in relation to the bench)
- basic steps
- basic step patterns
- variations possible, using basic steps and basic step patterns (see Figure 8.12)

These step techniques are photographed and described by the "mirroring technique" for all *front* views shown (actual left of the model is your right). Natural photography is used and described for all *side* and *rear* views, including traveling patterns that have a side or rear-view portion. The words and the movements, therefore, are to be performed *exactly* as shown.

If you're following the movements of an instructor, position the bench for maximum visibility.

## Warm-Up

The warm-up begins with active, low-level, rhythmic, limbering, standing, range-of-motion types of exercises that raise the body's core temperature slightly, initiate muscular movements, and prepare you for more strenuous moves to come. Involve the step/bench by performing moves that integrate the floor and the bench.

Example: Perform bench step taps, with bicep curls (Figure 8.13). Use low-impact moves that allow you to adjust to the height and contour of the bench, such as stepping up and down at half the tempo, marching on top of the bench, or straddling the bench and alternating tapping on top of the bench (Figure 8.14). The timeframe is approximately 5 minutes.

After the muscles, tendons, ligaments, and joints are loose and pliable, exercise takes the form of slow, sustained, static stretching. Static stretching, probably the most popular, easiest, and safest form of stretching, involves gradually stretching a muscle or muscle group to the point of limitation, then holding that position for approximately 15 seconds. The stretch is repeated to the opposite side. Several repetitions of each stretch are performed. Static stretching is recommended when muscles are warm (after the initial active phase of the warm-up and later after intense physical activity).

Stretch all major muscles from head to toe. Chapter 6 presents ideas with special consideration for the major muscle groups in the legs (the thighs, hips, and calves), as step training is lower-body intensive. When step training, the bench can be used as a fixed object to enhance stretching (Figures 8.15–8.18).[26]

---

## *Goal-Setting Challenge*

 Set a short-term goal to develop at least one new 16-count pattern you enjoy each week. Then set a course goal to use your created new patterns together in a sequence that lasts as long as your favorite step training song. Write this Step Training Goal for Chapter 8 following the four steps presented in Chapter 2, Exercise 2.3, then recording it in your Fitness Journal.

**Figure 8.12**

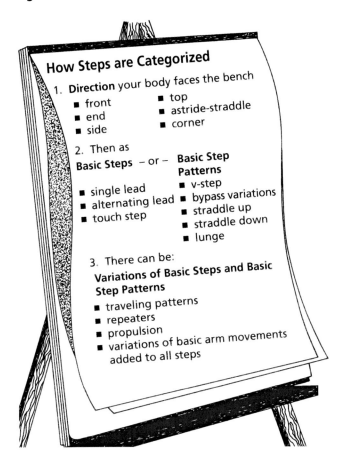

How Steps are Categorized

1. **Direction** your body faces the bench
   - front
   - end
   - side
   - top
   - astride-straddle
   - corner

2. Then as
   **Basic Steps** – or – **Basic Step Patterns**
   - single lead
   - alternating lead
   - touch step
   - v-step
   - bypass variations
   - straddle up
   - straddle down
   - lunge

3. There can be:
   **Variations of Basic Steps and Basic Step Patterns**
   - traveling patterns
   - repeaters
   - propulsion
   - variations of basic arm movements added to all steps

## Breathing Technique

Breathe continuously. Your entire system, especially your working muscles, constantly needs oxygen. Holding your breath and turning red is never appropriate. While performing the warm-up and cool-down stretching (or any strengthening exercise), exhale when you stretch by puckering your lips and breathing out, and inhale when you relax your muscles. Cue yourself: "Breathe out and stretch"; "breathe in and relax." The timeframe for the warm-up stretching segment is approximately 5 minutes.

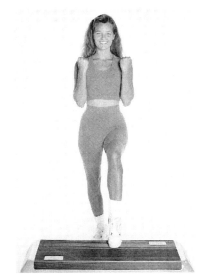

**Figure 8.13** Bench Step Taps with Bicep Curls

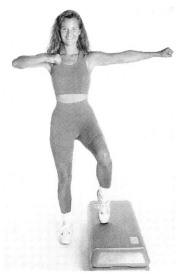

**Figure 8.14** Alternate Tapping on Top from the Straddle Position

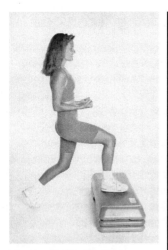

**Figure 8.15** Hip Flexors—Facing the Bench

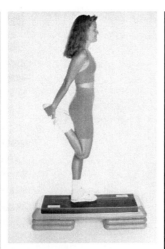

**Figure 8.16** Quadricep Stretch—Standing on the Bench

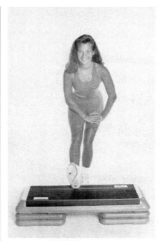

**Figure 8.17** Hamstring Stretch—Facing the Bench

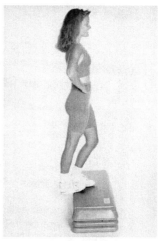

**Figure 8.18** Calf Stretch—Standing on Top of the Bench

## Bench/Step Directional Approaches and Orientations

Initial movement onto the bench can begin from one of the following directions (the direction your body *faces* the bench), Figures 8.19–8.24:

- front
- end
- side
- top
- astride/ straddle
- corner

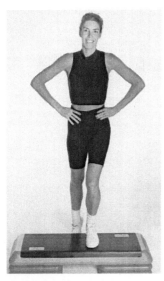

Face the bench squarely.

**Figure 8.19** From the Front

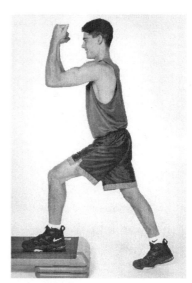

Face the end of the bench.

**Figure 8.20** From the End

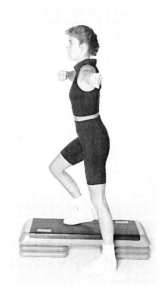

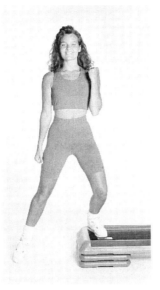

(a) Stand with your side next to the side of the bench.

(b) Stand with your side next to the end of the bench.

For both (a) and (b), step up with the foot that is closest to the side of the bench.

**Figure 8.21** From the Side

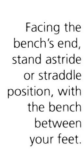

Facing the bench's end, stand astride or straddle position, with the bench between your feet.

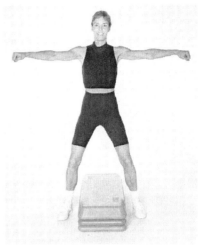

**Figure 8.23** Astride / Straddle Orientation

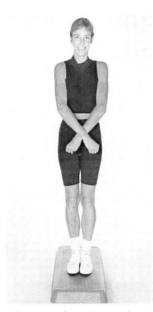

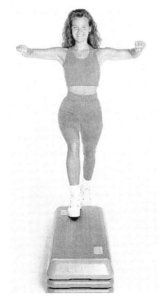

(a) Atop, face the end of the bench with feet together (shown), or feet in a forward/ backward stride.

(b) Atop, stand at the back end of the bench, and step off the back in a forward/backward stride.

**Figure 8.22** From the Top

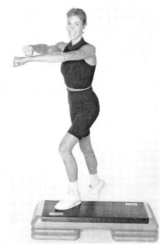

Face the corner of the bench. If facing at an angle to the left, step up with the right foot first; if facing at an angle to the right, step up with the left foot first.

**Figure 8.24** Corner Orientation, Facing the Corner

## Basic Steps

Three basic steps may be performed using a variety of directional approaches/orientations. They are identified as:

1. *Single* lead step, in which the *same* foot leads *every 4-count cycle*. (Figure 8.25)

2. *Alternate* lead step, in which the right and left foot both serve as the lead foot, *alternately initiating every 4 counts*, requiring a complete cycle for the alternating patterns to *take 8 counts* (both the right foot and then left foot lead a 4-count portion of the cycle). The examples, shown in Figures 8.26–8.28, are Bench Tap, Floor Tap, and Lunge Back.

3. *Touch step*, performed by touching the *same* toe or heel on the floor or bench (*2-count* move), (Figure 8.29), or by *alternating* legs. Touch step moves often are used during the warm-up segment to familiarize you with the bench, or as transition moves during the aerobic segment.

For both safety and variety when using the single-lead step, 4-count cycle patterns, lead with the right foot for a *maximum of 1 minute*, then change to a left-foot lead. To accomplish this change in lead foot (for single-cycle 4-count step patterns), perform a *non-weight-bearing, transitional, hold/touch/tap/heel* move as the last step of the cycle, initiating the change with that foot.

---

***Note:*** **Within the figure descriptions, only the moves typeset in boldface are shown in the figures.**

---

### Single Lead Step

**Figure 8.25** Single Lead Step

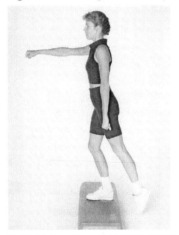 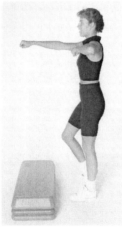

**Bench approach:** Front (shown), top, end, and straddle/astride.

|  | R | L | R | L |  |
|---|---|---|---|---|---|
| Right Lead: | **Up** | up | down | **down** | (4 counts) |

|  | L | R | L | R |  |
|---|---|---|---|---|---|
| Left Lead: | Up | up | down | down | (4 counts) |

**Arms shown:** Long-lever punching on up, up; pull, punch, on the down, down.

---

### Alternating Lead Step

You can alternate the lead leg with a Bench Tap up (on bench), or a Floor Tap or Lunge Back down (on floor).
**Bench approach:** Front (shown), top, end, or corner.

R   L   L   R
Up **bench tap** down down

Alternate: Up *L*, bench tap *R*, down *R*, down *L*.

(8 counts)

**Arms shown:** Forward punching.

**Figure 8.26** Bench Tap

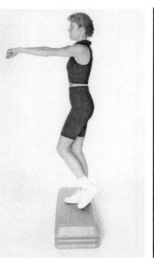 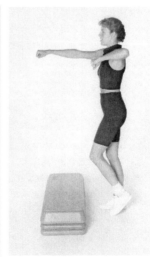

R   L   R   L
Up up down **floor tap**

Alternate. (8 counts)

**Arms shown:** Opposite arm long-lever punching; same arm flexing, elbows kept shoulder high.

**Note:** The Floor Tap also can be a non-weight-bearing lunge back.

**Figure 8.27** Floor Tap

**Alternating Lead Step**

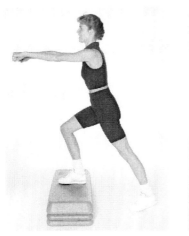 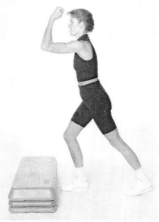

| R | L | R | L |
|---|---|---|---|
| **Up** | up | down | **down and back** |

Alternate. (8 counts)

**Arms shown:** Arms punching forward and parallel on up, up; bicep curls keeping elbows still high on the down, down.

**Figure 8.28** Lunge Back

---

### Touch Step
You can do the same or alternate the lead leg, touching toe or heel.
**Bench approach:** Front (shown), top, end, astride.

| R | R |
|---|---|
| **Bench-tap** with toe | down (a) (2 counts) |

Repeat with right or left foot.

**Arms shown:** Elbows shoulder-high, fists together on tap; fists apart on down.

**Options:**
Try tapping the bench using the **heel** (b), instead of the toe.

**Arms shown:** Arms extended to the side at shoulder level, alternating punching to the side.

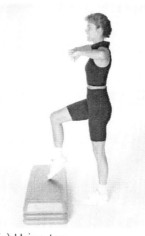  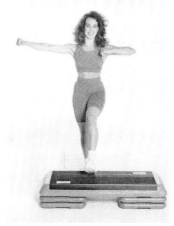

(a) Using toe.                    (b) Using heel.

**Figure 8.29** Touch Step

---

## Basic Step Patterns[27]

Basic step patterns may be performed as single lead steps (4-count pattern) or alternating lead steps (8-count pattern).

When performing a single lead basic step pattern, the fourth count of the cycle is weight-bearing.

In alternating lead steps, the two options are:

1. When the first three steps are weight-bearing, the fourth is non-weight-bearing.
2. When the first three steps contain a bypass move, the fourth step is weight-bearing.

The basic step patterns shown here are the V-step (Figure 8.30), Bypass Variations (Figures 8.31–8.34), Straddle Up or Down (Figures 8.35–8.36), and Lunge Side or Back (Figures 8.37 and 8.38).

## Basic Step Patterns

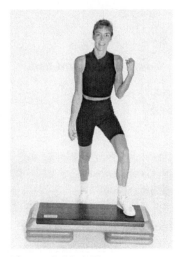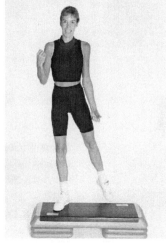

**Bench approach:** front (shown)

|  | R | L | R | L |
|---|---|---|---|---|
|  | **Up-wide** | up-wide | **down-center** | down-center |

Usually cued: "out" "out" "in" "in."

**Arms shown:** Same-side single bicep curls.

**Figure 8.30**  V-Step

---

**Bench approach :** front (shown)

| L | R | R | L |
|---|---|---|---|
| Up | **knee lift** | down (to floor) | down (to floor) |

(bypasses the
bench and lifts)

**Arms shown:** Initiate
from arms fully extended
out to the sides shoulder
high with palms up: Single
short-lever curls on the up
and knee lift; return one
at a time to long-lever,
shoulder-high initial
position on the down,
down.

**Options:**
Bench approach
side, top, end, a
stride/straddle, corner.

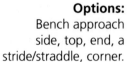

**Figure 8.31**  Knee Up Bypass[28]

**Bench approach:** front (shown)

| L | R | R | L |
|---|---|---|---|
| Up | **kick forward** | down (to floor) | down (to floor) |

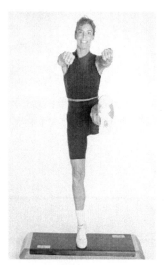

**Arms shown:** Arms
sweep up from sides,
together and parallel on
up, kick; sweep together
and parallel back down to
sides on the down, down.

**Options:**
Bench approach side, top,
end, astride/straddle,
corner.

**Figure 8.32**  Kick Forward Bypass

## Basic Step Patterns

**Bench approach :** front (shown)

L        R

Up    **kick back**      ("**long lever** raising" motion)

R                L

down (to floor)     down (to floor)

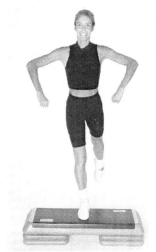

**Arms shown:** Initiate from the arms fully extended down at sides: Raise elbows out wide to shoulder high with fist ending at the waist, for the up and kick back; lower to the initial position at the side with each down, down.

**Options:**
Bench approach side, top, end, astride/straddle, corner.

**Figure 8.33** Kick Back Bypass

**Bench approach:** front (shown)

L        R

Up    **side leg lift**    (knee pointing forward position),

R                L

down (to floor)     down (to floor)

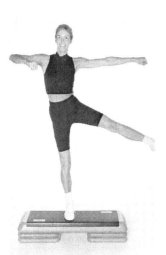

**Arms shown:** Raise both arms simultaneously to bent-arm lateral raise position for up; same side arm extends out to side shoulder high for side leg lift (shown); return extended arm to bent-arm lateral raise on the down; lower both arms simultaneously on the last down.

**Options:**
Bench approach side, top, end, astride/straddle, corner.

**Figure 8.34** Side Leg Lift Bypass

---

**Bench approach:** astride (shown)

R        L

**Up**    **knee lift** (bypasses bench, lifts waist high),

L                R

straddle down (to floor)     straddle down (to floor)

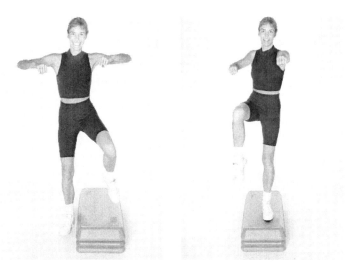

**Arms shown:** Same initial position as last pattern; opposite arm punches forward on lift.

**Options:**
For variety, try the other *bypass moves* (Figures 8.32–8.34), incorporating one or more accompanying arm movements that will keep your balance atop the bench. Straddle Up also can be a non-bypass basic step pattern.

**Figure 8.35** Straddle Up

## Basic Step Patterns

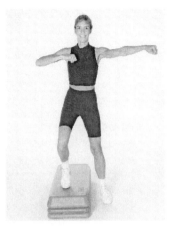
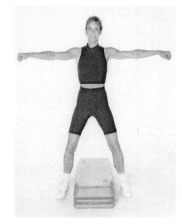

**Bench approach:** top (shown)

R

**Straddle down** (on R side of bench)

L

**straddle down** (on L side of bench)

| R | L |
|---|---|
| up | up |

**Arms shown:** Shoulder high, short levers, and fists together at center. Extend the same long-lever arm out to the side as the same leg steps out. Return one arm at a time back in to center on each up, up step.

**Figure 8.36** Straddle Down

---

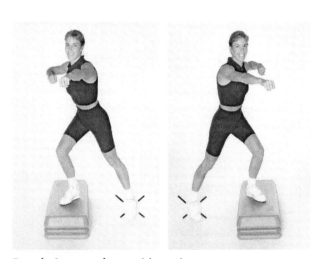

**Bench Approach:** top (shown)

| R | R | L | L |
|---|---|---|---|
| **Touch down side** | up | **touch down side** | up |

**Arms shown:** When the right leg lunge-steps to the side, punch the right arm in front at an angle; when the left leg lunge-steps to the side, punch the left arm in front at an angle.

**Figure 8.37** Lunge Side

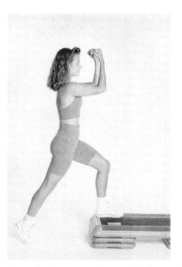

**Bench Approach:** end (shown)

| R | R |
|---|---|
| **Touch down back** | up |
| L | L |
| touch down back | up |

**Arms shown:** Arms parallel at shoulder level; bicep-curl touch down back; and punch forward on the touch up on bench.

**Figure 8.38** Lunge Back

## Variations of Basic Steps and Basic Step Patterns

To add interest to basic steps and basic step patterns, a number of variations can be implemented.

These are categorized here as:

- Traveling (Figures 8.39–8.44)
- Repeaters (Figure 8.45)
- Propulsion (Figure 8.46)

---

### Traveling Patterns

**Bench approach:** side (shown)

Single lead: 4 counts    Alternating lead: 8 counts

| L | R | L | R |
|---|---|---|---|
| **Up** | **body 1/2 turns left and up** | **down** | **tap-down** |

**Arms shown:** Shoulder high, alternating punch and pull back.

> **Note:**   Keep your eyes on the platform. Also, this pattern is shown using natural photography and descriptive words, as it could not be photographed, and therefore described, from a "mirrored" perspective.

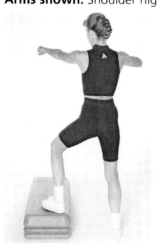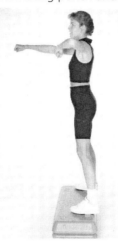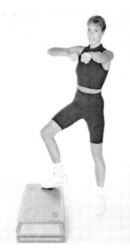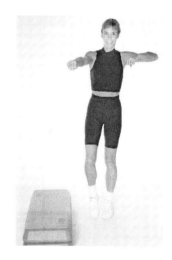

**Figure 8.39** Turn Step—Length of the Bench

---

**Bench approach:** side (shown)

Single lead: 4 counts    Alternating lead: 8 counts

| L | R | L | R |
|---|---|---|---|
| **Up** | **up** | **down on the left side of bench/platform** | **touch-down** |

Alternate. Cued: "up," "over," "down," "tap."

**Options:**

For variety on the *fourth* step, instead of tapping the floor, touch the heel on the bench; knee up; or kick front.

**Arms shown:** Elbows pointing skyward and shoulder high, with arms wide open on the first, third, fifth, and seventh steps—(a) and (c); and arms low and crossed in front on even-numbered steps—(b) and (d).

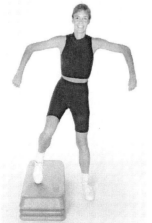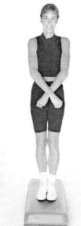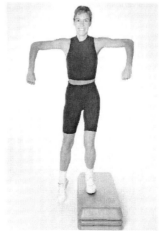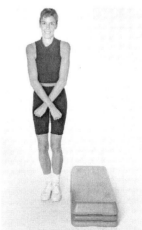

(a) Arms wide.    (b) Arms crossed.    (c) Arms wide.    (d) Arms crossed.

**Figure 8.40** Over the Top—Width of the Bench

## Traveling Patterns

**Bench approach:** end (shown)

Single lead: 4 counts     Alternating lead: 8 counts

  R  L                R                        L

**Up   up   down on the right side of bench   touch-down**

Cued: "up," "across," "down," "tap"

**Arms shown:** Arms at shoulder level; when the legs are apart, the arms are straight out to the side—(a) and (c); bend the arms into the chest when the feet are together—(b) and (d).

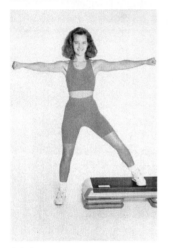 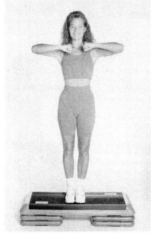 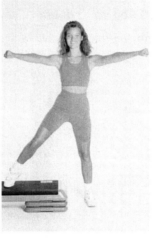 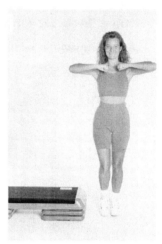

(a) Arms out.         (b) Arms in.         (c) Arms out.         (d) Arms in.

**Figure 8.41** Across the Top—Length of the Bench

---

**Bench approach:** corner (shown)

Alternating lead step: 8 counts

  L     R       R                      L

**Up   knee lift   down   down turning body (on diagonal) facing left corner**

**Options:**
For variety on the second and sixth steps, use any bypass move (knee, kick front/back, side leg lift, hamstring curl, adductor).

**Arms shown:** Arms at shoulder level, row position (a), punch the opposite arm forward as the knee comes up (b), pull-punch in on down (c), and both arms punch forward when the body turns to the corner (d).

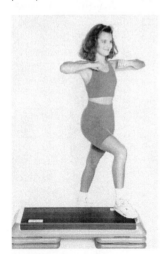 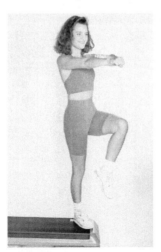 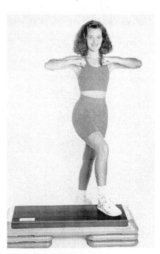 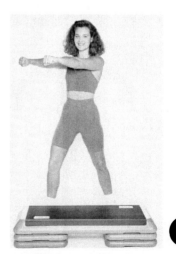

(a) Row position.      (b) Punch.        (c) Pull-punch.      (d) Both arms punch forward.

**Figure 8.42** Corner to Corner

## Traveling Patterns

**Bench approach:** side (shown)

Single lead step: 4 counts

> L            R            L            R

**Up-forward    up    down-forward    down**

Cued: "up," "to the middle," "down," "tap."

> **Note:** Because you never approach the bench with your back to it, the next steps must use either the close end of the bench or all floor patterns, to realign your body so your front or your side is facing the bench.

**Arms shown:** Arms to the side at shoulder level and angled in the direction the body is traveling.

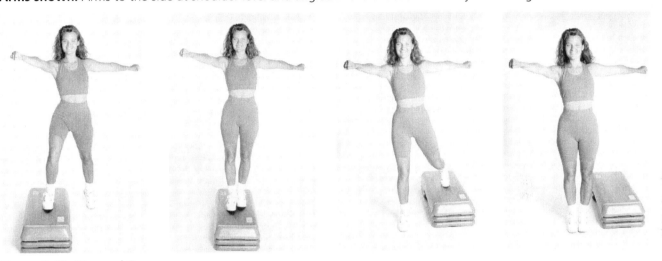

**Figure 8.43** Diagonal Over

---

**Bench approach:** side (shown)

Single lead step, 3 cycles each: 4 counts

> R       L              L              R

Up   **side leg lift**   down (to floor)   tap (on floor)

> **Note:** This variation shows natural photography, as it is a traveling sequence that can't be mirrored.

Repeat from the **end** (b) and on the **other side** (c) of the bench.

**Arms shown:** Both arms raised to the side when the leg lifts to the side, and lowered when stepping down to the floor.

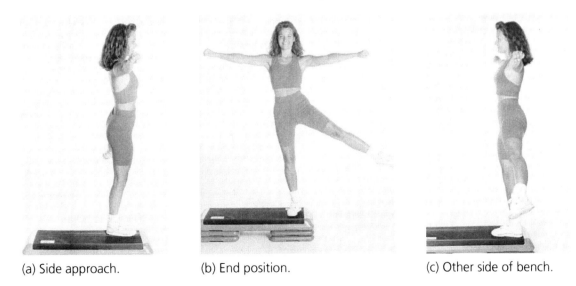

(a) Side approach.          (b) End position.          (c) Other side of bench.

**Figure 8.44** Around the Corner

## Repeaters[29]

*Repeaters are repetitions of any non-weight-bearing move* and can be a single or an alternating lead step.
Limit the number of repeaters to a maximum of four.

**Options:**
Use knee-lifts, forward kicks, kick-backs, side leg-lifts, or similar moves.

**Bench approach:** corner front (shown)

    L      R          R

**Step up**, **tap up**, **tap down and back,** tap up *R*, tap down and back *R*, tap up *R*, step down *R*, step down *L* squarely facing front of the bench; or the other corner and alternate stepping up *R* and tapping *L*.

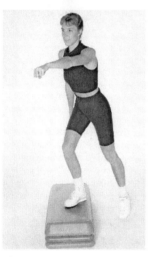
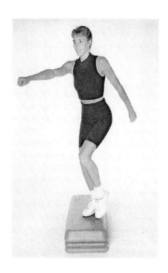
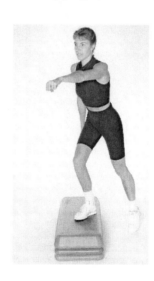

**Figure 8.45** Repeaters

---

## Intermediate / Advanced Variations

In propulsion, both feet push off the floor or bench, exchanging positions during the airborne phase of the pattern. Propulsion steps are commonly used with touch and lunge steps.[31] Propulsion moves also can be used when performing bypass or traveling moves by adding a hop or pushing off the foot on the bench.

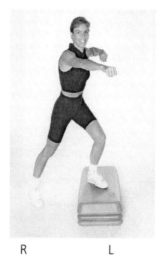
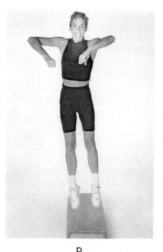
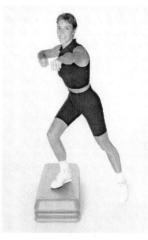

R             L
Up     **lunge down and back**
(2 counts)

R
Push off (with propulsion into this airborne position)
(1 count)

L
Landing on opposite foot up and other foot (R)
**lunging down and back**
(1 count)

**Figure 8.46** Propulsion[30] Steps

## *Variations of Basic Arm Movements*

Varying the arm movements adds *significantly* to the variety of your workout. Before adding any arm movements, be sure you are comfortable with the basic steps and basic step patterns.

Participants can then add less intense, low-range motions (elbows kept low, near the waist), and gradually incorporate more intense, middle-range motions (elbows are chest-to-shoulder high). Finally, movements progress to the highly intense upper-range arm movements (elbows at and above shoulder level).

### Low-Range (Elbow) Arm Movements (#1–5)

1. **Bicep Curls**   With elbows *fixed* at the sides, *palms up*, flex both elbows, forearms moving toward shoulders.

   **Alternating Bicep Curls** Alternate right and left forearms.

2. **Hammer Curls**   With elbows *fixed* at the sides and the *palms facing* each other, flex both elbows, moving forearms toward the shoulders.

   **Alternating Hammer Curls** Alternate right and left forearms.

3. **Low Wide 'n Cross**   Begin with elbows at sides and forearms wide. Criss-cross the arms at waist level in front of the body, keeping the palms up. By rotating both elbows forward, low punches can be performed by extending both elbows forward away from the body (palms still up).

   **Alternating Low Punches** Extend one forearm at a time.

4. **Row Low**   Begin with forearms (only) extended in front of the body, waist-level. Pull the elbows backward until the fists are *next to* the waist (Figure 8.47); return to the starting position.

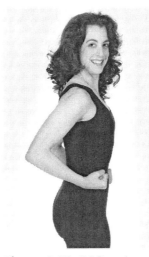

**Figure 8.47** #4 Row Low

5. **Triceps Kick-Back**   With the elbows *fixed* behind the shoulders and the fists next to the sides (Figure 8.47), extend both elbows, forearms now moving backward.

   **Alternating Triceps Kick-Back** Alternate right and left arms. Palms can face up/in/down.

### Mid-Range Arm Movements (#6–12)

6. **Criss-Crossover**   Keeping elbows at chest height, criss-cross arms over each other, palms facing down. Alternate arm that crosses over the top, for each repetition.

7. **Cross and Lateral Raise** Begin with arms crossed low in front of the abdomen, palms facing the body. Uncross palms and laterally raise elbows up pointing skyward to shoulder height, keeping arms wide open.

8. **Double and Single Side-Out** Begin with fists under the chin at shoulder level, palms down, elbows directly out. Extend both arms wide out to the sides, keeping elbows at shoulder height. Pull fists back into the chin.

   **Single Side-Outs**   Alternate the right and left arms.

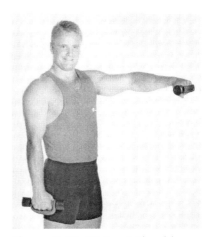

**Figure 8.48** #9 Front Shoulder Raise

9. **Front Shoulder Raise**   Begin with palms together in front of thighs. Keeping elbows soft, raise both arms straight up to the front to shoulder level, palms down.

   **Alternating Front Shoulder Raises** (Figure 8.48). Alternate right and left arms.

10. **Shoulder Punch**   Start with hands lightly resting on shoulders. Extend one arm forward *or* diagonally across the body, at shoulder height. Pull back and return to shoulder.

11. **Side Lateral Raise**   Start with fists together in front of thighs. Lift arms up and out wide, palms facing down, always leading with the elbows, keeping them slightly bent.

12. **Upright Row**   Begin with palms in front of thighs. Keeping fists close to the body and elbows wide, raise hands up to the chin.

## Upper-Range Arm Movements (#13–18)

13. **Butterflies**   Begin with fists and forearms together and parallel in front of face, elbows pointing down. Keeping elbows shoulder-high, open them wide and out to the sides.

14. **Front-L**   Start with fists resting on the shoulders—see Figure 8.49. Simultaneously extend one arm straight out in front of you, shoulder height, while extending other arm upward above the head. Pull both fists back to shoulders and repeat, other direction.

15. **Overhead Press**   Start with fists resting on shoulders—see Figure 8.49. With palms facing, extend arms upward over head, keeping elbows close to ears.

    **Alternating Overhead Press** Alternate right and left arms.

16. **Side-L**   Begin with fists resting on shoulders—Figure 8.49. Simultaneously extend one arm straight out to the side at shoulder height while extending the other arm upward above head. Pull both fists back to shoulders and repeat, other direction.

17. **Slice**   Begin with fists facing and resting on shoulders, elbows low at the sides. Simultaneously extend one arm upward straight above head while extending other arm downward, along side of the leg. Pull both fists back to the shoulders, and repeat with other side high/low.

18. **Triceps Extension**   Begin with elbows fixed high, near ears and fists on shoulders. With palms facing, extend arms high and parallel overhead.

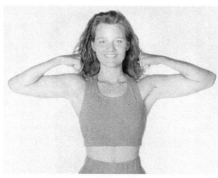

**Figure 8.49** Starting Position for #14, #15, #16

## *Applying the Techniques*

All basic steps and basic step patterns can be used to create an 8- or 16-count step pattern that incorporates *all three sides* of the bench, beginning from the end of the bench. When you get creative, your back should never face the bench while you are stepping up. Only three sides of the bench are available for any one pattern, for safety reasons.

Steps from the end use multiple bench-approaches and multiple basic step patterns. Try the sample pattern diagrammed in Figure 8.50, Double "T" Step.[32]

The figure illustrates an empty bench with sequential placement of each foot. Beginning from the end of the bench and with your weight on your *right foot* on the floor, step up on bench to the #1 location with your *left foot*. Continue with the pattern, placing your next foot on top of the bench, or on the side, or at the end, and on the floor, wherever the sequential number indicates foot placement.

When alternating the pattern, final step #16 takes the *weight* onto the *left* foot. The next move is up (right). When repeating the pattern, or when changing to create a totally new pattern, final step #16 is a non-weight-bearing move (like a "tap"), with the next weight-bearing step on that same ("tap") foot, either in place on the floor, or up, on the bench.

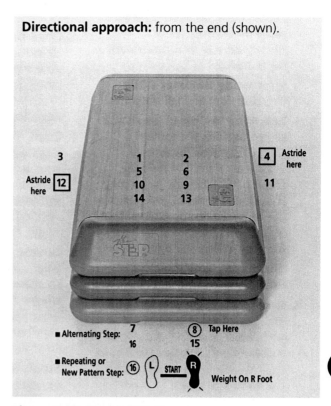

**Directional approach:** from the end (shown).

**Figure 8.50** Double "T" Step

## *Exercise 8.1  Creating Your Own Step Training Combinations*

**Directions:**

Following all of the guidelines you have been given (see summary, Figure 8.51), create your own patterns. For safety reasons, only three sides of the bench can be used in a pattern. Start with a bench approach from the end, front, side, top, or corner, and proceed, incorporating multiple basic step patterns and multiple bench approaches.

- Indicate the location of the weight-bearing foot (WBF) to start the pattern, freeing the other foot to then be step #1. The bench and floor have been divided into six sections for your convenience in placing the number locations.

- Begin the pattern by locating a "1" up on the bench (or down on the floor), followed by the location of the next step, identified as "2."

- Continue locating steps 3–8, then 9–16, identifying any step that has a key directive (for example, ⑧ is a tap non-weight-bearing move; ⑫ is an astride position).

- Identify any bypass step movement with a double circle around the non-weight-bearing foot location and labeling the type of bypass move (e.g., ⑤ forward kick).

- List arm gestures to accompany each step movement, plus any additional technique pointers (sounds, etc.) below at right. Enjoy being creative!

As you begin to develop an individualized program, you can incorporate your favorite step training moves in the combinations you choose.

## Steps:

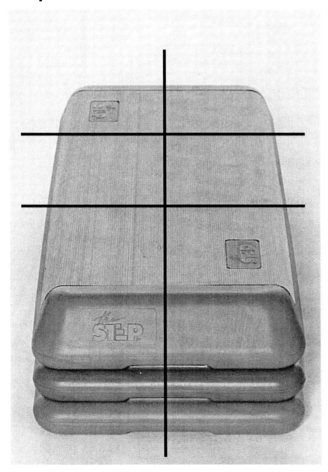

## Arm Gestures to Step #:

1. _____
2. _____
3. _____
4. _____
5. _____
6. _____
7. _____
8. _____
9. _____
10. _____
11. _____
12. _____
13. _____
14. _____
15. _____
16. _____

**Figure 8.51** Summary of Step Training Techniques[33]

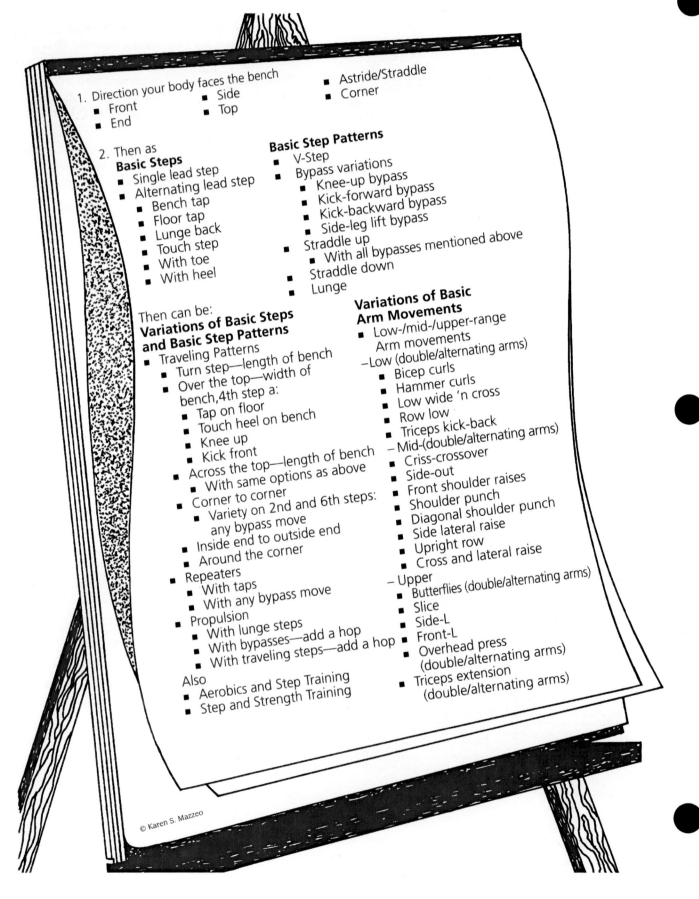

1. Direction your body faces the bench
   - Front
   - End
   - Side
   - Top
   - Astride/Straddle
   - Corner

2. Then as

**Basic Steps**
   - Single lead step
   - Alternating lead step
     - Bench tap
     - Floor tap
     - Lunge back
     - Touch step
     - With toe
     - With heel

**Basic Step Patterns**
   - V-Step
   - Bypass variations
     - Knee-up bypass
     - Kick-forward bypass
     - Kick-backward bypass
     - Side-leg lift bypass
   - Straddle up
     - With all bypasses mentioned above
   - Straddle down
   - Lunge

Then can be:

**Variations of Basic Steps and Basic Step Patterns**
   - Traveling Patterns
     - Turn step—length of bench
     - Over the top—width of bench, 4th step a:
       - Tap on floor
       - Touch heel on bench
       - Knee up
       - Kick front
     - Across the top—length of bench
       - With same options as above
     - Corner to corner
       - Variety on 2nd and 6th steps: any bypass move
     - Inside end to outside end
     - Around the corner
   - Repeaters
     - With taps
     - With any bypass move
   - Propulsion
     - With lunge steps
     - With bypasses—add a hop
     - With traveling steps—add a hop

Also
   - Aerobics and Step Training
   - Step and Strength Training

**Variations of Basic Arm Movements**
   - Low-/mid-/upper-range Arm movements
   –Low (double/alternating arms)
     - Bicep curls
     - Hammer curls
     - Low wide 'n cross
     - Row low
     - Triceps kick-back
   – Mid-(double/alternating arms)
     - Criss-crossover
     - Side-out
     - Front shoulder raises
     - Shoulder punch
     - Diagonal shoulder punch
     - Side lateral raise
     - Upright row
     - Cross and lateral raise
   – Upper
     - Butterflies (double/alternating arms)
     - Slice
     - Side-L
     - Front-L
     - Overhead press (double/alternating arms)
     - Triceps extension (double/alternating arms)

© Karen S. Mazzeo

# Aerobic Exercise: #3 Fitness Walking

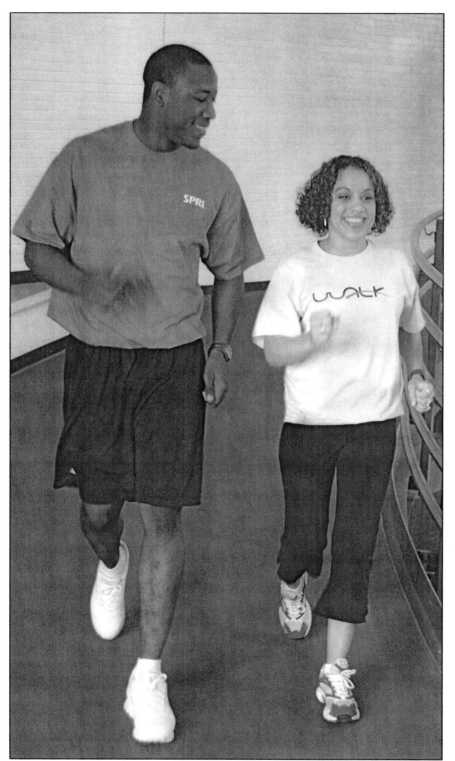

9

itness walking is probably the easiest of all aerobic options because it can be done anywhere with no need for equipment or direction from someone else. Because it takes three times as long to get the same aerobic benefits from walking as from running,[1] *time* is a key factor. Exercise action taking *14 minutes or longer per mile is classified as walking*, taking 9 to 12 minutes per mile is labeled *jogging*, and taking less than 9 minutes per mile is *running*.[2]

## Shoes and Apparel

Supportive walking or running shoes are important to cushion and absorb the impact that walking provides. Make sure you have walking shoes with a low, rounded heel and flexible sole. They should support your arches, cushion your feet, and be lightweight and ventilated.[3] Because one foot is always on the ground, fitness walking is classified as a low-impact activity.

Clothing worn is loose and comfortable, the pants not too baggy or too long to interfere with motion and ground contact. When temperatures are 40°F or below, the air passages are always covered appropriately.

## Principles and Techniques

The initial body position is the same as it is for standing (see Figure 4.3 in Chapter 4), except that as the legs swing forward, a new base of support is established with each swing and the center of gravity moves forward, over the base. The body weight is

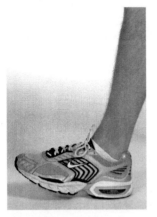

**Figure 9.1** Heel Makes First Contact

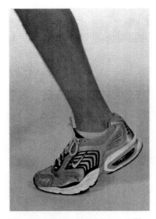

**Figure 9.2** Pushing Off with Ball of Foot

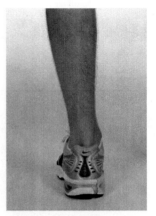

**Figure 9.3** Shifting Weight Through Outer Half of Foot

balanced, *slightly forward*. The breathing pattern is easy and continuous while you move quickly.

## Mechanics

The sequence of movements follows.

1. Swing legs forward with hip/thigh leading until heel strikes the ground (with a minimum of lateral or vertical movement).

2. As heel touches down (Figure 9.1), push off the back leg from the ball of foot and big toe area (Figure 9.2), transferring weight to the first foot.

3. Swing back leg easily under the body as the base of support is formed. Keep the body in a balanced position so you can change direction.

   The balanced position is supported by strong leg muscles, which allow the shift in weight to heel of first foot to be smooth and controlled. Many people incorrectly use the back muscles instead of the leg muscles to lead and support the body. The center of gravity (center of your weight) then is ahead of the base of support, which puts the trunk in an unsupported position and leads to early fatigue and back pain. Think *relaxed lower back*.

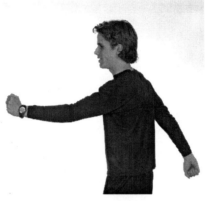

**Figure 9.4** Long-Lever Position

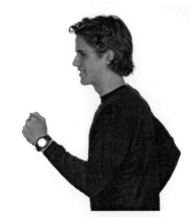

**Figure 9.5** Short-Lever Position

4. Position and make ground contact with feet as follows:

   a. Touch center of the heel first.

   b. With a rolling action forward, shift weight through center and outer half of foot (Figure 9.3).

   c. Push off from ball of foot and big toe.

   d. Point feet straight ahead and place them just to the left and right of an imaginary center line.

5. Keeping shoulders level and parallel, swing arms freely and naturally and in opposition to the forward leg, in one of these two positions:

   a. Hold arms in a *long-lever*, relaxed-elbow position (Figure 9.4), with a forward and backward controlled swinging motion that also involves upper-torso conditioning.

   b. Hold arms in a *short-lever* position, elbows flexed and held near sides (Figure 9.5).

Hold the hands in a relaxed fist with either arm position.

## Pedometer Use

Do you need *motivation* to add fitness walking, or just more movement and activity into your life style? If so, try adding the use of a pedometer and watch how your interest in integrating more movement into your day suddenly becomes an *all day* exciting challenge![4]

## Intended Design

Pedometers measure physical activity. They don't measure *every* type of movement activity and exertion. Therefore, if you're interested in keeping an accurate journal of your activity (your overall daily expenditure of energy), you'll have to understand a pedometer's intended purpose, and its limitations.

Pedometers measure the number of steps you take and the movement you accumulate throughout the day.[5] Pedometers aren't waterproof so they can't measure swimming activity. They don't accurately measure activity *on wheels* such as bicycling, skateboarding, and rollerblading.[6] Since most of the activity you accumulate in a day is over land and directly on your feet, pedometers are one of the best ways to measure physical activity, whether you are young, old, or at an age in between.

## How It Works

Pedometer technology at present is digital and detects movement through a spring-loaded, counter-balanced mechanism (fulcrum) that records the vertical acceleration at the hip.[7] Having this design, you can understand then how it only records the movement for which it is intended—direct foot contact, impact-related activity.

Currently an abundance of research on pedometer usage has been reported because of its sustained popularity as a motivational tool. Professional fitness agencies and exercise science educators (including professionals working in various agencies of the U.S. Government) are aware of the trend toward a lack of physical movement and exercise, and

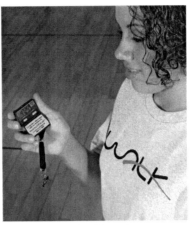

**Figure 9.6** Checking Steps Displayed on the Walk4Life, Inc.™ DUO-2 Function Digital Pedometer

are all getting on board to reverse the alarming statistics that are surfacing, especially regarding obesity. The result is an overwhelming "let's get moving" spirit, using pedometers to provide that motivation.[8]

## Selecting and Using a Pedometer

Select a model that research has shown to be both valid and reliable. (Validity in research studies means that the pedometer measures what it purports to measure, accurately. Reliability is a measure of consistency of data collected, and usually found in test-retest comparisons.)

The Walk4Life, Inc.™ models have been found to be both one of the most valid and reliable pedometers on the market today.[9] W4L™ offers a variety of pedometer models that can measure numerous criteria you may want to track. The pedometer functions presented here are two: Step Counts and Exercise/Activity Time.

The Step Counts function records foot contact with the ground. The Exercise/Activity Time function, however, is probably the best measure of daily activity. Every time a

person moves, the pedometer starts recording activity time. When the person stops, the timing function stops. This is the most accurate measure by pedometers because it is not affected by stride length or movement speed. At the end of the day, the total amount of exercise/activity time accumulated is displayed in hours and minutes. This may be the best measure to use for monitoring activity as it corresponds to most of the activity guidelines for adults and children.[10]

Figure 9.6 displays the Walk4Life, Inc.™ DUO-2 Function Digital Pedometer ~ a perfect match for this total fitness course and your walking program. It features:

- Both functions mentioned ~ Step Counts and Exercise/Activity Time.

- An extra-large digital display; it's easy to read.

- A delayed reset button, so you purposefully must shut it off ~ it can't lose your steps counted or activity time by accidentally bumping it.

- It records up to 1 million steps, so if you're into long-term "tracking your mileage," you can. (In the top right corner, the one digit changes after every 100,000 steps from 0–9, continually.)

- The hinged protective covering will not allow it to operate unless it is *closed.*

- Its battery operates for approximately 1 to 2 years before needing replacement ($1.00); the display will begin to fade when it needs replacement.

- The loss prevention strap clips firmly onto your clothes to doubly secure its placement at your waist area.

- It has a 1-year warranty.[11]

## Placement and Attachment to Insure Accuracy

- Starting point: *On waist in line with the middle of the kneecap* (see Figure 9.7). This works for 80% of people.
  - First Adjustment: Just in front of hip is often better for females
  - Second Adjustment: Near belly button
  - Third Adjustment: On the back, over the kidney area
- The following impacts accuracy:
  - not finding an accurate placement
  - speed of walking; a number of pedometers measured accurately at speeds less than 3.0 mph (less than a 20-minute mile)
  - become less accurate with increasing age, weight, and BMI[12]
  - must be snug to minimize excessive movement of the pedometer
  - must move up and down in unison with the body—loose clothing and body fat will absorb the small vertical movement (and make it less accurate)
  - must be parallel to the body and not open or angled away from the vertical plane of the body
  - designed for the waistband; sometimes a watch pocket (on jeans) will work, so test it
  - do not place in pocket or on shoe (however, at present research is developing one to fit onto shoe)
  - can place on underwear, or reversed with the face toward the body so it "sticks" to the skin

Basically, test the placement of your pedometer with a 100 steps test. Take 100 steps and see if it records accurately by your placement. It should be within +/− 5 steps.[13]

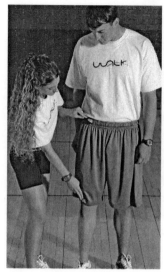

**Figure 9.7** Pedometer Placement on Waist in Line with the Middle of the Kneecap

## The Value of Activity Time over Counting Steps

- All national exercise guidelines are listed in minutes.[14]
- Walk4Life™ Pedometers measure activity time, which negates stride length differences.[15] Just a few other companies provide this key feature.

## *Designing Your Pedometer Walking Program*

In order to set goals that encourage continual change and improvement, you'll first need to establish a starting point. Since activity levels are individual, the goals you set will be based upon determining your "personal baseline of activity." Establishing this baseline can be accomplished by adolescents and adults with 8 days of monitoring and recording your activity level (or 4 days for children, grades K-6)[16] using the following method:

1. Set the pedometer at "0" in the morning before you put it on. This will set both the Step Counter (recording the number of steps you take in one day) and the Activity Time (recording the total minutes of movement and exercise you experience in 1 day, provided it followed the criteria mentioned earlier for foot contact and impact with the ground).

2. At the end of the day before retiring, open the case and record the step count you engaged in that day using Exercise 9.1, Recording Baseline Step Count. Continue this process of monitoring and recording your data for 8 days (4 days for children).

3. At the end of 8 days of recording, add the column of data, to establish your total steps taken in 8 days.

4. Divide by 8 (days of monitoring) to establish your daily average baseline steps taken per day.

5. You can now set personal goals for improvement. Your first goal to set: Try increasing your baseline step count by 10%. *Example:* If you used 6000 steps per day, you'll now add 10% (600 steps) and try for 6600 steps per day. This will be the personal goal to strive for over the next 2 weeks. If the goal is reached for a majority of the days during this 2 week period, another 10% (600 steps) is added to the goal and the process repeated.

6. For most people, a top goal of 4000 to 6000 steps *above their baseline level* is a reasonable expectation. Using the example of 6000 steps, a goal of 10,000 to 12,000 steps per day would be the ultimate goal.[17]

This baseline and goal-setting approach allows individuals to customize personal goals that are attainable for all levels of walkers. As you increase your step total, your

## Exercise 9.1 Recording Pedometer Baseline Step Count

Day:   Total Steps Taken Today:

1  _____
2  _____
3  _____
4  _____
5  _____
6  _____
7  _____
8  _____

**8 Day Total:** _____

**÷ 8 Days  =** _____
### Average Steps Per Day*

*This is your baseline step count and your *starting point*. Now add 10% to this total:

_____

This is your first **goal** to achieve daily, for 2 weeks

activity time will increase, making the goal of 30 minutes of continuous activity more attainable.[18]

## Fitness Walking Program

Fitness power walking, wearing a pedometer (see Figure 9.8), is fun and energizing! Table 9.1 presents a Level I, 10-Week Walking Program.[19] It is easy to follow and can be enjoyed anywhere. Note that proper warm-up and cool-down ("warm down") are required for a safe program.

## Lifetime Walking Program

If you have access to a recreational facility that has a *pace trail*, you can add another element to your fitness program: challenging yourself to improve your cardiovascular and respiratory fitness continually by using the permanently visible measurement device built into the trail that quantifies time and distance covered.

This trail has outdoor safety lighting poles at premeasured distances. Each is equipped with a bank of mechanized, color-coded, flashing lights. These colored lights have been synchronized to flash at regular timed intervals, reflecting specific minutes-per-mile covered (see Figure 9.9). Arriving at a pole at the time the specific colored light you've chosen to follow is flashing reflects that you are covering a predetermined distance in a predetermined time. It is a helpful means to stay focused on fitness results and continued improvement.

## Research Data to Assist with Setting Goals

Research conducted at the Cooper Institute in Dallas[20] demonstrated that walking at a moderate pace of 3 miles per hour (a 20-minute mile) increased cardiovascular and respiratory fitness and reduced the risk of heart disease by increasing the HDL ("good") cholesterol (see Chapter 13). Walking a 12-minute mile resulted in a greater improvement in fitness levels than for the 20-minute-per-mile group but similar increases in HDL cholesterol. This demonstrated that you don't have to do vigorous activity to get a health benefit.

Also, you don't have to do all your activity in one session. Studies show that you can get almost the same benefit from three 10-minute exercise bouts as one 30-minute exercise bout of equal intensity. Most people can find time to take a brisk power walk for 2, 5, or 10 minutes several times during the day. Minimum amounts of exercise to achieve results are given in Table 9.2.

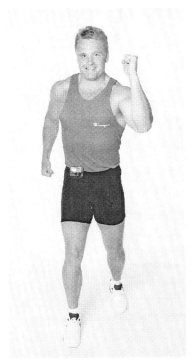

**Figure 9.8** Fitness Power Walking, Wearing a Pedometer

*Table 9.1  Level I:  Walking Only\**

| Week | Session | Warm-Up | Exercise | Warm-Down | Goal (Distance) |
|------|---------|---------|----------|-----------|-----------------|
| 1 | 1 | yes | 15–20' | yes | 0.5 to 0.8 mi. |
|   | 2 | yes | 15–20' | yes | 0.9 to 1.0 mi. |
|   | 3 | yes | 20' | yes | 0.9 to 1.0 mi. |
| 2 | 4 | yes | 20' | yes | 0.9 to 1.0 mi. |
|   | 5 | yes | 24' | yes | 1.1 to 1.2 mi. |
|   | 6 | yes | 24' | yes | 1.1 to 1.2 mi. |
| 3 | 7 | yes | 28' | yes | 1.3 to 1.4 mi. |
|   | 8 | yes | 28' | yes | 1.3 to 1.4 mi. |
|   | 9 | yes | 32' | yes | 1.4 to 1.6 mi. |
| 4 | 10 | yes | 32' | yes | 1.4 to 1.6 mi. |
|   | 11 | yes | 36' | yes | 1.7 to 1.8 mi. |
|   | 12 | yes | 36' | yes | 1.7 to 1.8 mi. |
| 5 | 13 | yes | 40' | yes | 1.9 to 2.0 mi. |
|   | 14 | yes | 40' | yes | 1.9 to 2.0 mi. |
|   | 15 | yes | 44' | yes | 2.1 to 2.2 mi. |
| 6 | 16 | yes | 48' | yes | 2.3 to 2.4 mi. |
|   | 17 | yes | 48' | yes | 2.3 to 2.4 mi. |
|   | 18 | yes | 48' | yes | 2.3 to 2.4 mi. |
| 7 | 19 | yes | 52' | yes | 2.5 to 2.6 mi. |
|   | 20 | yes | 52' | yes | 2.5 to 2.6 mi. |
|   | 21 | yes | 56' | yes | 2.7 to 2.8 mi. |
| 8 | 22 | yes | 56' | yes | 2.7 to 2.8 mi. |
|   | 23 | yes | 60' | yes | 2.9 to 3.0 mi. |
|   | 24 | yes | 60' | yes | 2.9 to 3.0 mi. |
| 9 | 25 | yes | 58' | yes | 3.0 mi. |
|   | 26 | yes | 58' | yes | 3.0 mi. |
|   | 27 | yes | 56' | yes | 3.0 mi. |
| 10 | 28 | yes | 56' | yes | 3.0 mi. |
|   | 29 | yes | 54' | yes | 3.0 mi. |
|   | 30 | yes | 54' | yes | 3.0 mi. |

\*Program written by Dr. Richard Bowers, ACSM certified Program Director

# Adding Variety Encourages Adherence

Incorporating variety (using pedometers, mechanized pace trails, or even participating in charity walkathons) into your fitness walking program can reduce boredom and increase adherence to the lifetime commitment to fitness you're making.

If you are a candidate for high-impact aerobic exercise, try adding more variety to your program by incorporating at least one **rope jumping** segment to your workouts. Varying your speed of jumping, floor contact at impact with one or two feet, and feet positioned close together or wide stride are all ways to make this particular exercise challenging.

Or, if low impact is your choice, one of the most popular cardiovascular exercise machines capturing exercise enthusiasts' interest at fitness facilities today is the Elliptical Trainer (see Figure 9.10).[21]

Elliptical Trainers engage the legs in a movement pattern that combines the motion of stair stepping with cross-country skiing, providing a low-impact workout. Some elliptical machines also include poles that can be maneuvered with the arms while the legs are in motion, similar to cross-country machines. This option increases the amount of muscle mass used to perform the exercise.[22]

# Using an Elliptical Trainer

- Be sure to select a machine to suit your size and range of movement.

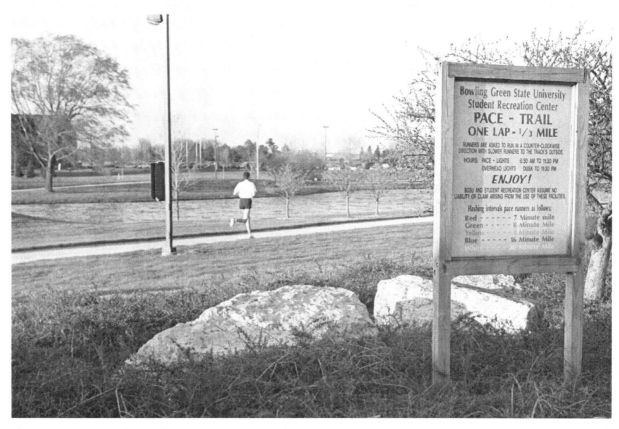

**Figure 9.9** Pace Trail to Help Keep Focus on Goals

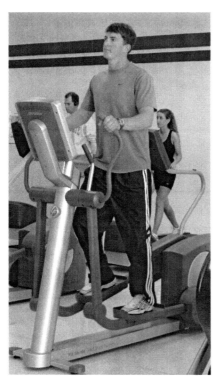

**Figure 9.10** Elliptical Trainer Adds Low-Impact Variety

- Get comfortable with any new programming features such as exercise time, distance goal, resistance level, speed level, and caloric expenditure.

- Before you start exercising on the Elliptical Trainer, make sure that you are familiar with the controls that increase speed and/or the resistance. Make sure that the emergency shut-off switch or button works.

- When exercising, maintain the correct posture by keeping your shoulders back, head up and slightly forward, chin up and straight, your abdominal muscles tight, and arms relaxed. Do not lean forward, or grab and grip the balance bars/handrails too tightly.

- Make sure that your weight is evenly distributed and that your lower body supports the majority of your weight.

- A good stride should be relaxed and maintained while going through your normal range of motion.

- Set a specific time of day and number of minutes, then make using an Elliptical Trainer a regular part of your exercise/fitness routine.

- Start out slowly and make sure that you have checked with your doctor before beginning this or any new exercise program.[23]

## *More Variety*

If jumping rope and using an Elliptical Trainer are not aerobic options you're choosing to use, select one of the many other exercise modalities that are popular today like spinning, cardiokickboxing, or inline skating. Or, how about the traditional jogging and endurance swimming? Variety is the spice of your program!

*Table 9.2  Minimum Exercise Needed*

|  | **Women** | **Men** |
|---|---|---|
| For "moderate" exercise | Walk 2 miles in less than 30 minutes (a 15-minute mile) at least 3 days per week, or walk 2 miles in 30 to 40 minutes (a 15- to 20-minute mile) five to six times per week. | Walk 2 miles in less than 27 minutes (13½-minute mile) at least 3 days per week, or walk 2 miles in 30–40 minutes (a 15- to 20-minute mile) six to seven times per week. |
| For "high fitness" | Walk 2 miles in less than 30 minutes 5 or 6 days per week. | Walk 2½ miles in less than 37½ minutes 6 to 7 days per week. |

> *Younger people probably need to do a bit more, and older people could do a bit less than the typical program.*

## Goal-Setting Challenge

 Set a short-term and long-range fitness walking goal in order to incorporate variety in your total fitness program. Write these Fitness Walking Goals for Chapter 9, following the four steps presented in Chapter 2, Exercise 2.3, then record them in your Fitness Journal.

 Using Exercise 9.2, Fitness Walking Log (shown below) as a sample of the columns to monitor, record your fitness walking exercise entries in 10-minute increments, which you include in your schedule every day. If your program includes the use of a pedometer, record your daily Step Count and Activity Time (total minutes per day). Do this monitoring either separate from or in conjunction with the Fitness Journal (Exercise 5.4) for at least 3 weeks. This daily monitoring of 10-minute increments a day (or for as long as you fitness power walk) or recording the Step Count and Activity Time registered on your pedometer each evening, will significantly help you develop the pattern of enjoying moving, as well as encouraging your positive self talk. You'll hear, "I love to move! Fitness walking is so refreshing, for just 10 minutes a day, or for 10,000 steps a day!"

## Exercise 9.2  Fitness Walking Log~

| Today's Date | Route Covered | Mileage Distance (miles) | Total Time | Comments or Variables (heat, detours, well-being) | Step Count | ~Pedometer~ Activity Time Minutes |
|---|---|---|---|---|---|---|
|  |  |  |  |  |  |  |

*Note: Here is a sample of the columns of information to log into your Fitness Journal or on separate paper.*

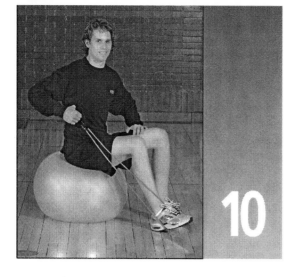

# Strength Training

**10**

Although all of the muscles of the body are strengthened during vigorous aerobic exercise, a strength training program included within an aerobic fitness class setting provides the opportunity to develop strength and endurance of *specific skeletal muscle* groups. Actually, your overall physical function is improved. Research indicates that adults who perform properly designed strength training programs can slow bone loss, preserving bone density.[1] Your body needs weight bearing exercise using all of the major muscle groups (that both aerobic exercise and strength training provide), to keep your bones in an ideal state of health.[2] Added to these benefits is the aesthetic transformation that will happen. You're going to look much better!

## Primary Training Goal Determines Your Program Order

According to the training goals established for a course, the strength training segment can come before, during, or after the aerobic segment. Because this is a beginning fitness class and aerobic conditioning is the primary goal, strength training usually is offered at the conclusion of the aerobic segment and before the final cool-down, flexibility training,

and relaxation segments. This is true at least in the initial stages of the class, until the class as a whole becomes sufficiently aerobically fit. (If your *primary* course goal is fat weight loss, the aerobic segment *follows* the strength training segment.)

For the novice exerciser, the reasoning for this program order is simple. With an increase in the resistance (weight) that must be applied to any movement for significant change to occur, the workload placed on the heart, lungs, and vascular system also increases, placing the beginner more readily in a breathless "oxygen-debt" state. During the aerobic phase, your goal is *not* to be in a breathless state. You want to be working continually in a breathe-easy state, steadily pacing your intensity.

Strength training (also called weight training) is performed in a steady, controlled (more static and less dynamic) manner and usually concentrates on the areas not adequately worked during the aerobic segment of class. Because aerobics, step training, and fitness walking usually are lower-body intensive, this segment focuses primarily on the muscles in the upper body and the abdominals.

Strength training exercises are included to more quickly define, tone, shape, and make more dense (thicken) the muscle fibers. They also

allow for longer periods of work to be accomplished during the exercise program, and later in daily work tasks. To incorporate variety into the strength training segment, different forms of resistance, such as hand-held weights, resistance bands and tubing, medicine balls, and stability balls can be used. Principles, guidelines, and suggested exercises for safe, effective strength training follow.

## Principles of Strength Training

Because the focus now is on resistance work, which is best done when the body is thoroughly warm, the timeframe becomes optional and follows your priorities in your workout session. If possible, plan to use approximately 15 to 20 minutes[3] for strength training during your fitness class, following these principles:

- Precede and follow muscle-strengthening exercises by stretching exercises specific for the muscles that are made to work against resistance. Any muscle group strengthened by exercise also should be stretched regularly to prevent abnormal contraction of resting length.[4]

- Of key importance, stabilize your joints and your spine before beginning each exercise.

- The exercise must induce muscular overload so that the body senses a stimulus (overload) and responds to the stimulus by becoming stronger.

- Perform each movement using a smooth, continuous, full range-of-motion action for the joint/muscle group involved, and keep the timing of the movement (usually slow) totally under your control. *Ballistic* (rapid or jerky) *movements* increase the risk of injury.

- Take approximately 1–2 seconds to perform the overcoming-resistance (concentric phase of the muscle you're training) and 2–4 seconds (at least the same time, or up to twice as long) during the release or lowering (eccentric phase of that same muscle being trained) to return to the starting position of each exercise.[5]

- Exhale during the lifting, overcoming-resistance-action move; inhale during the release or lowering and return. (Exception: During overhead pressing movements, inhale as you lift.)[6]

- Engage in visualization and self-talk (see Chapters 2 and 12). Plan your concentrated thoughts to accompany your lifting/exhale and lowering/ inhale movements.

- For general fitness of healthy adults, include in a strength training session a minimum of one set of at least one exercise for all major muscle groups. This recommendation is for healthy adults desiring minimal fitness, and not for athletes, because multiple sets do result in greater strength gains than single-set programs.[7]

- Therefore, for this class, follow a progressive resistance format that suggests beginning with one[8] to three sets of 8–12 repetitions for most exercises. (Exception: For abdominal work, begin your program by performing two sets of 15–30 repetitions per set.) Work with weights or resistance that

fatigues the muscles for those 8–12 repetitions. If your muscles start getting larger than you would like, simply decrease the resistance (weights) or frequency that you use them.[9]

- Select 8–10 exercises that condition the major muscle groups of your body and perform them for preferably three,[10] or at least two, of your fitness class sessions per week, if you have no other separate strength training program.

- A common mistake of beginning exercisers is not lifting enough weight.[11]

- Or, use *circuit programs* as good alternatives if you have a limited amount of training time. This means that everyone is working at once, with their own light resistance (tube or band), and the circuit consists of a series of resistance training exercises performed one after the other with minimum rest (15–30 seconds) between exercises. Participants perform approximately 10–15 repetitions[12] of each exercise per circuit (using a tube that represents resistance of 40–60% of 1 repetition maximum, the amount you can smoothly and safely lift just one time).

- If you become jerky, are not smooth, continuous, and rhythmical in the move, and are not using the full range-of-motion possible around your joints, stop. You've completed your lower limit for that set. This lower limit becomes your *baseline*, to which you attempt to add more repetitions as soon as possible.

- Add resistance in increasingly greater increments (1–4 pounds if using hand-weights, or thicker rubber if using bands/tubing). In the fitness class setting, don't go over the 4-pound limit for hand-held weights if this is your choice of resistance equipment.

- It is important for everyone to work their fast twitch muscle fibers.

These are the muscle fibers that make up about 50% of your total muscle mass, and are worked using compound lifts (more than one muscle and movement from more than one joint). *Heavier weight* is used and *fewer repetitions* are performed. You should have strength training experience before going through a fast twitch phase. It is a great way to build muscle and strength and should be done about four times per year.[13]

- Traditionally, allow one day of recovery between training sessions for a given muscle group,[14] so perform strength training of isolated muscle groups *every other day*. Your muscles need a day to recover, so don't incorporate a program to strength train with resistance (weights/bands/tubing) daily. As an alternative to this program, perform strength training exercises with resistance (weights/bands/tubing) for the upper half of your body one day and for the lower half of your body the next day. Thus, you are alternating the days that the muscles are strength training.

- Allow brief rest periods between bouts of vigorous exercises. The timeframe for *rest* is defined as *regaining a normal breathing pattern*.

- To incorporate variety into your program, try using all of the forms of resistance illustrated in this chapter:
  1. Your own body (or parts) lifted and lowered against gravity as the weight resistance used, as in push-ups or curl-ups. To progressively increase the resistance involved in lifting your body's weight against gravity, use a strategically placed free-weight (on the sternum for a curl-up, Figure 10.21a, or between the shoulder blades for a push-up, and so on).
  2. Hand-held weights (not wrist-weights) in controlled movement

or placed on the body in the key locations to add weight resistance to the body part being lifted and lowered.

3. Rubber resistance *bands*, 9", 12", or 16" long, in widths of ¼–1½ inches. The length and width are selected according to whether the exercise works the upper or lower body, and your current strength fitness level in the muscle group being trained.

4. Rubber resistance *tubing*, approximately 3–4½ feet long, so you can adjust it according to your height, in a range of light-to-heavy thickness that you select according to your current strength level.

5. For optimal performance, you must learn to use your body and muscles as an integrated unit. This will get you away from the one-muscle-at-a-time concept of strength training that has dominated fitness for decades… Using a stability ball (see Figure 10.1a) in conjunction with a normally structured resistance training program will facilitate greater gains in movement quality (movement becomes easier and feels more fluid), with no additional training time necessary. There is also a greater amount of muscle stimulated per minute of the workout.[15]

6. All the above combined, using a step bench in a level position, or in the gravity-assisted incline or decline positions. Note: The bench is not designed for using free-weights of more than 10 pounds.[16] For comfort and safety, place a towel on the bench platform when lying on it.

From the exercises presented in this chapter, you will begin to realize that the possibilities for variety in your strength training segment are fun, exciting, inexpensive, and unlimited.

Options 1 to 6 just mentioned are all illustrated in Figures 10.1a, b, and c. Following are the principles for using these unique pieces of equipment.

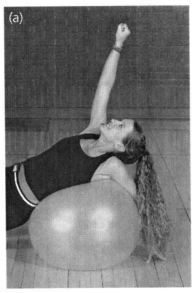

(a)

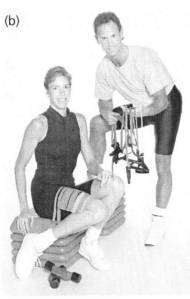

(b)

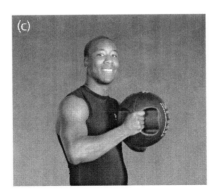

(c)

**Figure 10.1** Various Equipment Used for Resistance

**(a)** Stability Ball

**(b)** Resistance Bands, Tubes, Free Weights

**(c)** Medicine Ball with Handles

## Using Resistance Bands and Tubing

General principles for using either resistance bands or tubing include the following:

- Select bands and tubing based on your fitness level.

- Before each use, inspect the bands and tubing for nicks and tears that may arise from continued use.

- Never, under any circumstances, tie pieces of band and tubing together.

- Always exhibit proper body alignment and posture while exercising, as illustrated in the figures in this chapter.

- Keep your face turned slightly away from the direction of movement, for safety.

- While performing single-limb, upper body movements, always anchor the band between one hand and the thigh, hip, side, or shoulder, depending on the movement.

- Always anchor the tubing under the ball of one foot or both feet, depending on your level of fitness and the desired amount of tension.

- Always control the bands and tubing, especially during the return phase of the movement. Do not let them control you.

- Perform 8–10 repetitions of each exercise. When using one arm or one leg, switch sides so the same muscle group is worked an equal number of repetitions on the opposite side of the body. Be sure to work all muscular groups with equal intensity and repetitions at each session, to avoid muscular imbalance.[17]

## Specifics of Bands

Bands (Figures 10.2 and 10.3) are available in a variety of sizes to change the intensity of your workout.[18] Suggested sizes are:

- **Beginner**
  3/8" upper body (pink)
  3/8" (pink) or 5/8" (light blue)
    lower body

- **Intermediate**
  5/8" upper body (light blue)
  5/8" lower body

- **Advanced**
  3/4" upper body (dark blue)
  3/4" lower body

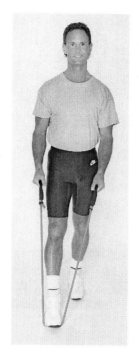

**Figure 10.4**
Beginner: One Foot
on Tubing

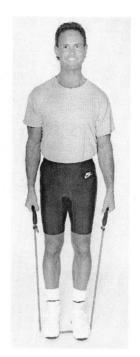

**Figure 10.5**
Intermediate: Both
Feet on Tubing

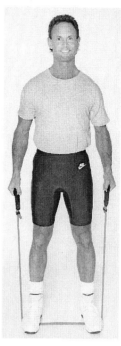

**Figure 10.6**
Advanced: Feet
Spread on Tubing

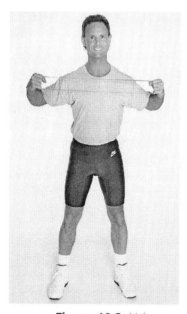

**Figure 10.2** Using
Resistance Bands for Upper
Body (deltoid press-away)

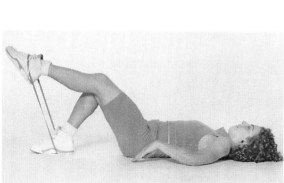

**Figure 10.3** Using Resistance Bands for Lower
Body (leg extension for quadriceps)

## Specifics of Tubing

Tubing is also available in a variety of sizes to change the intensity of your workout.[19] Suggested sizes are:

- **Beginner**
  Very light (yellow) and light
    tubing (green)

- **Intermediate**
  Light (green) and medium
    tubing (red)

- **Advanced**
  Heavy tubing (blue) (purple)

All of the tubing exercises described in this chapter are designed for the beginner and intermediate exerciser. This means that one foot always will be placed on the center of the tubing to create resistance. You can use the other foot to anchor the tubing if you like. Participants who want to create more resistance stand on the tubing with both feet. The wider you spread your feet, the more resistance you will create (Figures 10.4–10.6).[20]

## Stability Ball Training

Using stability balls can provide all of the following.

✔ Add an element of *fun* to your strength training session.
✔ Add a challenge to exercises already in use by experienced exercisers.
✔ Provide an opportunity for newer exercisers to enhance their comfort level with resistance training, by using one piece of equipment.
✔ The most important benefit in using a stability ball is that any exercise performed with it *forces the individual to learn dynamic stabilization* ~ a precise combination of muscular contractions to maintain balance while using the ball.[21]

With endless options available, it is *initially* easier and safer to incorporate stability ball training moves into a more conventional program routine with guidance from a fitness instructor or personal trainer who is knowledgeable with this piece of equipment and can provide professional direction.

Typically, you would first add a few basic movements to develop a comfort with the ball, and over time add more options into your program. You can also use a stability ball in the same way you use a weight bench (see Figure 10.7 when working with dumbbells[22] or an Xerball® (a medicine ball with handles, by Spri™).

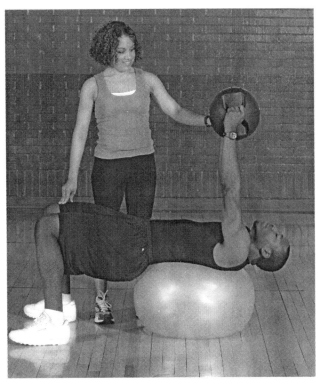

**Figure 10.7** Use the Stability Ball the Same Way You Use a Weight Bench

## *Guidelines for Strength Training*

Because strength and endurance are considered together as a vital component of total physical well-being, most fitness classes today include a 10- to 20-minute segment on strength training the skeletal muscles. Guidelines from the American College of Sports Medicine state:

Strength training of a moderate intensity, sufficient to develop and maintain fat-free weight, should be an integral part of an adult fitness program. One set of eight to twelve repetitions, of eight to ten exercises that condition the major muscle groups, at least 2 days per week, is the recommended minimum.[23]

Thus, the prescription for more fully developing your lean (fat-free) weight is:

| Set | Reps | Varieties of Exercises | Minimum Days/Week |
|-----|------|------------------------|-------------------|
| 1 | 8–12 | 8–10 targeting major muscle groups | 2 (with maximum 4 days per week, or every other day) |

You'll be focusing on the following isolated muscle groups of the upper, mid, and lower body.

■ Upper body: chest, upper back, shoulders, and arms.

■ Mid-section: abdominals, lower back.

■ Lower body: hips and buttocks, thighs, and lower legs.

The exercises illustrated and described here have been categorized according to the location of the muscle group(s) benefited (upper body/mid-section/lower body) using a variety of equipment. Breathe evenly on all strength-training exercises. Do not hold your breath. Your working muscles need oxygen constantly. Figure 10.8 illustrates the major muscle groups to be strength-trained,[24] and Table 10.1 identifies, in the order of their presentation, the exercises that will accomplish the training.

Your body is very adaptive so it constantly needs a new stimulus. Variables that can be manipulated are the sets, reps, exercises, grips, rest time, tempos, and frequency.[25]

**Figure 10.8** Major Muscles to Be Strength-Trained

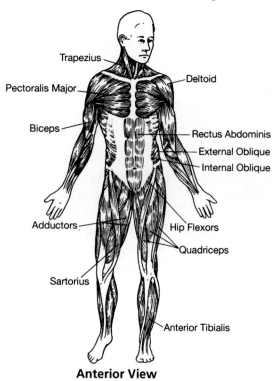

**Anterior View**

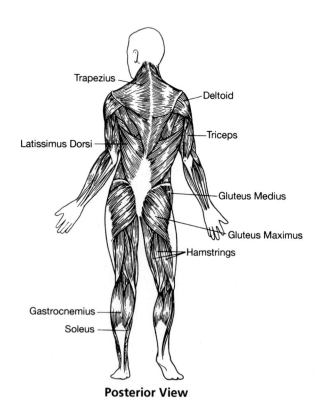

**Posterior View**

*Table 10.1* **Strength Training Exercises Using Various Forms of Resistance**[26–28]

---

**UPPER BODY—Chest/Upper Back/Shoulders/Arms**

- **Chest Press-Away** (Xerball®) (Figure 10.9ab)
- **Push-Up Variations** (Figure 10.10a;b;c)
- **Flyes Variations** (weights/tubing) (Figure 10.11ab; c)
- **Seated Lat Row** (tubing) (Figure 10.12ab)
- **Lat Pull-Down** (tubing) (Figure 10.13ab)
- **Deltoid Lateral Raise** (weights/tubing) (Figure 10.14a; bc)
  - **Half Raise** (bench/tubing) (Figure 10.14d)
  - **Variety** (tubing) (Figure 10.14bce)
  - **Stability Ball** (stability ball/tubing) (Figure 10.14f)
- **Upright Row** (bench and tubing) (Figure 10.15)
  - **Tubing** (not shown)
- **Biceps Curls** (tubing/double tubing/weights/band/bench) (Figure 10.16ab; c; d)
  - **With Squat** (bench and tubing) (Figure 10.16ef)
- **Triceps Kick (Press) Back** (tubing) (Figure 10.17ab)
- **Triceps Extension** (tubing) (Figure 10.18ab)
- **Overhead Press** (tubing/bench and tubing/Xerball®) (Figure 10.19ab; c; d; ef)

**MID-SECTION—Abdominals/Low Back**

- **Back Extension** (incline bench) (Figure 10.20)
- **Gravity-Assisted Curl-Up** (weight/incline bench) (Figure 10.21a)
  - **Reverse Curl-Up** (decline bench) (Figure 10.21b)
  - **Curl-Up Variation** (Figure 10.21c)
  - **Curl-Up with Xerball® and Trunk Rotation** (Xerball®) (Figure 10.21def)

**LOWER BODY—Hips and Buttocks/Thighs/Lower Legs**

- **Squats** (bench/weights) (Figure 10.22a; b)
- **Buttocks/Heel Lift** (band) (Figure 10.23)
- **Side Leg Raise** (band) (Figure 10.24)
- **Leg Curl** (band) (Figure 10.25)
- **Seated Lower Leg Flexor and Extensor** (tubing) (Figures 3.6–3.7)

Xerball® (Pectorals)

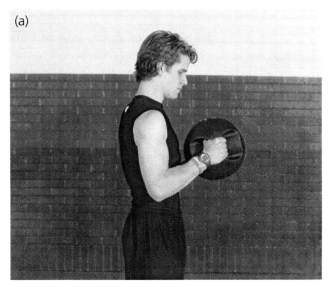

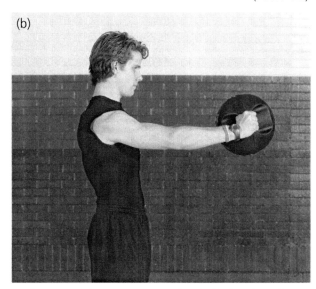

**Position:** Stand, holding the Xerball® close to the chest with both hands in the handles. (a)

**Action:** Straighten arms, pressing ball directly in front of you, keeping Xerball® shoulder high. (b)

**Figure 10.9** Chest Press-Away

---

Floor Space (Pectorals)

**Option 1:   Static Push-Up**

**Position:** Men and women alike perform a static push-up for as long as possible. This is done by lowering the body until the arms are flexed to 90° or less (2" or 3" above the floor) (a). Keep the entire body straight and off the floor, with the exception of the hands and feet.

**Action:** Using a timer, record the *number of seconds the position is held in this position*. (Exercise is over when abdomen drops or arms straighten.)

**Option 2:   Push-Up**

**Position:** Perform as many continuous push-ups as possible. Keeping the body straight, the chest must touch the floor each time, and the arms must be fully extended at the end of each repetition (b).

**Action:** Count one rep each time you complete a cycle and return up to full-arm extension. Record the *number of continuous reps* (in good form, until muscle exhaustion) as one set.

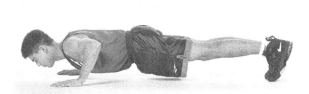

(a) Arms flexed to 90° or less.

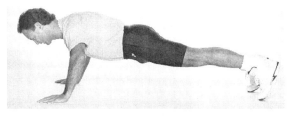

(b) Arms fully extended at end of rep.

**Option 3:   Bench Push-Up**
**Position and Action:**
Perform (c) same as Option 2 here.

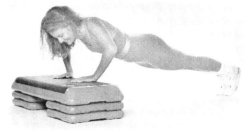

**Figure 10.10** Push-Ups

(c) Keep abdomen tightly contracted for all push-ups.

1-4 lb. Hand Weights                                    (Pectorals; Anterior Deltoid)

### Option 1:    Floor Flyes

**Position:** Lie on back, holding 1-lb to 4-lb hand-weights in each hand above shoulders, arms slightly bent (a).

**Action:** Inhale as you move weights away from each other and lower them toward the floor (b).

**Action:** Exhale as you return hand weights to starting position above you.

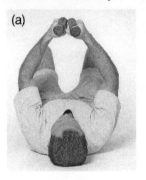
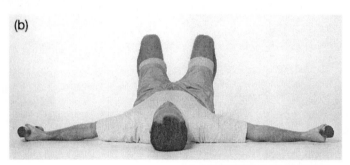
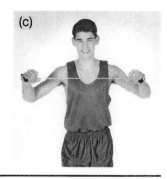

Tubing and Music

### Option 2:    Tubing and Aerobics

**Position:** Stand with bent knees, one heel forward and one foot back. The tube is in front of the chest, rolled up around your hands, for correct tube length (not shown).

**Action:** Pull the hands horizontally apart (as wide as possible with the resistance tubing you're using (c)). Return to the starting position, shifting your weight and repeating with a heel or tap to opposite side.

**Figure 10.11** Flyes

Tubing

(Lats/Trapezius/Rear Deltoid)

**Position:** Seated, with both knees bent, toes pointed forward, abdominals contracted (to protect lower back). Hands at waist level, fists facing, arms away from body (a).

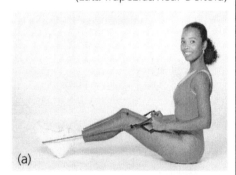

**Action:** Pull the elbows behind the body, fists facing sides; keep head and spine stationary (b).

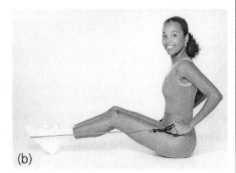

**Figure 10.12** Seated Lat Row

Rolled-up Tubing                                    (Latissimus Dorsi)

### Option 1:    To One Side

**Position:** Grasp the tubing with *R* hand and place overhead. *R* elbow is slightly bent, and tubing is anchored above/behind center of your head (a).

**Action:** Grasp the tubing with *L* hand, keeping hand away from *L* ear, slowly pull down so *L* elbow comes toward *L* side of body (b). Control the return.

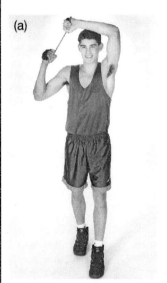
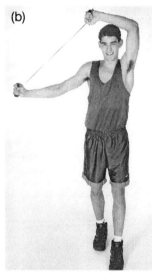

### Option 2:    Down and Back *(not shown)*

**Position:** Stand astride, arms high and wide, above your head, with tube rolled in your palms to a 3' length.

**Action:** Bend elbows, lowering tube *behind your neck* and upper back; hands will be wide and shoulder high, with elbows down near sides. Return to the position high above your head.

**Figure 10.13** Lat Pull-Down

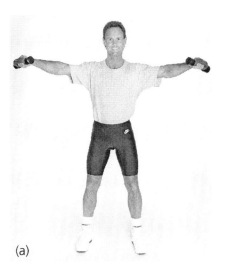

(a)

## Option 1:   1-lb to 4-lb Hand Weights

**Position:** Standing astride, with hand-weights resting on side of the thighs.

**Action:** Raise one arm, or both together (a) to the shoulder-level position. Control the return.

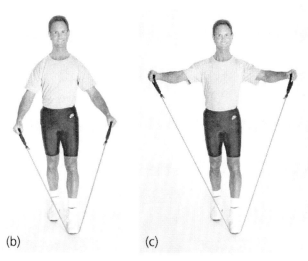

(b)   (c)

## Option 2:   Tubing

**Position:** Step on the tubing with R foot while L foot is behind and L of midline, knees and elbows slightly bent (b).

**Action:** Raise the elbows away from sides up to shoulder level while keeping the wrists/forearms locked, and hands slightly higher than the elbows (c).

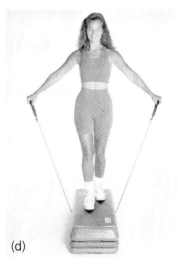

(d)

## Option 3:   Bench and Tubing Half-Raise

**Action:** If fatigued, raise the arms just halfway (d).

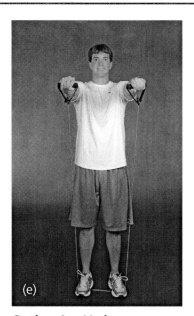

(e)

## Option 4:   Variety

**Position:** For variety, start with arm position (b); tube is now under *both* feet, astride.

**Action:** Lateral raise (c) position.

**Action:** Bring hands and arms directly forward, still shoulder high (e).

**Action:** From this forward position (e), return arms either: wide (c) and then down (b); or directly down (b).

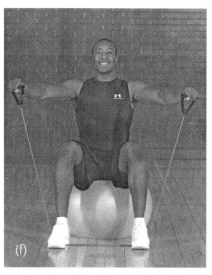

(f)

## Option 5:   Stability Ball/Tubing

**Position:** Sit on stability ball with feet in advanced, wide-stride position. Place tubing under both feet, hands lowered at sides. (not shown)

**Action:** Raise both arms to the sides to a '9 o'clock–3 o'clock' position (f).

**Figure 10.14** Deltoid Lateral Raise

Bench and Tubing/Tubing                                                      (Deltoids/Trapezius)

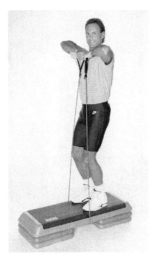

**Option: Bench and Tubing**

**Position:** Place both feet together on bench, bend knees, tube under bench, hands/fists together, and resting on thighs (not shown).

**Action:** Raise handles up to the chin, flaring out elbows slightly, keeping spine firmly erect.

**Option: Tubing** (not shown)

**Position:** Perform the Upright Row using just the tubing (without the bench). Stand on the tubing with two feet, close. Place both handles together (both hands holding both handles together).

**Figure 10.15** Upright Row

**Action:** Raise handles together up to the chin, flaring out elbows, keeping abdomen pulled in.

> **Note:** Bent knees in some of these illustrations assist in keeping a target heart rate so these exercises also *can serve as 1-minute strength-training intervals* in aerobic step training with strength programs.

---

Tubing/Hand Weights/Bench and Tubing                                          (Biceps/Brachialis)

**Option 1:**

**Tubing**

**Position:** Step on the tubing with one or two feet, slight bend in the knees, and fists/palms facing the body, wrists locked, elbows kept at the sides throughout (a).

**Action:** Curl both arms toward the shoulders (b).

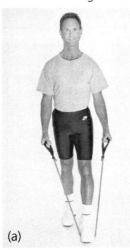
(a)

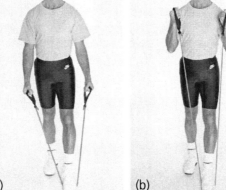
(b)

**Option 2:**

**Double Tubing (advanced)**

**Position:** Same as Option 1 except place both tubing handles in one hand (c).

**Action:** Curl arm with tubing (use other hand as a stabilizer).

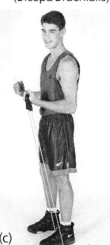
(c)

(d)

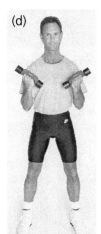

**Option 3:**

**1-lb to 4-lb Hand Weights**

**Position:** Resting weights near thighs, palms up.

**Action:** Raise one arm, or both together (d). If using just one arm, alternate.

**Figure 10.16** Biceps Curls

(e)

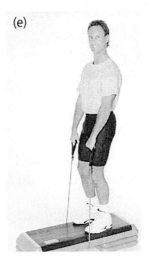

(f)

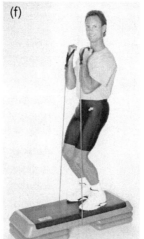

**Option 4:   With Squat on Bench**

Bench and Tubing

**Position:** Stand on top of bench with tubing under center and have hand/fist position facing thighs (e).

**Action:** Curl up to sky, rotating palms on the way up so they face the shoulders. Reverse the rotation for the return. Bend knees to increase heart rate (f).

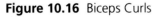

Tubing (Triceps)

**Position:** Stand in forward/back stride position and grasp the handles with palms facing up/in, elbows cocked (a).

**Action:** Press both arms backward, rotating the wrists so palms are facing rear, firm wrists, arms fully extended (b).

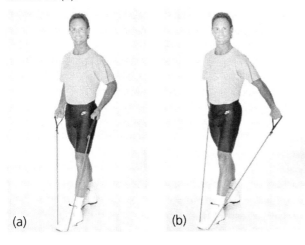

(a) (b)

**Figure 10.17** Triceps Kick (Press) Back

Tubing (Triceps)

**Position:** Stand on one handle with *L* foot. Take other handle in *L* hand; grab tube midway with *R* hand behind your back at the waist area. Raise *L* elbow, pointing skyward, lowering *L* hand to atop shoulder (a),

**Action:** Extend *L* forearm skyward (b).

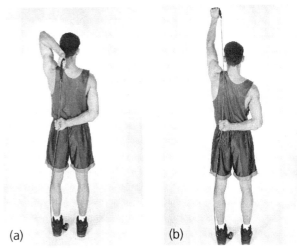

(a) (b)

**Figure 10.18** Triceps Extension

Tubing/Incline Bench and Tubing/ Xerball®

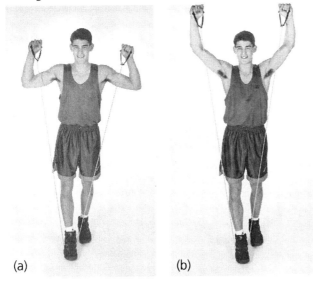

(a) (b)

**Option 1: Tubing**

**Position:** Stand with tubing under one foot; hands are holding tubing, with elbows shoulder high (a).

**Action:** Press upward to full extension, keeping elbows slightly flexed (b).

**Figure 10.19** Overhead Press

(Deltoids/Triceps)

**Option 2: Tubing**

**Position:** Sit on tube, bending knees, feet flat on the floor (c); continue hand position and arm movement as in (a) and (b).

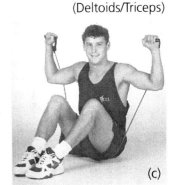

(c)

**Option 3: Incline Bench and Tubing**

Adjust bench so two blocks are at the low end and four blocks are at the high end.

**Position:** Prone, with tubing in back of the groove in the second block, hands starting at sides, wide, and chin resting on incline bench top (d).

**Action:** Press up and forward, ending with thumbs in and facing each other (not shown).

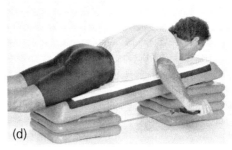

(d)

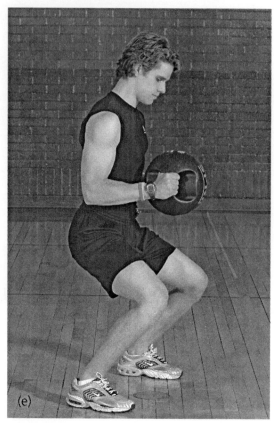

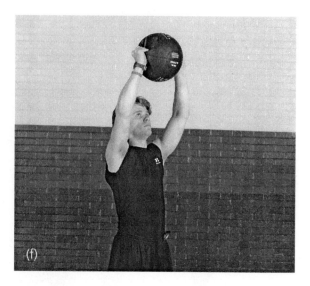

**Option 4:   Xerball® (14lb.\* medicine ball with two handles)**

**Position:** Stand, 12″ astride, holding Xerball® at chest.

**Action:** Bend your hips and knees and lower into a squat position, keeping your head erect, your back flat, and your elbows at your sides (e).

**Action:** As you are straightening your hips and legs, raise the Xerball® skyward, to a full extension of your arms above your head (f).

**\*Note:** Spri™ Xerballs® are available in 8-20lb. weights, in two pound increments (#8/10/12/14/16/18/20).

**Figure 10.19** Continued

---

Stability Ball                                                   (Erector Spinae)

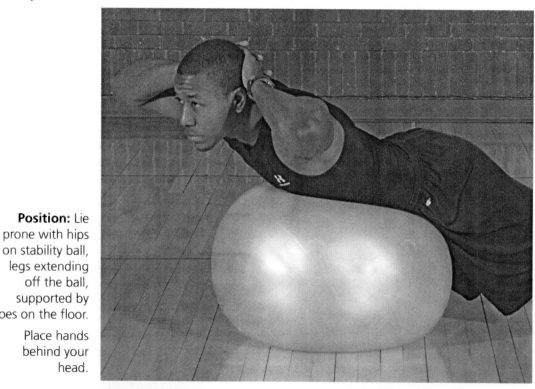

**Position:** Lie prone with hips on stability ball, legs extending off the ball, supported by toes on the floor.

Place hands behind your head.

**Action:** Contract low back, stretch and raise upper chest, looking up. Lower.

**Figure 10.20** Back Extension

Incline Bench and 1-4 lb. Hand Weights/Decline Bench/ Xerball®                    (Abdomen)

Incline Bench and 1-lb to 4-lb. Weights

### Option 1:  Gravity-Assisted Curl-Up

**Position:** With bench in incline position, straddle and *sit on lower third*. Place a free weight\* on sternum (breastbone), with knees flared out wide and heels together, flat on floor.

**Action:** Keeping your lower back on bench at all times, curl up, head looking forward (a). This is all as far as you go; release and curl back down to lying position.

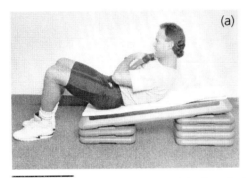

(a)

---
\* Adding more weight resistance is optional, but if you do, this is where it should be done. Maximum hand-weights to use while on the bench is 10 lb.

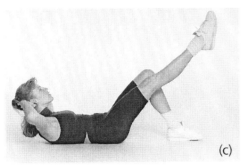

(c)

### Option 3:  Curl-Up Variation

**Position:** Lie on back, with fingers spread behind head, elbows wide. Bend *L* knee, placing foot flat on floor, *R* leg lying on floor. (not shown)

**Action:** Keeping mid-to-low back on floor at all times, contract abdominals and curl up, head looking forward and up, while raising *R* leg to a thigh-parallel position (c); toe is extended and skyward.

**Action:** Lower head and *R* leg simultaneously. Repeat with *L* leg.

Decline Bench

### Option 2:   Reverse Curl-Up

**Position:** Place bench in a decline position, lie on bench, face up with *head at lower end* of bench. Grasp the lip of the platform and top block, over your head. Legs are skyward, with hips, knees, and ankles bent loosely.

**Action:** Contract abdominals and raise buttocks up, keeping lower back on the platform (b). Lower.

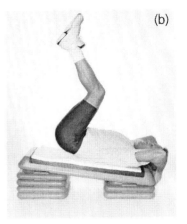

(b)

Xerball®

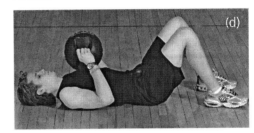

(d)

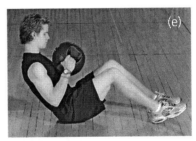

(e)

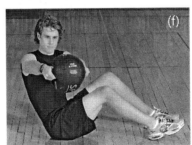

(f)

**Figure 10.21**  Curl-Ups

### Option 4: Curl-Up with Xerball® and Trunk Rotation
~Advanced Only~

**Position:** Lie on back, hold Xerball® slightly above breastbone, with your knees bent and feet flat on the floor (d).

**Action:** Slowly Curl-Up to the "10 o'clock" position, with Xerball® still close to the breastbone (e), pressing your heels to the floor for stability, or keeping your feet flat on the floor.

**Action:** Twist **slowly,** turning your trunk to one side. **Slowly** extend arms using a Chest Press Away movement with the Xerball®, keeping it shoulder high and directly in front of your chest (f).

**Action:** Bring Xerball® *close* and return to the center position (e), then back down to the floor (d).

**Action:** Repeat slowly to the opposite side.

**Note:** Reps for abdominal work can be 15–30, and two sets—one *before* the first program segment and one *before the cool down*—because the muscle tissue located here responds better to more repetitions for definition than do other groups of the body. These exercises are used specifically to help strengthen the sensitive lower back; the low back is supported completely during the abdominal contraction.

Bench/ 1-4 lb. Hand Weights/ Xerball®

(Buttocks)

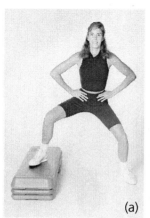

**Option 1:   Bench**

**Position:** Stand with your side next to side of bench. Place *L* foot on center of bench, *R* foot on floor in wide stance; hands on hips.

**Action:** "Wide-sit," flexing knees and lowering buttocks until knees are over, but not beyond, toes (a). Raise.

(a)

**Figure 10.22** Squats

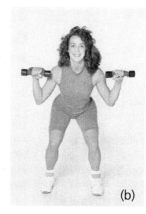

**Option 2:   1-lb to 4-lb Hand-2 Weights**

**Position:** Stand with feet shoulder-width apart, holding 1-lb to 4-lb hand-weights near shoulders, elbows at sides.

**Action:** "Sit," flexing knees and lowering buttocks until knees are over (but not beyond) toes (b). Raise.

**Option 3:   Xerball®**

**Position and Action:** See Figure 10.19 (e).

(b)

---

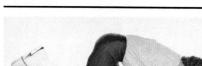

Band                                                                       (Gluteals)

**Position:** Assume an all-fours position, resting on forearms, knees wider than hips, abdominals tight. Place band atop *L* instep (shoe strings) and *R* sole/instep (not shown).

**Action:** Bend *R* leg with heel pointing to ceiling, lifting heel without bending knee any farther, going as far as band will allow. Lower. Alternate legs to achieve balance.

**Figure 10.23** Buttocks/Heel Lift

---

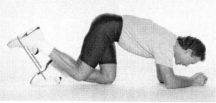

Band                                                                (Thigh Abductors)

**Position:** Place band just above knees. Lie on your side, with your head resting on bottom arm, which is straight overhead. The top arm is in a bent-arm support in front of chest, with legs either slightly bent or knees bent to 90°.

**Action:** Raise top leg (bent as shown) 6"–12" toward the ceiling. Control body position during raising and lowering. After reps, change position and alternate, to strengthen both legs.

**Figure 10.24** Side Leg Raise

---

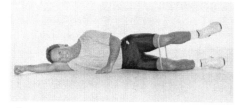

Band                                                                   (Hamstrings)

**Position:** Lie face down with band around your ankles (not shown).

**Action:** Bend *R* leg, bringing heel toward and within 12"–18" of buttocks, keeping hips down firmly on the floor. Return. Alternate.

> **Note:** An excellent exercise for the quadriceps, as a balance to this exercise, is shown in Figure 10.3. The hips again are held firmly on the floor, and the action is alternated after the reps.

**Figure 10.25** Leg Curl

---

**Seated Lower Leg Flexor and Extensor (see Figures 3.7–3.8)**
Tubing
(Anterior Tibialis)

**Position:** Sit tall, chest raised, shoulders down, holding handles near thighs, palms down, with tubing around ball/toe area of both feet held close together.

**Action:** Without moving your body or hands, point toes away from you.

**Action:** Now, without moving your body or hands, point toes toward you, flexing your ankles. (This is a great exercise for preventing or relieving shin splints.)

**Note:** Securing the tubing firmly around your toes while holding the tubing firmly in place will prevent it from rolling off your toes and toward your face/chest area for this exercise.

## Implementing Your Program While Traveling

Various equipment can be used to train the muscle groups, so whatever your preference or whatever is available to you, take advantage of at least one way to strength-train each muscle group (see Figure 10.8). Are you traveling? No problem! Even while on the road, your workout sessions can continue, with a minimal amount of preparation or equipment. You can easily pack the light resistance tubing or bands and continue your strength training program, uninterrupted.

The following is a sample calisthenics-based routine that can be performed daily, for those individuals who already have a moderate level of fitness, and who have no accompanying orthopedic problems.[29]

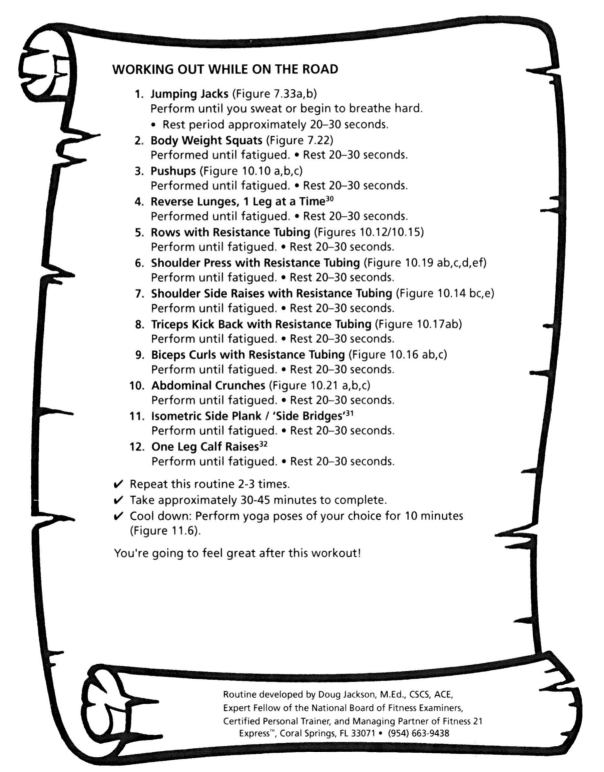

**WORKING OUT WHILE ON THE ROAD**

1. **Jumping Jacks** (Figure 7.33a,b)
   Perform until you sweat or begin to breathe hard.
   • Rest period approximately 20–30 seconds.
2. **Body Weight Squats** (Figure 7.22)
   Performed until fatigued. • Rest 20–30 seconds.
3. **Pushups** (Figure 10.10 a,b,c)
   Performed until fatigued. • Rest 20–30 seconds.
4. **Reverse Lunges, 1 Leg at a Time**[30]
   Performed until fatigued. • Rest 20–30 seconds.
5. **Rows with Resistance Tubing** (Figures 10.12/10.15)
   Perform until fatigued. • Rest 20–30 seconds.
6. **Shoulder Press with Resistance Tubing** (Figure 10.19 ab,c,d,ef)
   Perform until fatigued. • Rest 20–30 seconds.
7. **Shoulder Side Raises with Resistance Tubing** (Figure 10.14 bc,e)
   Perform until fatigued. • Rest 20–30 seconds.
8. **Triceps Kick Back with Resistance Tubing** (Figure 10.17ab)
   Perform until fatigued. • Rest 20–30 seconds.
9. **Biceps Curls with Resistance Tubing** (Figure 10.16 ab,c)
   Perform until fatigued. • Rest 20–30 seconds.
10. **Abdominal Crunches** (Figure 10.21 a,b,c)
    Perform until fatigued. • Rest 20–30 seconds.
11. **Isometric Side Plank / 'Side Bridges'**[31]
    Perform until fatigued. • Rest 20–30 seconds.
12. **One Leg Calf Raises**[32]
    Perform until fatigued. • Rest 20–30 seconds.

✔ Repeat this routine 2-3 times.
✔ Take approximately 30-45 minutes to complete.
✔ Cool down: Perform yoga poses of your choice for 10 minutes (Figure 11.6).

You're going to feel great after this workout!

Routine developed by Doug Jackson, M.Ed., CSCS, ACE,
Expert Fellow of the National Board of Fitness Examiners,
Certified Personal Trainer, and Managing Partner of Fitness 21
Express™, Coral Springs, FL 33071 • (954) 663-9438

## Goal-Setting Challenge

 Giving definition (shaping/toning/sculpting) to your muscles makes you look better and also can provide you with more strength and endurance to perform all of your daily tasks. These are two good reasons to set a goal to strength-train regularly, using your favorite resistance from the variety presented.

"Only about 9% of adults regularly engage in muscular fitness-promoting behaviors, a percentage that is well below the national goal of 30%."[33] Make the choice now not to allow this current national statistic to describe you. Write one Strength (or Endurance) Training Goal for Chapter 10, following the four steps presented in Chapter 2, Exercise 2.3, then record it in your Fitness Journal.

## Recording Your Strength-Training Program

Recording your strength-training progress will prove to be a motivational tool for you to continue your program after the formal structure of a fitness class setting ends. Record the following on Exercise 10.1, and then continue recording in your Fitness Journal, (or on Exercise 5.4):

- Specific exercise techniques you are choosing for your program.
- Number of sets and reps of each exercise you perform.
- Types of weight resistance used.
- Date of the workout.

Begin the strength-training segment of your program slowly, methodically, and in absolute control of the amount of resistance or weights you are using. Strength-fitness training, which develops muscle strength and endurance more fully, is a long-term project.[34] It calls for a dedicated personal commitment of many hours, just as the programs of stretching for flexibility improvement and aerobics for aerobic capacity improvement are. *All fitness programs are for life!*

## Exercise 10.1  Recording Form for Strength Training

**Strength Training with Bands, Tubing, Light (1-lb. to 4-lb.) & Heavy (8-20 lb.)
Free-Weights and Tubing with the Bench**

| Name | | | | | |
|---|---|---|---|---|---|
| **Date** | | | | | |
| **Exercise** | **S/R/Res*** | **S/R/Res*** | **S/R/Res*** | **S/R/Res*** | **S/R/Res*** |
| **UPPER BODY Chest/Upper Back/Shoulders/Arms** | | | | | |
| 1. Chest Press-Away (Xerball)® (Figure 10.9ab) | | | | | |
| 2. Push-Up Variations (Figure 10.10a;b;c) | | | | | |
| 3. Flyes-Variations (weights/tubing) (Figure 10.11ab;c) | | | | | |
| 4. Seated Lat Row (tubing) (Figure 10.12ab) | | | | | |
| 5. Lat Pull-Down (tubing) (Figure 10.13ab) 6. - Behind Neck/Back (not shown) | | | | | |
| 7. Deltoid Lateral Raise (weights/tubing) (Figure 10.14a; bc;e) | | | | | |
| 8. - Half Raise (bench/tubing) (Figure 10.14d) | | | | | |
| 9. - Variety (tubing) (Figure 10.14bce) | | | | | |
| 10. - Stability Ball (stability ball/tubing) (Figure 10.14f) | | | | | |
| 11. Upright Row (bench and tubing) (Figure 10.15) | | | | | |
| 12. - Tubing (not shown) | | | | | |
| 13. Biceps Curls (tubing/double tubing/weights) (Figure 10.16ab;c;d) | | | | | |
| 14. - With Squat (bench and tubing) (Figure 10.16ef) | | | | | |
| 15. Triceps Kick (Press) Back (tubing) (Figure 10.17ab) | | | | | |
| 16. Triceps Extension (tubing) (Figure 10.18ab) | | | | | |
| 17. Overhead Press (tubing/bench and tubing/Xerball®) (Figure 10.19ab;c;d;ef) | | | | | |
| **MID-SECTION Abdomen/Low Back** | | | | | |
| 18. Back Extension (incline bench) (Figure 10.20) | | | | | |
| 19. Gravity-Assisted Curl-Up (weight/incline bench) (Figure 10.21a) | | | | | |
| 20. - Reverse Curl-Up (decline bench) (Figure 10.21b) | | | | | |
| 21. - Curl-Up Variation (Figure 10.21c) | | | | | |
| 22. - Curl-Up with Xerball® and Trunk Rotation (Xerball®) (Figure 10.21def) | | | | | |
| **LOWER BODY Hips and Buttocks/Thighs/Lower Legs** | | | | | |
| 23. Squats (bench/weights) (Figure 10.22a; b) | | | | | |
| 24. Buttocks/Heel Lift (band) (Figure 10.23) | | | | | |
| 25. Side Leg Raise (band) (Figure 10.24) | | | | | |
| 26. Leg Curl (band) (Figure 10.25) | | | | | |
| 27. Seated Lower Leg Flexor and Extensor (tubing) (Figures 3.6–3.7) | | | | | |

***S/R/Res = Sets, Repetitions, and Resistance (e.g., 3/8/GT = 3 Sets of 8 Repetitions with Green Tubing).**

## *Exercise 10.1  Recording Form for Strength Training ~ Continued*

| Date | | | | | |
|---|---|---|---|---|---|
| **Exercise** | **S/R/Res*** | **S/R/Res*** | **S/R/Res*** | **S/R/Res*** | **S/R/Res*** |
| **UPPER BODY Chest/Upper Back/Shoulders/Arms** | | | | | |
| 1. | | | | | |
| 2. | | | | | |
| 3. | | | | | |
| 4. | | | | | |
| 5. | | | | | |
| 6. | | | | | |
| 7. | | | | | |
| 8. | | | | | |
| 9. | | | | | |
| 10. | | | | | |
| 11. | | | | | |
| 12. | | | | | |
| 13. | | | | | |
| 14. | | | | | |
| 15. | | | | | |
| 16. | | | | | |
| 17. | | | | | |
| **MID-SECTION Abdomen/Lower Back** | | | | | |
| 18. | | | | | |
| 19. | | | | | |
| 20. | | | | | |
| 21. | | | | | |
| 22. | | | | | |
| **LOWER BODY Hips and Buttocks/Thighs/Lower Legs** | | | | | |
| 23. | | | | | |
| 24. | | | | | |
| 25. | | | | | |
| 26. | | | | | |
| 27. | | | | | |

*S/R/Res = Sets, Repetitions, and Resistance (e.g., 3/8/GT = 3 Sets of 8 Repetitions with Green Tubing).

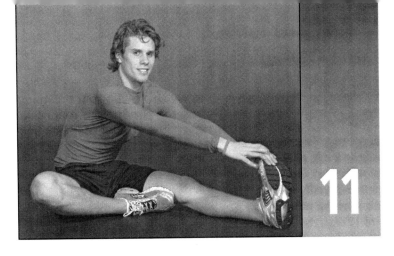

# Cool-Down and Flexibility Training

## 11

The final segment of a total fitness program consists of the cool-down and flexibility training. Because they are complementary, these two types of activity are presented together in this chapter. *Linking* the standing, moving, cool-down positions to the stationary, seated, on-the-floor, stretching exercises, is a classic 12-position yoga routine for beginners. After the yoga positions and the final static stretching exercises have been completed, you'll easily transition to a position of lying on the floor (or mats) and begin relaxation techniques.

Physiologically throughout this entire process, you'll experience a steady lowering of your heart rate, a slowing down of your rate of breathing, and a curbing of profuse sweating. Your body will have totally recovered from the workout, become energized, emotions calmed, and your mind rested.

## Cool-Down

The purpose of the cool-down portion of your fitness session is to give your body time to readjust to the preactivity state in which you began. This will allow the large quantity of blood now in your working muscles, primarily in your arms and legs, to gradually return to your head and brain, trunk, and vital organs.

Stopping a highly strenuous activity session abruptly can cause the blood (primarily in your legs) to pool or to stay in the extremities. This happens because the veins of the legs are not being forcefully squeezed now by strenuously working the leg muscles. The result of pooling can cause cramping, nausea, dizziness, and fainting, because the needed quantity of oxygen and blood is not being delivered to the brain and other vital organs.

Depending on whether you have just finished aerobic exercise or a strength-training segment and also your ability to recover from exertion usually will determine how long your cool-down period will have to be. A minimum of 5 to 10 minutes is essential, however, for two reasons:

1. To curtail profuse sweating
2. To lower the heart rate to below 120 beats per minute

Give yourself time to readjust your pulse, breathing, profuse sweating, and other physiologies. Research tells us that most of the problems occur *after* an intense workout, so be sure to take this needed time to readjust (*5 minutes minimum*). You'll begin your cool-down by slowing all large muscle activity. Tapering off the activity level can be done in various ways, using lower intensity and lower impact moves that gradually lower your heart rate.

The exercises are still active and rhythmic, using a full range of motion, but they now are low-level and slower, half-the-tempo moves, with arms changing from big moves to smaller moves. Examples of cool-down moves are:

- pressing and lunging "The Heiseman" (Figure 11.1)
- two-foot bouncing, with a variety of mid/low arm gestures (Figure 11.2)

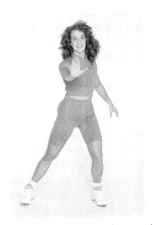

**Figure 11.1** Pressing and Lunging

- a step tap (toe or heel) facing the bench using various directional approaches and arm gestures (Figure 11.3)
- wide-stride standing, upper- and lower-body strength conditioning moves (performed *without* weights) such as a squat with biceps curls (Figure 11.4); or
- slow-paced walking (Figure 11.5)

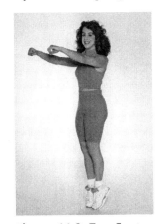

**Figure 11.2** Two-Foot Bouncing

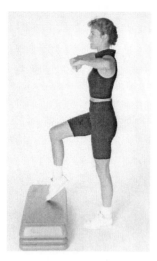

**Figure 11.3** Step Tap (toe or heel)

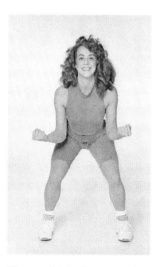

**Figure 11.4** Squat and Curls

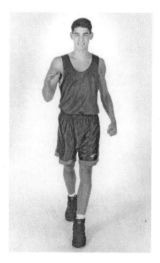

**Figure 11.5** Slow-Paced Walking

## Continuing the Transition Using Yoga

A 12-Position Yoga Routine (Figure 11.6, Positions 1-12) with classic moves for beginners is accessible to everyone and easily learned. It is a complete exercise routine and is made up of 12 successive movements, repeated one after the other, which serve to bring the whole musculature into play.[1] For our purposes, it provides a focused and calming link between dynamic movement and a stationary position. At this time, you'll want to remove your shoes and place them at your station on the floor.

You'll notice that it is made up of just six movements, to be repeated in reverse. Start by learning the first four, then repeat backward (performing positions 9,10,11,12). Next, try only positions 5,6,7 returning to 8. When you have mastered positions 1 to 4 and 9 to 12, then positions 5 to 8, it's time to combine the 12 positions together into the routine.

Work through each position separately for a few days. You'll be adding the rhythm of the movements when your technique has been accomplished. When you have a thorough knowledge of the entire 12 positions, you will be able to rhythmically complete the 12 movements within 20 seconds.[2] A short-term goal to set is to be able to complete 15 repetitions of these 12 positions, in about 5 minutes.[3]

*Concentration* is absolutely essential, and the conscious mind must play an active part in every movement. Try thinking of, and concentrating on, the sun. It energizes all of life! Focus on your energy used in this routine. Image that the amount of energy you have now multiplies as it is touched by a sunray. Your own creativity can suggest many images for this yoga routine.

Finally, it is essential to synchronize *breathing* with the movements. When you coordinate your movements with your breathing, you can perform this routine without running short of breath and energy.

## Correct Positions:

**1 / 12** Attention to your body in full alignment, imaging giving an acknowledgment or salutation.

**2 / 11** Link thumbs in position overhead and stretch arching backward, looking up and backward.

**3 / 10** Bend forward, reach for the floor, pushing your head toward your slightly bent knees.

**4 / 9** Place right knee backward on the floor, with weight maintained on both the base of the right toes and on the left foot, as the left knee bends forward and upward. Balance, keeping weight on fingertips that are on the floor beside forward knee, as chest and head are raised. (Position 9: Then, since it is not easy to bring the forward foot backward to the starting point at back, settle the weight of your body onto your right hand and foot. This allows your pelvis to tilt slightly, thus easing the return of your left foot to the back position, ready for Position 10.)

**5 / 8** Keeping hand(s) on the floor, weight is on both hands now, raising buttocks. Heels *touch* the floor as body forms an inverted 'V,' eyes focusing on the *navel* area. Stretch your back, and contract your stomach.

**6** Stretch out long and low, keeping your hands and your toes on the floor. Stomach is raised slightly off the floor. (Once extended, your feet will remain in the same place on the floor until they are brought back to their starting point, at the end of the routine. This is accomplished with practice over time.)

**7** Keeping the weight of your body *firmly on your hands* and bent toes, raise head and chest up, skyward.

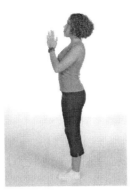

**1** Breathe Out

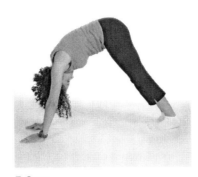

**5** Stop

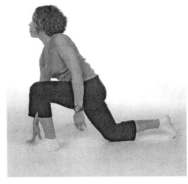

**9** Stop

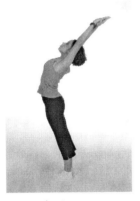

**2** Breathe In

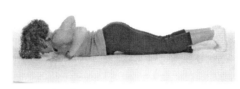

**6** Breathe Out

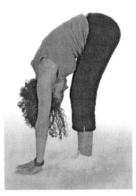

**10** Breathe Out

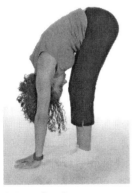

**3** Breathe Out

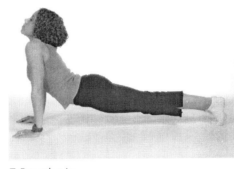

**7** Breathe In

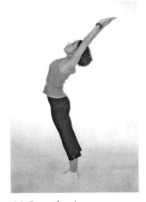

**11** Breathe In

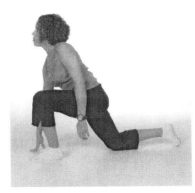

**4** Breathe In

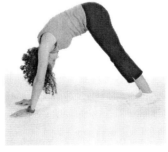

**8** Stop

**Figure 11.6** Breath Rhythm during 12-Position Yoga Routine

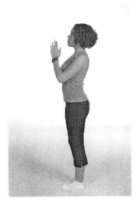

**12** Breathe Out

## Flexibility Training

Flexibility refers to the range of motion of a joint and its corresponding muscle groups. It is influenced genetically, is highly specific, and varies from joint to joint within an individual. Flexibility training, or stretching, is a widely accepted means of effectively increasing joint mobility, improving exercise performance, and reducing injuries.[4] When stretched repeatedly, muscles can be lengthened by approximately 20%.[5] Tendons can increase in length much less, about 2% to 3%.

Stretching programs follow the principle of *specific adaptation to imposed demands* (SAID), which states that an individual must stretch the soft tissues around a joint slowly and progressively to and slightly beyond the point of limitation but not to the point of tearing.

The two most widely accepted methods of stretching to improve flexibility are static stretching and proprioceptive neuromuscular facilitation (PNF). Both follow the philosophy that flexibility is increased and risk of injury is prevented when the muscle being stretched is as relaxed as possible.

> *The highest incidence of problems comes after an intense workout, so be sure to take this needed time (5 minutes minimum) to readjust.*

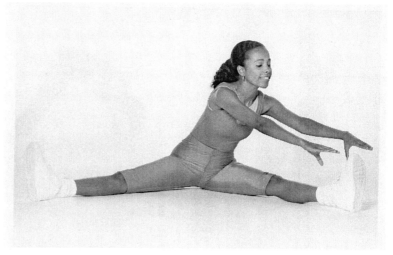

**Figure 11.7** Static Stretching

## Static Stretching

Static stretching is slow, active stretching, with the position held at the extremes of the joint. The aim is to *ease gently into a controlled, stretched position and hold it as you press gently* (Figure 11.7). You push or press to the point of tightness, "stretch pull" (not painful, but a tight feeling) so you feel the muscle working. You continue to stretch slightly beyond this point, without any motion. Then, mentally, you relax your mind and hold the position for approximately 15 seconds, allowing the muscle also to relax and feel heavier.[6] Performing the same stretching on the opposite side of your body always follows.

At present, static stretching is considered one of the most effective methods of increasing flexibility. Research has shown that significant gains can be achieved with a training program of static stretching exercises. This type of continuous stretching produces greater flexibility with less possibility of injury than other modes of exercise, probably because it stretches the muscles under controlled conditions.

## PNF Stretching

PNF stretching techniques, in which muscles are stretched progressively with intermittent isometric contractions, also offer an effective method of increasing flexibility. Like static stretches, they are used when the muscles are warm. Two of the most commonly used modified PNF stretches are:

1. *Contract-relax technique:* In phase one, perform a 5- to 6-second maximum voluntary contraction in the muscle to be stretched. The contraction is isometric because any motion is resisted. In phase two, relax, then stretch, the previously contracted muscle.

2. *Agonist contract-relax technique:* In phase one, maximally contract the muscle opposite the muscle to be stretched against resistance (a partner, the floor, or other immovable object) for 5 to 6 seconds. In phase two, relax the agonist muscle and stretch the antagonist muscle.[7]

An example of a forward PNF contract-relax exercise for the hamstrings and spinal extensors, shown in Figure 11.8, is performed with a partner's assistance.

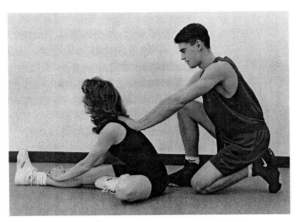

**Figure 11.8** Forward PNF Contract-Relax Stretching

**Position:** In a modified hurdler stretch position, the performing partner leans forward to the point of limitation while keeping the back straight and the toes of the extended leg facing upward to stretch the hamstrings correctly.

**Action:** To begin the action, the performer pushes her back against the partner (contracting the spinal extensors) and pushes the extended leg against the floor (contracting the hamstrings) for a 6-second isometric contraction. The partner, gently but firmly, resists any movement.

**Action:** Releasing the contraction, the performer stretches to a new point of limitation, holding a static stretch for 12 seconds or longer, while the partner maintains light pressure on the performer's back.

## Static-Stretching Sequence (on floor)

Stretching to increase your flexibility and range of motion is crucial, at this point in your session. It is the time when your muscles are *warm* (full of blood, oxygen, and nutrients) and your joints are pliable from vigorous exercise, so take full advantage of the next 5 to 10 minutes to static (or PNF) stretch.

Many stretching techniques are presented in Chapter 6 (Figures 6.2–6.14). Refer to any of them to incorporate into this flexibility training segment. Add the sitting and lying-down stretches sequenced and presented in the opening photo to Chapter 11 and Figures 11.9–11.12.

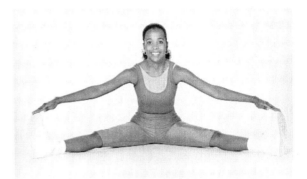

**Figure 11.9** Hips/Groin/Calves Stretch

**Position:** Sit tall with your feet comfortably apart, arms shoulder high over the legs, keeping your kneecaps and toes pointing skyward.

**Action:** Flex toes back toward you as you bend forward at the hips, placing the hands on shins/ankles/toes (whatever you can reach), leaning forward and stretching. Hold 8/16 counts. Relax and recover to start.

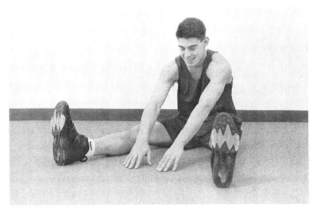

**Figure 11.10** Groin/Hips Stretch

**Position:** See Figure 11.9. Then bring hands inside the "V."

**Action:** Lean forward from the hips, and reach forward as far as you can, keeping your head in line with your spine. Hold 8/16 counts. Relax and recover to start.

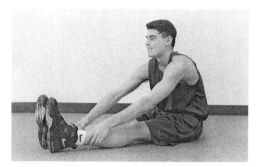

**Figure 11.11** Lower Back Stretch

**Position:** See Figure 11.10. Then slide legs together and grab ankles/calves.

**Action:** Lean forward slowly from the hips, keeping chin parallel with your knees. Hold 8/16 counts. Relax and recover to start.

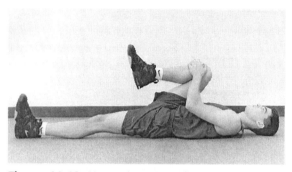

**Figure 11.12** Hamstrings Stretch

**Position:** See Figure 11.11. Now bend your knees, round your back, and lie down. Stretch long (not shown), arms overhead.

**Action:** Bring one knee up to chest, encircling it with hands. Pull knee to chest, keeping other leg long-stretched on the floor, foot flexed. Hold 8/16 counts. Relax and recover to start. Repeat with other leg, 8/16 counts.

## Static Stretching with Relaxation

At the conclusion of your workout, enjoy the natural high your beta endorphins are giving you, by beginning relaxation techniques to accompany the final stretching segment. This is an excellent time to develop rich images and affirmations for yourself (see Chapters 2 and 12), starting with visualizing your energized muscles now becoming *"wider-and-longer-and-warmer-and heavier."*

Your breathing is sequential with the pictures and affirmations. Breathe in deeply for 8 counts, hold your breath, and exhale and stretch for 8/16 counts (Figures 11.13 and 11.14).

Continue relaxing, imaging, and silently self-talking for several more minutes when stretching is completed. These are the re-energizing, mental training moments of your session. A complete program of relaxation techniques is presented in Chapter 12 to finalize your total physical fitness workout session. You'll set a program ending goal *there*!

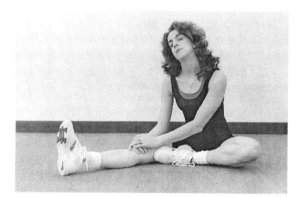

**Figure 11.13** Lateral Neck Stretches

In half-hurdler position (sole of *R* foot against *L* inner thigh), drop head to *L* side. Hold 8/16 counts. Switch leg positions now dropping head to *R* side. Hold 8/16 counts. Relax using recovery and re-energizing images and silent self-talk throughout.

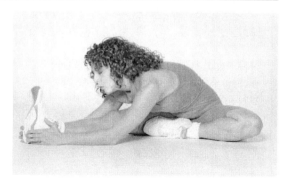

**Figure 11.14** Stretching, Relaxing, Imaging, and Self-Talking

In half-hurdler position, lean forward and press, holding 8/16 counts. Continue to image and self-talk. Sit up, round your back, and lie on the floor. This concludes your *physical* program.

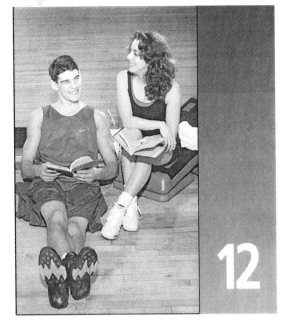

# Stress Management and Relaxation

## 12

*The quieter I can make my mind, the more I can perceive the link between my thoughts, and how I feel.*

*To the possession of the self, the way is inward.*
— *Plotinus*

*We each must, therefore "come of age" by ourself. Each must journey to find our true center, alone.*
— *KSM*

The physical training (workout) portion of your program is in place. Now is the time to reconsider the *mental* training aspects, to put completion to understanding how to establish a lifetime fitness program. Mental training provides the link of understanding between having a *desire* (velleity—wish without the slightest action) to change and improve your body, and actually *achieving* that goal by taking action. It also provides the link of understanding between experiencing the stress caused by life's difficulties and becoming aware of the direct positive effects (training effect) that exercise, and relaxation afterward, provides your wellbeing.

## Mental Training

Now is the time to continue traveling within your thinking process, for it is ultimately there, within the development and enrichment of your mental training skills that program consistency, compliance, and enjoyment reside. And, after all, one of the major goals set forth in this course and textbook is to develop an enjoyment of and understanding for how to *continue* your program long after the 10- to 15-week course is over. To understand this important final step requires you to make a decision. It's no small choice this time. It's time to make a huge leap-of-faith *commitment* to yourself to be open to the possibilities available within you to solve problems.

The commitment you make first requires *ownership* on your part (discussed in Chapter 2), *to keep the power to change*. By not blaming other people or circumstances, you are empowered to use the creative potential within you. Your potential

and answers for problem solving reside there. When you believe that the creativity to solve problems lies within you, you find a way. It simply has to be awakened, called upon, and invited into action.

For example instead of blaming, "That *gym* is too hot/cold to work in" or, "That *instructor* goes too fast/ slow for me," keep ownership of a problem by thinking, "How can I make the best of (or change) this unpleasant situation?" Take a moment now and consider the Goal Setting Challenge on the next page.

Continue this self-awareness process by now turning to Exercise 12.1, My "Top 10" List, at the end of this chapter. Read the content areas of life found to be most stressful to your peers and ask yourself, "Which areas are causing *me* the most difficulty and are taking up too much mental energy?" This exercise serves as a pretest (or survey) to make you more aware of the factors that currently are most stressful to you.

## Goal-Setting Challenge

 Make a choice to update any thoughts you have that you "cannot accomplish, improve, or master" something. Ask yourself, "What is the biggest problem that I currently own?" — *something that up until now has eluded you.*

Can you then practice accomplishing this problem by visualizing the idea of becoming a role model to others in this problem area? Try it! You have everything to gain. Translate this mid-chapter, powerful idea into a Goal Script *now* and write it here:

'Biggest Problem':_____

Action/Goal Script:_____

## Setting a Standard

To understand our own unlimited capabilities, we each must begin by setting a *standard*—establishing a mental training starting point, or basis from which to grow. A balanced state of well-being (seeing life as a "bowl of cherries"—your life and stress in balance) expresses this ideal condition. Next, by taking apart the concept of balance and labeling its parts, and then by understanding imbalance ("the pits"!), you are made aware of both ends of the continuum of life management.

## Establishing the Foundation

All of our world and universe is based on balance. Personal wellness is your life in balance. It requires an awareness of your beliefs, attitudes, emotions, actions, will, and power-source—all of which must be kept in mind and utilized when solving problems. Figure 12.1 illustrates life balance and wellness as six components ("balls") that we need to keep juggling in the air, all at once. These six components are: physical, emotional, social, spiritual, intellectual, and talent expression. Each contributes equally to the total balancing act we must engage in every day.

When any wellness component being juggled and kept in balance gets overlooked temporarily, or is

totally forgotten, it falls out of this balanced alignment and drops out of sight. We then are out of sync with life, or get the feeling of not being a whole person. This is understandable because we aren't! We've allowed one or more components of our life to take over and receive all or most of our attention, disregarding other equally vital parts.

For example, if the *expression of our talent* (our job, career pursuit, or volunteering) takes an inordinate amount of our mental and physical energy every day, little time is left to participate in a *physical* fitness program, to develop a *social* network of friends, or to *intellectually* pursue other interests that can provide positive release of our stress. Our physical, social, or intellectual "ball" drops. We soon experience the results—a decline in physical fitness and the loss of a well-rounded social network of friends, with an accompanying boring, one-dimensional focus in our daily conversations.

## Success

How do you know if and when you are truly balancing the six areas of your life? Developing a working definition for success is one way. Take some quiet time to develop your own definition of success or borrow part, or all, of this one:

*Success* is the ongoing process of striving and growing to become more, in each of the

dimensions of wellness (physical, emotional, social, spiritual, intellectual, talent expression), while positively contributing to others' needs.

By accepting a definition such as this, you can believe unconditionally that you are successful in anything you attempt in life if you (a) attempt and grow from it, (b) continually make more distinctions about what you're doing, and (c) accomplish it for the purpose of contributing positively what you've learned, to your own and others' needs. Adopting a broad definition for success such as this makes it difficult, if not impossible, to feel like a loser or a failure in any dimension of your life.

Therefore, you experience your daily successes (or failures) as steps in a journey rather than as the destination. Life is an ongoing process, and wellness and success (or failure) are intermittent landmarks in the journey. Life has no one port or station—no one place to arrive at once and for all. The true joy of life is the trip! A port, station, or lifetime goal should only evoke a mental image to be held as a *possible* solution, to enable us to be continually free to tap into our creativity—our unlimited potential for what can be possible. (You can accomplish far more than you ever have envisioned!)

Accessing our creative problem-solving skills allows us to use various paths and answers to solve an issue or the task at hand. Life must be

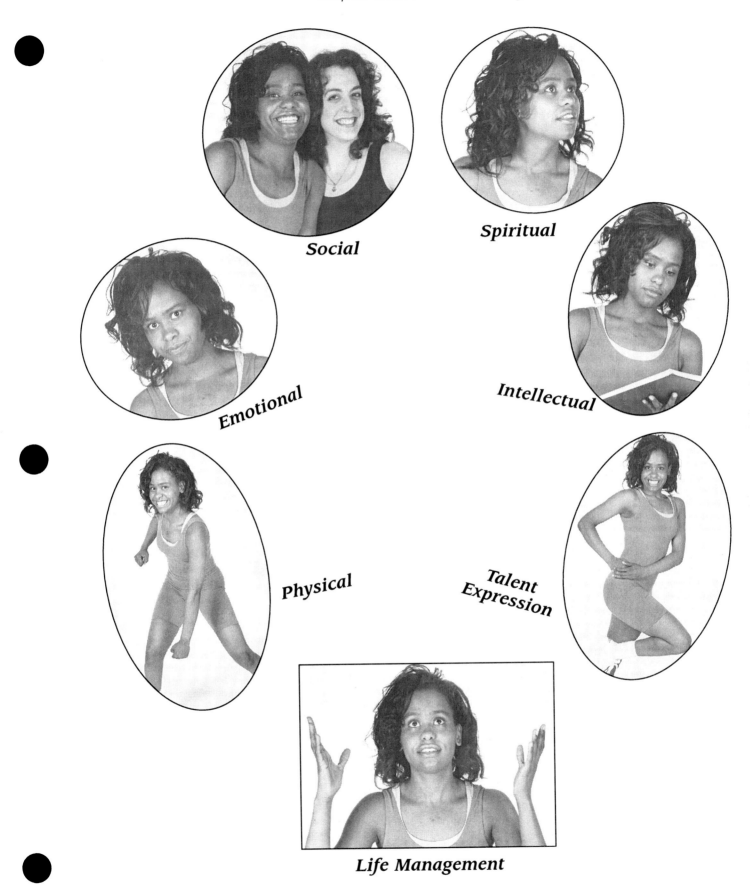

**Figure 12.1** Life Management Requires Balancing Six Key Dimensions of Your Life

lived and enjoyed in the *present moment* and accomplished as daily steps as we go along. The "final port" (and the accompanying eulogy of your successes) will come along soon enough!

## Balancing the Six Wellness Dimensions

We experience the *physical wellness* component by participating in a regular program of the expenditure of physical energy for increasing one's flexibility, heart and lung capacity, and muscular strength and endurance; maintaining good posture (for safety reasons) while exerting this physical effort; selecting the proper intake of food and liquid; maintaining recommended body weight; and providing for restorative relaxation and restful sleep. (Individuals in the personal counseling profession believe that *the most effective, natural reliever of stress and depression*—which they prescribe to their clients—is participation in a regular physical exercise program.)[1]

The *emotional wellness* component (see Figure 12.2) deals with gaining pleasure and avoiding pain. It looks at the distinctions or labels for pleasure (joy) and pain (sadness, anger, fear) and the mixed neuro-associations we feel when these two driving forces are blended (we feel confusion first, then distinctive other emotions surface). Becoming aware of the precise emotions we feel and then understanding what we *link* to pleasure and what we *link* to pain will assist us in being thinking and rational (rather than just emotional), and then capable of choosing productive behavioral responses to stressful life situations. This awareness process develops patience and lengthens our (emotional) fuse, provides ideas for positive outlets for stress that enhance our lives, and educates us on how to change our need to participate in negative, risky behaviors if these exist.

*To reveal myself openly and honestly takes the rawest kind of courage.*[2]

The *social wellness* component means creating balance in the time you spend with others and the time you need to spend alone. You could choose to be independent and achieve alone every goal you set. You would discover, though, that the most mature and successful people, who tap into their creative potential regularly, are *inter*dependent. They choose intentionally to interact with other people regularly even when they could fully accomplish their goals alone. They are able to stretch themselves to unbelievable heights because they constantly draw upon other people as a network of key resources to use.

Inherent in the social wellness component is to become more aware of your communication skills. Sharpening your invitational, assertiveness, and confrontational skills with others will assist you in becoming a victor instead of a victim in life.

The *intellectual wellness* component challenges you to become a lifelong learner, to never become complacent and satisfied with past learning and all of your

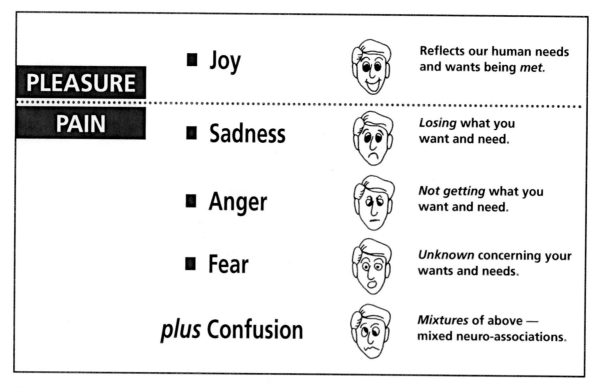

| | | | |
|---|---|---|---|
| **PLEASURE** | ■ Joy | | **Reflects our human needs and wants being *met*.** |
| **PAIN** | ■ Sadness | | ***Losing* what you want and need.** |
| | ■ Anger | | ***Not getting* what you want and need.** |
| | ■ Fear | | ***Unknown* concerning your wants and needs.** |
| | *plus* Confusion | | ***Mixtures* of above — mixed neuro-associations.** |

**Figure 12.2** The Four Big Emotions

accomplishments. Keeping an *open mind* to growth and change in the world at large will help us realize that our potential, individually and collectively, has no boundaries. The only boundaries or limits to our potential are those we self-impose inside our heads.

The *spiritual wellness* component challenges you to investigate the balance you must maintain between relying on your own self-energy source (your will power or how you uniquely solve problems if you are free to be yourself) and that which ultimately fuels you. You'll find a clarity of purpose or meaning for your existence when you make a connection or bond between yourself and the source of power that fuels your will and your existence.

This process is assisted or hastened by developing a consistent belief system, which is the foundation for your values. You express your spirituality as the beliefs and philosophies by which you live your life daily (through the actions, reactions, and responses you make) as you interact with others, the environment, and your inner self.

The *talent expression* component of balance refers to your natural and trained abilities and interests that become translated into your career path or jobs, the volunteer giving of your time to others, and many times the activities you engage in to relieve your stress. Because it usually has a significant impact on self-worth and prestige, this probably is one of the most difficult components for us to keep in perspective and balanced with the other five dimensions of wellness and life management.

The foundation of your life, then, is based upon balance (an ideal wellness state) of six dimensions: physical, emotional, social, spiritual, intellectual, and talent expression. To stay balanced, each of these areas of your life has to receive your regular attention.

## Needs

Why do we need to keep our wellness in balance—for what reasons, purposes, intentions? The five clearly defined survival *needs* we all must have met, supported by the wellness components of our lives, are:

1. I need to live and be healthy.
2. I need safety and security.
3. I need to be loved.
4. I need prestige (self-worth) and power (the ability to take action).
5. I need variety and change in my life.

These needs are *birthrights* that we all require for survival and never should be taken away or used as ways to manipulate others.

## Wants

In addition to our five basic needs are a wide variety of wants. *Wants* are the privileges and comforts we attempt to attain by being responsible and accountable for the actions we take in life. We should begin to label not only what we require for survival (our *needs,* which we also call our ends or ultimate goals) but also what gives us additional pleasure and joy in the process (our *wants,* also called the means to our ends or priorities). When we clearly understand both our basic needs and our wants, we can pinpoint the purposes of and intentions for our various wellness decisions and choices.

## *Defining and Managing Stress*

What happens when we become imbalanced and stress enters our life (our "bowl of cherries" becomes "the pits")? We must be realistic and aware that life will not be continually, perfectly balanced, because life is not static and unchanging. Change is a constant. Thus, we must consider how to deal with imbalance in our life.

Demands. Problems. Challenges. Change. Whatever you choose to call it, imbalance happens within the journey of life. We cannot control our world and all it presents to us. Drunk drivers injure us permanently. Fire and floods destroy our homes and belongings. Death takes our loved ones. A close friend moves far away. We win the lottery! Imbalance asserts itself daily and throughout our life, and we are left to react.

*Stress* is our response. We cannot control the changes, demands, problems, or even the dirty deals we encounter, but we can learn how to manage certain situations so they are less offensive to us.

Probably the most noted modern scientific researcher on the topic of stress and its effect on the human body is the late Viennese-born endocrinologist Hans Selye. In his words: *Stress is the nonspecific response of the body to any kind of demand that is made upon it.*[3]

Selye established the groundwork in defining stress, which recently has been updated. Stress now is believed to be specific, as a result of the scientific findings of the unique body of information called psychoneuroimmunology. A new definition to consider is the following:

> **Stress:** *a series of positive or negative physiological responses and adaptations your body undergoes when any kind of demand is made upon it.*

## *Physiological Responses to Stress*

The physiological response of your body to the positive or negative stressful demands impinging upon it from life situations includes:

- Increased sugar in the blood
- Faster rate of breathing
- Faster heart rate
- Higher blood pressure

- Activation of the blood-clotting mechanism to mitigate effects of injury
- Increased muscle tension
- Cessation of digestion and diversion of blood to the brain and muscles
- More output of perspiration
- Less salivation
- Loosening of bladder and bowel muscles
- Outpouring of various hormones, including adrenalin
- Dilation of pupils of the eyes
- Heightening of all senses

In effect, your body goes into a "Red Alert" and you are ready to fight or flee. This has been aptly named the *fight or flight* response to stress.

Many times you can't do either —fight or flee. You stay in the situation and "stew." If this response, as characterized by the above list, is long enough or severe enough, your bodily systems will undergo wear and tear. This leaves you open to the invasion of some sort of illness. Once a person becomes ill, the illness also becomes a stressor. This increases your stress response (again, as described in the list of bodily changes) and you are caught in a double-bind. Good or bad, stress is our response to any kind of imbalance resulting from demands, problems, challenges, or changes. Therefore, scientifically and physiologically, the overall concept of stress is a neutral term.

Good or positive stress, called *eustress*, is exemplified by running a marathon or seeing our loved one after 7 months of being apart. Negative stress, called *distress*, occurs, for example, when we are in a car accident or our home is vandalized. The goal in managing either kind of stress is the same as with all of life: to return to and achieve a balanced state.

This can be understood more easily using the analogy of playing a guitar. To play the guitar, we must use strings that come in a package,

*The foundation of life is grounded in balance or a wellness state, composed of six dimensions: physical, emotional, social, spiritual, intellectual, and talent expression.*

limp and with no tension on them (no demands or challenges). Without tension or stress on the strings, we can make no sounds. The same comparison goes for our lives. If we have no stress, we have no challenges, no risks, no growth. Life is boring, and so are we, because not enough is going on in our life. But if we stretch those strings to their potential by placing them on the instrument with just the right amount of tension on them and add the human touch, we will make beautiful sounds—harmony. If we place too much tension on the strings (too many commitments on our time), even the slightest pressure will cause the strings to pop—and so will we.

To experience life with continual growth, *imbalance must occur to create room for new possibilities.* Change is one of the certainties of life. It is a given. If we approach change from a positive perspective, it can open the doors to unlimited possibilities and growth. If we take the negative view and see it as a threat to our comfortable stability, change can imprison us in the depths of despair and result in stagnation. The choice of perspective, and our subsequent reactions, is ours to make.

## Coping Skills

In the past, how have you chosen to use your resources to cope (regain balance) when life has dealt you an imbalancing experience? Have you begun to realize that, to stay mentally balanced, we all do *something* to cope with the stress in our lives? Some of these coping mechanisms are positive, and some are negative and detrimental to our total well-being. How do you habitually cope with stress? What are your positive

means, and what are your negative detrimental means?

For instance, if a depressing event is anticipated, you can use *desensitization* in advance, to lighten the impact. Try looking at alternative options to offset the event from happening, or planning ahead ways to deal with the situation after it occurs. The worst coping is to deny it is going to happen.

Have you ever considered going to a health resort, taking time to improve *all* areas of your life?[4] The benefits to be had are numerous. Most health resorts specialize in providing full body massages. The benefits of a massage have been scientifically documented by more than 50 research studies in the past 20 years.[5] A full body massage can relax you, boost your immunity, improve your circulation, relieve back pain to name a few. To find a qualified massage therapist in your area, look on the Websites! section of this text.

At the end of this chapter, you'll be asked to establish a stress management or relaxation goal to work on to improve the one response to stress you make that seems most disabling to you.

You probably will come away from this reflection a lot less judgmental of other people and their abilities to cope with stress. Knowing that we all do something to relieve and cope with the stress in our lives can help you tolerate another person's choices that sometimes can affect you directly. You come away realizing that some people are not bad people because, say, they smoke cigarettes in your space, but they simply are making a bad choice in coping with the stress in their lives. (Bad choice?! About half of all smokers are killed by their habit.)[6]

Your success in adjusting to and managing your response to stress can provide you with growth and more confidence to continually meet your *next* challenge (life situation) and the one after that. We each learn how to adjust to everyday big and small problems and life situations by using our vast internal resources (life experiences from the past, and so on). We are not born adjusted. We learn how to adjust.

## Overview of Stress Management

We all would prefer to experience the feeling of harmony that life, in balance, provides. Reality, however, tells us that life will not always be that perfect bowl of cherries. The pits of imbalance are also needed, as they provide the seeds for growth and change. Realizing that you can't control all of the imbalancing, stressful events that life brings to you leaves you with a choice regarding the management of your stress. How you respond to a stressor is a *choice* you make. This course and text are designed to give you positive mental training ideas to consider when you're making those choices, as well as principles and techniques for safely releasing stress, physically.

## Relaxation: Making the Connection

> *People with an authentic style know what they are,*
> *but even more important,*
> *they know what they are* not....
> *The trick is to go deep enough*
> *to mine the core of your*
> *authenticity.*
>
> Sarah Ban Breathnach,
> *Simple Abundance*

To go deep enough to mine the core of your authenticity sounds challenging and rather mysterious. Yet, it actually holds the answer to the next step of your fitness journey—to ultimately know yourself and

to make the best choices consistently and enthusiastically for a lifetime.

## Stepping In— A Little Deeper

To intimately know yourself requires having the courage to ask crucial questions at the right moment and then staying open to receiving the answers or suggestions that surface from deep within. These answers or suggestions can provide you with a specific plan regarding how to proceed with future changes.

To go forward, we first must step back and reflect for a moment. You are familiar with the opposite of owning your problems—having others provide all of the answers/ solutions/suggestions for you, telling you what to do, when, where, why, and how.

External coaching, or *role modeling*, is the usual way by which instructors advise students to begin the educational process toward self-knowledge, self-improvement, and positive change. This state of others being responsible for your change must cease at some point along your fitness journey, to enable you to take the next step forward. The main ingredient in this key move is called *problem ownership*. When you decide to take this step, you'll find that it occurs internally and involves "teaming up" in accepting responsibility for your life and relaxing. It is initiated by becoming quiet, followed by internally listening to (or seeing, feeling) a problem you are experiencing, and allowing that experience to come up into your consciousness. Then, asking yourself the direct and difficult questions that have to be asked. And, finally, patiently waiting for a response, in a deeply relaxed state. (This "state" can be achieved more readily if you first imagine someone stroking your head or back, in time with your breathing, stroking *downward* with each exhale.)

What happens when you stop and in a contemplative way take the time to be open to new approaches

or solutions to a problem? *They come to you!* Your self-knowledge or self-wisdom is finally given the space and opportunity to surface, to be considered, to be looked at, heard, and felt! Answers will begin to come so fast and furious that you'll wonder why you've never before allowed yourself the time to experience this incredible gift of insight that is located deep within you! It just takes time and patience to dig deep enough to mine these resources, and an openness, then, to consider what you find ("Aha! That's it!") Most of the time we choose to run in life's fast lanes and not make quiet time to slow down long enough to reflect.

> *The key is stillness and patience to remain open, allowing the answers enough time to surface. You'll discover that your mind, body, and spirit "connection" is made here, at this level of your being.*

Your creative potential to solve problems and find answers to all of your total fitness program concerns is unlimited. Believe this and you will begin to experience it. Doubt these abilities and you'll find yourself back in a "blaming" mindset forever, never really taking charge of your life or achieving what you set out to accomplish. *Something* or *somebody* will invariably stop you, paralyzing your responses. Why let this happen?

## The Necessary Preparation

The relaxation techniques that follow are meant to provide you with mental tools or means to obtaining the answers that lie deep within you, waiting to surface. Four factors to keep in mind are:

1. *Time of day*. Consider using one or all of the techniques especially during these situations:
   - directly following physical exercise workouts to recover, refresh, and restore both your mental and physical energies (5–15 minutes)

- at the beginning of the day establishing a focused plan for using your time and energies
- at mid-day, as a "mini-vacation breakaway" from the pressures you're experiencing that day
- before a major performance, interview, presentation, or test
- at the close of the day before you go to sleep

2. *Conducive environment.* Explore finding a quiet location that has relaxing sounds from nature, or soft, slow-tempo instrumental music, and lighting that is dimmed, darkened, or candlelit.

3. *Body position.* Choose your positioning according to whatever your situation will permit (sitting comfortably or lying down).

4. *Open mind.* After emptying your mind of distracting entries and of past or future thoughts or tasks, focus on the present moment and experience images and sounds conducive to your short or lengthy relaxation needs.

## Guided Imagery

The guided imagery techniques that follow can evoke a sensation of total relaxation in 3 minutes (or less) if you speak the words in a soft, monotone voice using a low pitch and slow tempo. Have someone cue you by reading the steps slowly, or record them slowly onto a cassette tape and then play them to relax. They are meant to be used one at a time according to your needs, and each can take just a few minutes to complete.

Guided imagery techniques such as these have a cumulative effect. The more techniques you use together at one session, the more deeply relaxed you'll become during that time. If you simply need to lower your pulse rate—to slow your breathing and excessive sweating mechanisms after an intense work-out session before dashing off to another class—you or your instructor can use just one of the techniques for 3 to 5 minutes.

Follow any technique by immediately asking yourself a question regarding a fitness concern for which you need suggestions or answers. The question you ask when you are in the relaxed state is preceded by: How? Where? What? or When? (Forget asking "Why" questions!) Here are a few examples:

- *How* can I stay motivated to exercise regularly after this course ends?
- *Where* can I find nutritional snacks to eat mid-day between classes?
- *What* do I need to change in my lifestyle to drop excessive body fat?
- *When* is the best time for me to practice daily relaxation?

When you have more time available to practice relaxation techniques (for instance, at bedtime), use several of the techniques together, back-to-back. Then, when you are in a deeply relaxed state, specifically ask yourself a question that greatly concerns you. If you become still and your mind remains open, a multitude of great ideas will come forth for you to consider. The best ideas closely resemble a "time-honored recipe": they contain key *ingredients,* in defined measurable *amounts,* and are used in a *prescribed order* for consistently good results to occur.

Enjoy these classic guided imagery techniques. Then use your creativity to develop more of your own powerful images such as "taking a trip" to your favorite vacation spot, talking with the heroes and role models in your life, or other rich resources in your head. For your convenience, Exercise 12.2, "Creating Your Own Guided Imagery," at the conclusion of this chapter, presents seven easy steps for creating personalized scenes, seasons, and scenarios.

When you've completed this exercise, tape-record your guided imagery and use it for relaxation, whenever you need it. Add to your relaxation tape any of the following

guided imagery techniques that you believe can enhance your personal relaxation time.

---

*Ease the pounding of your heart by the quieting of your mind.*

---

## Total Body Scanning

Total body scanning will develop your life management skills through your imagination. Your mind seeks out and recognizes tension and eliminates it through your ability to imagine the relaxation. It requires no physical exertion or planned tensing of muscle groups. Total body scanning has four steps: (a) assuming the relaxation position, (b) establishing the breathing pattern and clearing your mental screen, (c) tuning in to various parts of the body, and (d) monitoring your heart rate, followed by simple static stretching to make you alert again (unless you use the technique prior to going to sleep).

### Step One: Assume the Relaxation Position.

1. Lie on your back (see Figure 12.3a). If you feel uncomfortable because your entire back is not in contact with the floor, raise one knee up with your foot flat on the floor approximately 1 foot from your buttocks (Figure 12.3b). Individuals with substantial buttocks or shoulder mass will find that this knee-up position will relieve the arched lower-back feeling.

2. Turn your head slightly to one side. When you become totally relaxed, your tongue will relax backward and cover your windpipe if you keep your head straight in line with the rest of you.

3. Place your arms on the floor at your sides, palms down, with

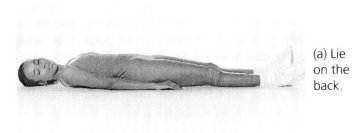

(a) Lie on the back.

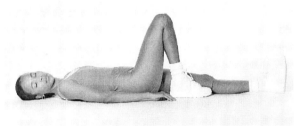

(b) Raise one knee if desired.

**Figure 12.3** Relaxation Positions

elbows slightly bent. Flexed joints are more relaxed in this position.

4. Place your legs apart (not crossed or in contact with one another). As the legs relax, your feet will tend to roll outward.

5. If you relax best with your eyes closed, close them. If you relax best with your eyes open, keep them open and focus continuously on one object above you.

### Step Two: Establish a Deep Breathing Pattern.

1. Take a deep breath and hold it in your lungs. Focus on the stretched-tight feeling you get in your chest by holding in the oxygen.

2. Now, slowly and purposefully breathe out through puckered lips in a long, steady exhale. Create an image in your mind to lengthen the exhale. For example, see yourself slowly blowing the fuzzy seeds off a dandelion that has gone to seed. Or blow a long, steady, calming note on a flute.

3. Repeat this inhale, holding it, and follow with another long, slow, steady, calming exhale. During this inhalation and exhalation, recognize that these next few minutes belong only to you. Do

not share them with anybody or anything. Whatever problems, worries, or cares you have, including whatever you are going to do next in your day, briefly think what they are and list them all, writing them on a mental chalkboard in your mind.

4. Then, again mentally, take out a big chalk eraser and wipe off each problem, one at a time, so you are looking at a blank chalkboard in your mind. Verbalize a thought to yourself ("This is my time now, and you [problem] are just going to have to wait"). Then forget it during your relaxation technique by focusing on the next thought given here.

5. Follow your breathing cycle, whether it is fast, slow, regular, or irregular. Mentally tune in and follow each inhale and each exhale. Picture yourself on an elevator on which each exhale is a ride down one more floor (each inhale is the brief pause for the floor stop, door opening and closing). Or imagine that your mind is on a slow roller coaster ride of up and down, up and down.

6. Don't interfere with your inhalation and exhalation. As you begin to relax, the exhalation

(breathing out) becomes longer and longer. Ride with it, and experience the longer ride out. This focusing on your breathing begins the relaxation process.

7. At various times during the entire body scanning relaxation technique, you will want to tune back in mentally to your breathing technique, since mastering this process requires slowing down, and this is the central focus of your relaxation to this point.

### Step Three: Tuning In.

1. Start at the top of your head, travel down to the tips of your toes, and return to your mid-section.

2. On the top of your head, mentally feel the "part" of your hair. Make it wide by relaxing your scalp.

3. Try to remember the mirror you look into each morning when you wash your face, brush your teeth, put on makeup, or shave your face. Look closely at your forehead. Is it tense and full of wrinkles? Make it flat and wide with no wrinkles. Feel the temperature of your forehead as cool, and picture it shiny and smooth.

4. Mentally envision your ears, and drop all tension to your ears. If you are wearing earrings, mentally feel them as heavy on your earlobes.

5. What is the space between your eyebrows doing? Is it grooved and full of wrinkles? Relax. Make a wide space between your eyebrows. This is one of *the* telltale locations of human stress. A person who is highly stressed seems to permanently tense the space between the eyebrows (contracted, wrinkled). Calm, serene people stand out because this small space is wide, relaxed, and untensed.

6. Relax your eyebrows as if heavy weights were pulling down the ends. This also will relax your temple area.

7. To this point, feel a *cool* temperature around the forehead

and top of the skull (keep a "cool head").

8. From now on, feel a temperature of *warmth* and a *lengthening* or a *widening* of all muscles, joints, and internal organs.

9. Relax the mandible joint (a hinge joint near your ear opening that regulates your lower jaw) by dropping your lower jaw. It will make your lips part. Relax your chin and lips. Top-notch musicians who play wind instruments know that the best sounds can be made when the jaw and lips are relaxed enough to allow sounds to f-l-o-w.

10. When you relax your jaw, mentally feel your tongue and teeth. When some people try to practice total relaxation, they press their tongue tightly to the roof of their mouth. Relax your tongue. Also, some people grind their teeth during the night—an audible sign of too much tension in the mandible joint (TMJ).

11. Relax your throat by thinking of the feeling you get with the second stage of swallowing (first a gulp and then a "wide" feeling). Performing artists who sing have been trained in this widening technique, to allow the best sounds to come from a relaxed vocal mechanism.

12. Drop your shoulders and chest to make a wide space between your ears and shoulders. We unconsciously tense this area throughout the day. Whether we are driving a car or walking in miserable weather, we tense the shoulders near our ears, encouraging neck aches and headaches. When you think about it next time, untense these muscles by cueing yourself, "Long, w-i-d-e, and warm."

13. Allow the weight of your chest to sink through to the floor. Think "heavy chest."

14. Drop all tension from your upper arms, elbows, lower arms, and hands until you can just feel your fingertips pulsating on the floor. You may feel a tingling in your fingertips.

15. Relax your buttocks. (This is what must occur when you go to the bathroom and sit. The feeling is one of wide and warm.) This is also a key to untensing the lower half of your body.

16. Relax your kneecaps. This joint connects your upper and lower leg, and many times we tense the knee area when we attempt to relax other body parts. When you relax the knees, the upper legs will relax and the heavy weight of your legs will begin to drop to the floor. Likewise, the lower legs respond almost automatically, with the feet rolling outward. Now, as you relax your knees, make a positive statement to yourself such as, "I am confident and *open* to new ideas."

17. Mentally feel what your toes are doing. Are they tensed and curled under? If so, stretch them out and then relax your toes.

What has been relaxed so far is rather easy because if you open your eyes, you can *see* each part. What comes next is more difficult because you must truly envision the internal location and then relax each part completely, totally through the power of your imagination.

18. Return to your central torso— the heart, stomach and intestinal areas—the most difficult place to relax.

19. Picture your heart beating— lub-dub-lub-dub. As you make it wider and warmer, it begins to beat s-l-o-w-e-r. Persons well trained in relaxation skills can do this. As an observer, you can experience this by first feeling their pulse, and then using a timepiece, count their pulse beating, and watch as it beats slower and slower, as they envision their heart becoming wider, warmer, and more relaxed.

20. Envision where your stomach is located. If you picture this "food tank" comfortably wide and warm, it *will* receive food and liquid. It is only when we're nervous and squeeze it tight to look like a dried raisin or prune, that we're too upset and can't eat or drink. So, relax your stomach and receive the life-giving food and liquid. Then realize when you've had enough nourishment. The stomach feels comfortable, light and yet full.

21. Focus your mind on the navel area and picture a wide, flat, picturesque pond. Envision a small pebble being tossed into the very center, creating a soft, rippling effect in which each ripple is a wave of relaxation. Feel the weight of your navel area sinking through, past your spine, onto the floor below you. Envision your intestinal area wide and warm, allowing all the absorption and elimination processes to complete their cycles and run smoothly.

22. Return to your breathing cycle, and follow it several times. Focus totally on the long, slow exhale.

23. Now rest awhile and enjoy the totally untensed feeling you are experiencing.

24. After a few moments *in this relaxed state*, ask yourself a question regarding a fitness program concern you have. Remain open, patiently waiting, and suggestions will surface for you to consider.

## Step Four: Monitor Your Heart Rate and Stretch.

1. In the lying-down position, feel for your pulse. Again, mentally picture and feel your heart beating, and again try to slow it down with your mind by cueing it to beat slower.

2. Take a deep breath and as you slowly exhale, count your pulse for 15 seconds and multiply by 4

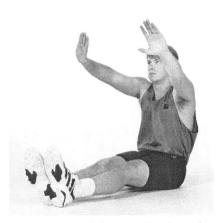

**Figure 12.4** Sitting Up Slowly and Stretching

for a full-minute heart rate count. How does this compare with your resting heart rate after 6–8 hours of sleep? Three minutes of relaxation does wonders for your body's recovery from exercise or daily stress.

3. Before you get up, sit up slowly and stretch your arms, legs, chest and back so you become rather alert. (Figure 12.4). You must do this 15-second stretch or you'll find yourself yawning for an hour afterward! Of course, if you do this relaxation procedure before going to bed, omit the stretch, stay in the present moment, and just let go.

4. When you are finished with the relaxation, write down the ideas or solutions that came to mind. Try to set at least one goal, starting today, using the Goal-Setting Challenge at the end of the chapter.

## Control Panel with One Large Dial

The Control Panel with One Large Dial (Figure 12.5) is used for rating or quantifying levels of tension and relaxation you feel within your body. First give a concrete label to each number on the control panel, from 0 to 10, as to what that level of relaxation/tension represents to you. Maybe "0" represents totally relaxed inner peace or lying on a warm beach, "5" represents balance and peak performance, and "10" means totally out of control, such as experiencing a death, divorce, or a debilitating disease. Write entries for what each number represents to *you*. Also assign a number to *today's* best and worst moments. Now that you have the idea of *quantifying stress*, visualize this second guided imagery technique.

1. Visualize yourself in a safe place that represents relaxation to you, possibly your bedroom. Envision yourself there, seated in front of a control panel that has one large dial.[7] Continue to hold onto that image in your mind's eye for the duration of the technique, and soon you will feel as if you were actually there.

2. Turn the dial to any setting from 0–10, which represents all the levels of relaxation and tension

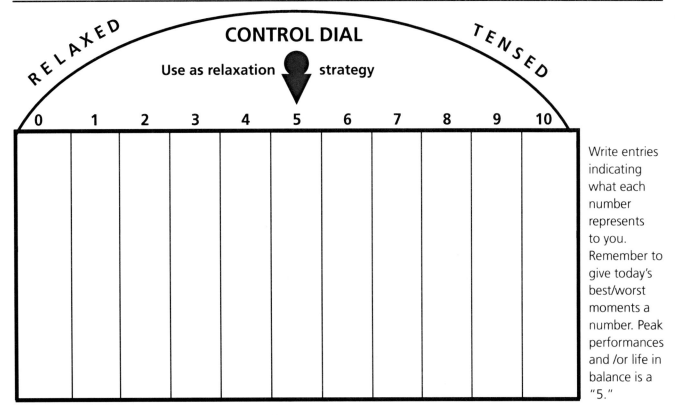

**Figure 12.5** Control Panel with One Large Dial

you are able to experience. Zero represents all of the relaxation that's possible for you to feel, and 10 represents as much tension as you are able to feel at one time.

3. Begin to look closely at this dial that directly monitors and controls the level of tension in your body. What is the reading on the dial at this moment (from 0–10)? Think for a long moment, then give it a number.

4. See yourself reaching over to turn down the dial. See yourself turning that dial down, v-e-r-y s-l-o-w-l-y, a little bit at a time. Feel your body relaxing more and more as you turn it down.

5. Feel the tension in your body lessening more and more as you turn the dial all the way down. As all of the tension in your body ebbs away, turn the dial all the way down to zero. Your entire body is as relaxed as it possibly can be. All of your previous tension is replaced with peaceful feelings of total relaxation and a centered calm. Currents of gentle tranquility soothe every muscle, every nerve, and every fiber of your being.

6. *In this relaxed state*, ask yourself a question regarding a fitness program concern you have. Remain open, patiently waiting, and suggestions will surface for you to consider. Stay there and consider each suggestion, weighing the "pros" and "cons."

7. Return now to the moment in your day and the location where you were at the beginning of this relaxation session. Open your eyes, continue to rest a moment, enjoying a fresh new beginning.

From now on, relax just like this, whenever you choose, by sitting or lying down, closing your eyes for a few moments, and visualizing yourself turning down the dial on this control panel. The more you

practice this new ability, the more easily and the more deeply you'll be able to relax and the longer these feelings of relaxation will remain with you.

You'll be able to sleep better at night, awaken more refreshed, work more efficiently without being bothered by people or situations during the day, feel rejuvenated to perform your very best when you need to, and enjoy your leisure-time activities to the fullest. Your unlimited potential awaits you in every aspect of your life. Whether it be rest, work, or leisure, every facet of your life will be improved and enriched considerably by your new ability to relax whenever you choose.

## Colorful Imaging

We all seem to be in search of the mind-body-spirit connection when it comes to our total fitness or wellness programs. Taking a ride through the following imaginary rainbow[8] is one method for you to make that connection. It allows you to *stretch* your creative imagination, opening up new pathways to explore when problem solving.

Now with your eyes closed, take one deep, "cleansing" breath. As you do, begin to erase the visual screen of your mind, similar to using a big eraser to remove entries on a chalk-board. Next picture yourself standing beside a sturdy and colorful hot air balloon, secured and resting on the ground in a favorite location that reminds you of total peace and relaxation.

Using a step bench, step over the side of the balloon's basket. Standing inside, take in a long, deep breath, and hold it momentarily before breathing out very slowly. Believe now that you are in for the most exhilarating and yet most relaxing ride of a lifetime.

You're watching as the hot air balloon's grounding devices are removed, and as they are, you ascend, slowly, ever so slowly,

upward. You're above your favorite area now, looking down from above, seeing it become smaller and smaller—like seeing a miniature version of it made to scale. The temperature is just right, and the breeze of the ascent softly blows across your face and scalp, and through your hair.

Because you are using the power of your imagination, things that usually are not possible are possible now. Carefully stepping out of your balloon, you now realize that, just as in your dreams, you have the ability to be suspended in air—moving about as you choose. You find yourself gently floating high above the ground now, drifting and dreaming and floating through patches of fleecy white clouds.

A sudden but refreshing shower has just passed. You breathe in the closest cloud's soft white color, filling your lungs and purifying them as you slowly inhale. Hold that image and breathe for several moments.

As you repeat this image of breathing in pure white color, begin to remove any darkness or sadness or grief that's been stored within. Fully appreciate the life-giving and energizing pure white air exchanged there.

Feel yourself moving on now, drifting slowly and gently, on and on, until you come to an indescribably beautiful rainbow. Shimmering brightly before you, you are drawn to the rainbow's brilliant colors of hearty red, creamy peach, golden yellow, cool mint green, aqua blue, and dusky violet. Begin to think how exhilarating and yet refreshing it is going to be to slowly drift on through the rainbow, experiencing each color one by one. You are ready to do just that, beginning with the outer band of hearty red.

Stepping in, you feel the band of red beginning to enter the soles of your feet, carrying with it a warm glow of energy, strength, and power. It spreads up quickly through your calves, and on up through the rest of your torso, bathing and massaging every muscle fiber and nerve with its warm, rosy glow of energy, strength, and power. Breathe deeply and slowly as you continue through the band of red, inhaling the warm energizing color, and stopping then to store it in every portion of your heart, along with the feelings of unconditional love and joy that it's carrying. Let yourself reexperience this image fully and completely, again and again, breathing in the hearty red color, saturating yourself with its warmth, retaining all of the feelings you have stored.

Now, as you continue slowly drifting deeper into the rainbow, the band of creamy peach appears. It begins to penetrate the soles of your feet and spreads itself throughout your body in the same way as the others did, bringing with it a calming sensation of complete and perfect peace. As you exhale, silently say to yourself the name of your role model for peace, very slowly. As this peacefulness progresses throughout your body with each breath, it blends with the pure thoughts, and the loving and joyful energy you already feel, and have stored inside, making you serenely more aware of everything you experience. You are calm, focused, and at peace.

Next the golden yellow band of the rainbow comes into view and begins to spread itself throughout your entire being as you breathe it in, filling and flooding you with its marvelous, smiling, golden glow. It brings to your consciousness an ever-increasing sense of happiness, well-being, and a new sense of *openness* that you've never before experienced. Flow with it and breathe it in as you allow yourself to merge completely with these rays of radiant openness . . . blending with them so completely that you now begin to automatically radiate back an openness of your own.

All worries and feelings of being stuck are gone. Openness to new ideas and possibilities has filled your mind, body, and spirit. Take a long pause to appreciate how open you are feeling at this very moment.

With great anticipation to continue on this wonderful journey through your rainbow, you observe that the green band is coming up next. You are entering the green band now, and beginning to experience a gentle tidal wave of kindness, giving first a large portion of needed kindness *to yourself,* and then, an abundance to others. This outpouring of growing kindness carries you even higher as you feel yourself giving kindness to others and also receiving kindness from others. All anger and resentment in your life has completely dissipated and has been replaced by wonder, and delight. Breathe in this cool green, and blend with it.

Savor and retain each of the emotions now being added to all of the other feelings you have gathered. Because this green band feels *so* refreshing, you are enjoying repeating the breathing and accompanying imaging several more times before moving on.

Approaching the rainbow's interior, the blue band is now in your sight. You are slowly drawn into the aqua blue color band and are storing it within. Storing this color causes you to feel as free and as fluid as the wind blowing above the aqua waters. In your imagination, feel yourself now blending with all of the wind and water everywhere in the world, gently rushing over the surface of the earth, and as you do, exhaling with a silent sound like a wind blowing. Continue on by moving gently over rocks and soft river beds, then gently cascading down cliffs, forming waterfalls, in a headlong but gentle rush to the sea. All of your fears and anxieties flow out of you completely and into the sea, where they are *swept* away. *You remain* and are again drawn up, windswept, to the sky above and back to the rainbow and to the blue band once more. You are ready to enter the next band of color. You retain the sensation of freedom that now has become

blended with all of the others throughout your being.

Finally, you enter the violet band on the inner side of the rainbow. Its soothing color fills your entire body silently as nightfall, extending your previous feelings of freedom to an almost infinite degree. You now feel strong enough to step away from all of your everyday thoughts and all of your customary roles. In this infinite violet stillness, you have discovered the location of your authenticity . . . the location of your soul. Slowly drifting to a stop within the violet band, you become filled with the stillness and peace of a comfortably warm, comfortably cool, summer night. You can feel within your own being the relaxing, tranquil color of the violet sky, long after the sun has slipped down behind the horizon.

It is here, while you remain within this violet band of color for what seems like an endless time, that you find the courage to ask your authentic self-questions concerning your life . . . and wait patiently for the suggestions to surface. You now openly receive suggestions from that infinite power source within you that guides you onto new paths of awareness and self-wisdom. You find that these new paths are richer and more rewarding than any of those you have ever known because they are answers that have been provided by an empowering source beyond your reasoning. Many names have been given to this deep well within each of us. What is your name for the infinite power source that fuels you within? If you haven't thought about this, stay with it now and consider it.

You have discovered the location of your personal mind-body-spirit connection and the location of your unlimited potential, where answers and solutions reside. What images have you seen, what questions have you heard yourself ask, and what sensations have you felt? The good news is that you can keep this location in your mind as long as you choose. No one can penetrate this intimate space. When you have finished posing questions and allowing answers to surface, create a "return trip" to the location from which you started. It then can be revisited at will, whenever you choose. It just takes a few moments to mentally walk over to your hot air balloon, step inside, and begin your exhilarating and peaceful ride.

## Summary—Making the Connection

Finding answers to continual life challenges can be enjoyable and relaxing. It requires that you take a quiet moment, find a conducive environment, get into a comfortable position, and be open to suggestions. These suggestions can come first in the form of guided imagery, used to induce a deeply relaxed state, and then, as answers that surface from deep within to the questions that you have posed while in the relaxed state. Openness to suggestions from within is the key to making the connection between life challenges and viable solutions.

---

### Goal-Setting Challenge

 Many novices to aerobic fitness and strength training programming omit the vital cooling-down and relaxation segment (presented in Chapter 11) from their program because they do not understand its physical and mental training importance. Be proactive regarding the conclusion of each fitness session by giving yourself a calm transition back into your busy, daily schedule. Write one Cool-Down, Yoga Positions and Flexibility Training Goal for Chapter 11, following the four steps presented in Chapter 2, Exercise 2.3, then recording it in your Fitness Journal. Include in the goal script a 5- to 20-minute time segment to conclude your aerobic fitness and strength training program, progressively slowing down your moves, transitioning to yoga positions, stretching, finishing with sitting or reclining and imaging your relaxation techniques.

 Set a goal regarding how to improve and manage your one response to stress that seems most disabling to you, the positive outlets you now choose to use, or set aside regular time to practice specific relaxation techniques. These are goals you'll enjoy setting and also experiencing, because of how helpful they can be for the rest of your fitness program. Write one of these goals as the Stress Management/Relaxation Goal for Chapter 12 following the four steps presented in Chapter 2, Exercise 2.3, then recording it in your Fitness Journal.

## Exercise 12.1  My Top "10" List: The Most Stressful Areas of Life

Have you ever wondered what areas of life and problem-solving are causing you the most stress? Experience tells us that our major stress management concerns can be grouped into the following ten areas.[9]

**Directions:** Take a moment to read through the entire list. Then choose, by placing in rank order (1–10), the most problematical areas you experience that stand in the way of your life management. Rank "1" as the most important to you (most stressful) and "10" the least important to you at this point in your life.

_____ *Taking ownership* of your internal resources to enable you to become the person you choose to be, vibrantly alive and free from both blaming others and the manipulation and control of other people.

_____ Understanding that what triggers your responses ultimately are your beliefs and attitudes, which directly reflect what you are picturing, hearing, and feeling inside, and that those can each be changed at will to improve your *motivation.*

_____ Knowing how to establish your *time* priorities; understand your moving toward pleasure values and your moving away from pain values; set short/intermediate/long-term goals; and manage your time using short cuts and principles that your role models use.

_____ Understanding your *beliefs*—the rules by which you live—and having the courage of your convictions to follow through and live by the parameters of behavior you've established and consider acceptable, and to soundly reject those you deem unacceptable.

_____ Labeling your strengths and weaknesses in terms of mental and physical energy (the will) you naturally and instinctively possess, which reflects directly *how you problem solve.*

_____ Openly expressing your wants, needs, thoughts, and feelings so you can consistently do your best, using intentionally inviting, assertive, and confrontational *communication skills.*

_____ Using your natural and trainable talents and gifts, the principles behind *peak performance,* and techniques of relaxed concentration and relaxation to manage stress and fully enhance your performance.

_____ Applying proper *exercise* principles and techniques to achieve specific goals such as achieving and maintaining aerobic fitness, increasing flexibility, gaining muscle strength and endurance, and developing good body positions for safety and efficiency.

_____ Understanding the principles for eating and drinking a *proper diet* in terms of selection of food/beverage; quantity of servings; caloric values; and the psychological implications, for both the general population and for athletes.

_____ Understanding the principles of *weight management* (gain lean, lose fat, maintenance, and body composition) and how to set goals to achieve your recommended ideal—one which is both safest for you, and one you can psychologically enjoy keeping managed for a lifetime.

My additions: Be specific. What else would you like to know more about that causes you stress?

_____

_____

_____

_____

## Exercise 12.2  Creating Your Own Guided Imagery[10]

**Begin by:**

- Finding a comfortable position in a quiet, dimly lit environment.
- Closing your eyes.
- Focusing on emptying the mental screen of your mind.
- Beginning to breathe slowly and deeply.

**Now:**

1. Imagine various locations (beach/woods/mountains/your home or bedroom), and a season of the year (spring/summer/fall/winter). From these scenes and seasons, choose a place to relax that is uniquely satisfying to you:

2. Consider:
   - What does it smell like?
   - What sounds do you hear?
   - What textures do you feel?
   - What parts of you are moving, and how?
   - What do you see?
   - What are you saying when you talk to yourself?
   - What emotions do you feel in your body?

3. Imagine being in a solitary, "do-nothing" activity such as:
   - Being at the shore, lying on a warm, sandy beach.
   - Being in a bubble bath, soaking by candlelight.
   - Being by a fireplace, sitting in a big, overstuffed chair.
   - Or:

4. Ask a question that currently concerns you regarding your total fitness program. Write a complete sentence, remembering to put it in the form of a question:

                                                                                                    ?

5. Slowly and with great patience, wait for an answer, or solutions, to surface.

6. After your relaxation session concludes, write down the detailed answer or the solutions that came to you:

### Creating Your Own Guided Imagery

Write out your own guided imagery on a separate page. Think it out slowly and completely. Use all five of your sensory modalities (sight, sound, taste, touch/feel, smell) and as many submodalities as possible. (A submodality further describes each of your senses with adjectives or adverbs—clear/loud/fast/sweet/fragrant and so on.) Underline each *sensory modality* used (*see, hear, taste, touch, smell*) and circle the descriptive submodalities used in your guided imagery (golden sky, crashing waves, sweet taste, soft touch, home-cooked smell). The more you use of each, the richer and more relaxing your imagery will be. Then tape record for personal use.

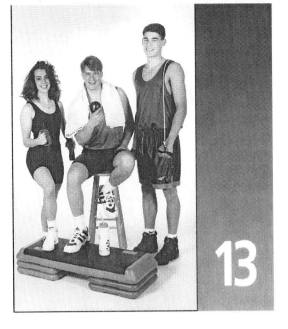

# *Nutrition*

*Choose what is best; habit will
soon render it agreeable and easy.*

—Pythagoras

This ancient principle for making choices hasn't really changed today. Better or best choices are available for you to make. The actions you take reflect whether you simply *have* the knowledge or whether you *apply* the knowledge. Enjoy making the best available choices, all day long.

## *Nutrients for Going and Growing*

Your body needs two basic types of nutrients:

1. Foods that satisfy your energy needs
2. Foods that meet your needs for growth, repair, and regulation of body processes

*Nutrients* are chemical substances that your body absorbs from food during digestion. Your body needs at least 40 nutrients. *Essential nutrients* are those your body cannot make or is unable to make in adequate amounts. You must obtain these nutrients from what you eat and drink. If your diet does not provide them adequately, your body cannot perform well, mentally or physically.

This is where choice comes in. You may know what the better choices of foods are (called *nutrient-dense* foods[1]), but if you don't eat the best choices available to you,

you aren't practicing good nutrition. Good health, optimum fitness, and good nutrition result from not just knowing what is best but actually choosing it 80 to 90% of the time.[2]

*Diet* here means *total intake of food and drink*. A well-balanced diet is one that contains these six basic nutrients:

1. Carbohydrates
2. Fats
3. Proteins
4. Vitamins
5. Minerals
6. Water

## *Dietary Plans*

Proper amounts of each nutrient have been established according to several variables. You cannot always take in all of the essential nutrients every 24 hours. What *is* important is that over a span of several days and weeks, you continually select from all of the food groups to meet your nutrient needs.

The food system that follows is not a rigid prescription but, rather, a general motivational and educational *guide* that lets you choose a healthful diet that's right for you. It calls for eating a variety of foods and beverages to get the nutrients you need and, at the same time, the proper number of calories to maintain a healthy weight.

Each of these food groups provides some, but not all, of the nutrients you need. Foods in one food group can't replace those in another. No one food group is more important than another. For good health, you need them all! A Fluid Replacement Pyramid [3,4] Figure 13.4, guides your planning for continual hydration.

## *A Personalized Dietary Plan*

As part of an ongoing effort to make Americans trimmer and healthier, every 5 years the U.S. Department of Agriculture updates its "Dietary Guidelines for Americans," considered the gold standard of nutrition advice[5] detailing the proper amount of each nutrient to consume.

Because a picture speaks a thousand words, accompanying the guidelines is a visual symbol that serves to market, promote, and give visibility to these dietary guidelines, making them easy to recall. In the recent past, this visual was called the Food Guide Pyramid. It focused on the food groups for all Americans to consume and recommended the servings to eat from those groups ... a "one pyramid guide fits all" concept.

The latest visual is also a pyramid; however, its design and its mission have greatly changed. *The Dietary Guidelines for Americans 2005* and accompanying image,

*"MyPyramid•Steps to a Healthier You"*[6] (Figure 13.1) is a much needed *personalized* approach to designing an eating plan for every American. (See Figure 13.2 for a sample 2000 calorie diet.) Just think! Now we each have our very own personal trainer for nutrition!

The suggested eating plans of what and how much to consume have been established according to three variables: age, sex, and the amount of physical activity a participant engages in daily. It is available to everyone via the Internet at the U.S. Government's web site http://www.MyPyramid.gov . When you access the site and enter your three variables, you are given one of the 12 eating plans to follow.

The following is a list of highlights for using this personalized *MyPyramid* Food System approach to eating.

## *MyPyramid* Highlights

- The *MyPyramid* Food System icon has vertical colored bands to depict six food groups to consume. The colors and associated food groups are:
  - Orange—Grains
  - Green—Vegetables
  - Red—Fruits
  - Blue—Milk
  - Purple—Meat & Beans
  - Yellow—Oils

- The most interesting aspect of the guidelines is the tough new goals set for *calorie intake* and for *daily exercise.*

  **Calorie Intake ~** Since the striped pyramid of colored bands instructs what food groups to eat, but does not offer guidelines on *how much* to eat, for actual advice on portions, you must go through several steps on the interactive *MyPyramid* web site to get your *customized eating plan* according to your age, sex, and physical activity. Your customized eating plan will advise you of the total number of calories to be consumed each day and the amounts to eat from all of the food

groups. Additionally, it provides your allowance for oils (*teaspoons* per day) and solid fats and sugars (*calories* per day). A caveat states, "This calorie level is only an estimate of your needs. Monitor your body weight to see if you need to adjust your calorie intake."

*Note:* To help you understand your body composition (ratio of lean weight you have to the appropriate level of fat weight to carry with it), see Exercise 14.5. It helps you to determine the number of calories you need to consume daily for weight maintenance (staying the same weight). If you then choose to lose fat weight, you will want to eat fewer calories than the weight maintenance number, and add more exercise to your day.

**Daily Exercise ~** *MyPyramid* includes an image of a figure climbing steps to reflect the advice that:

- All Americans should be active for a minimum of 30 minutes a day;

- For children, teenagers, or people trying to control their weight, it's 60 minutes a day;

- To sustain weight loss, up to 90 minutes of daily exercise is recommended.

- For those who don't use the Internet site provided, the government has a poster with pictures of food and serving sizes based on a 2000-calorie diet.

- *MyPyramid*'s visual advocates eating a variety of foods and watching calories, rather than focusing on one food group or another. It doesn't favor any commodity group or food company by showing foods we all should eat less of[7] to maintain good health. It treats all food groups equally [8] by telling you what to eat, and what allowances to consider, for the "Discretionary" category of foods (these are the foods that are high in salt, high in fat, or high in sugar).

- As you access the web site, you'll find these web-linked features particularly helpful:

✔ **MyPyramid Plan~** You'll be given an eating plan based upon the information you have provided, listing your daily recommended amount to consume from each food group.

✔ **Inside the Pyramid~** This link provides information concerning the individual food selections you can make within each food group. General principles, words, and phrases are also defined. (Note: A *Nutrient Density, 4-star* system of rating the best choices of foods in each group according to the most nutrition per calories, is not presented in *MyPyramid*. It is presented in depth, later in this chapter.) Advice on the amount of physical activity one needs is given for the first time since the government began educating on nutrition and eating patterns. Examples of *moderate* and *vigorous* kinds of activity are given.

✔ **Tips and Resources ~** Six general tips are provided, along with specific food tips for each of the food groups. Also present are: • sample menus • how to count mixed dishes when *MyPyramid* is used • tips for eating out, and • vegetarian diets.

✔ **Dietary Guidelines ~** These well-researched and documented guidelines are published every 5 years, the latest being in 2005. They are provided both in brief, and in depth, at the web site, www.mypyramid.gov.

✔ **Professionals ~** There is a section for professionals to access, providing both written and visual materials. The USDA mini poster (PDF) is presented in this *Fitness, Fourth Edition* to introduce the *MyPyramid* Food System.

✔ **Related Links ~** These provide answers to more nutrition questions you may have, and web sites to access.

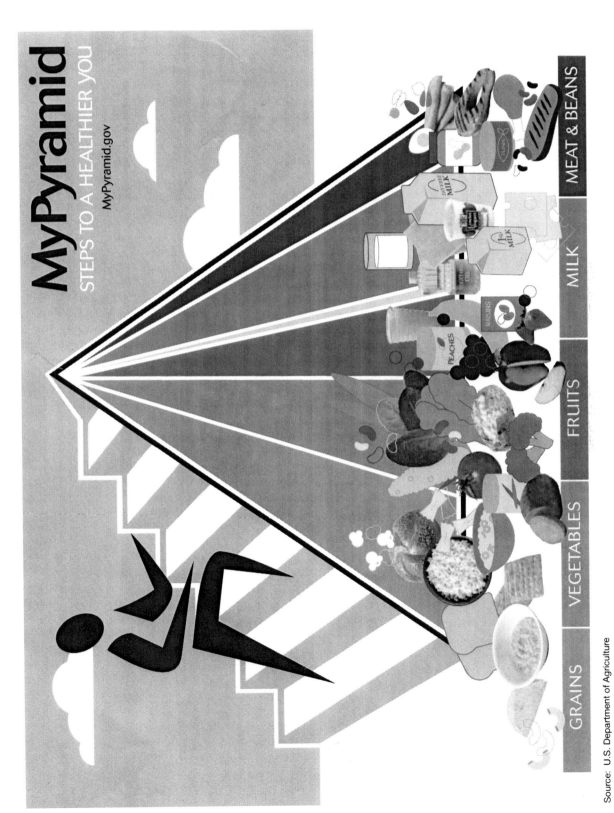

Source:  U.S. Department of Agriculture

**Figure 13.1**  MyPyramid

## GRAINS
### Make half your grains whole

Eat at least 3 oz. of whole-grain cereals, breads, crackers, rice, or pasta every day

1 oz. is about 1 slice of bread, about 1 cup of breakfast cereal, or 1/2 cup of cooked rice, cereal, or pasta

## VEGETABLES
### Vary your veggies

Eat more dark-green veggies like broccoli, spinach, and other dark leafy greens

Eat more orange vegetables like carrots and sweetpotatoes

Eat more dry beans and peas like pinto beans, kidney beans, and lentils

## FRUITS
### Focus on fruits

Eat a variety of fruit

Choose fresh, frozen, canned, or dried fruit

Go easy on fruit juices

## MILK
### Get your calcium-rich foods

Go low-fat or fat-free when you choose milk, yogurt, and other milk products

If you don't or can't consume milk, choose lactose-free products or other calcium sources such as fortified foods and beverages

## MEAT & BEANS
### Go lean with protein

Choose low-fat or lean meats and poultry

Bake it, broil it, or grill it

Vary your protein routine — choose more fish, beans, peas, nuts, and seeds

**For a 2,000-calorie diet, you need the amounts below from each food group. To find the amounts that are right for you, go to MyPyramid.gov.**

| Eat 6 oz. every day | Eat 2 1/2 cups every day | Eat 2 cups every day | Get 3 cups every day; for kids aged 2 to 8, it's 2 | Eat 5 1/2 oz. every day |

### Find your balance between food and physical activity

- Be sure to stay within your daily calorie needs.
- Be physically active for at least 30 minutes most days of the week.
- About 60 minutes a day of physical activity may be needed to prevent weight gain.
- For sustaining weight loss, at least 60 to 90 minutes a day of physical activity may be required.
- Children and teenagers should be physically active for 60 minutes every day, or most days.

### Know the limits on fats, sugars, and salt (sodium)

- Make most of your fat sources from fish, nuts, and vegetable oils.
- Limit solid fats like butter, stick margarine, shortening, and lard, as well as foods that contain these.
- Check the Nutrition Facts label to keep saturated fats, *trans* fats, and sodium low.
- Choose food and beverages low in added sugars. Added sugars contribute calories with few, if any, nutrients.

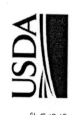

**MyPyramid.gov**
STEPS TO A HEALTHIER YOU

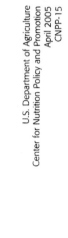

USDA

U.S. Department of Agriculture
Center for Nutrition Policy and Promotion
April 2005
CNPP-15

**Figure 13.2** A Sample 2000 Calorie Diet Plan

✔ **MyPyramidTracker~** This is an online dietary and physical activity assessment tool that provides information regarding your diet quality and physical activity status. The Food Calories/Energy Balance feature automatically calculates your energy balance; energy expenditure (exercise) is subtracted from your energy intake (food intake) to show you the relationship between good nutrition patterns and regular physical activity.

## Nutrient Density

In Tables 13.1 through 13.5, foods are listed according to *nutrient density*, the amount of nutrition per calorie each food provides.[9] Choose foods from the four-star groups (Figure 13.2), as they provide the most nutrition for the fewest calories. The categories are:

4 stars = most nutrition per calorie

3 stars = next-to-most nutrition per calorie

2 stars = next-to-least nutrition per calorie

1 star = least nutrition per calorie

They are also ranked *within* each starred group, and listed in descending order of nutrients per calories.[10]

## Milk Group

"Get your calcium-rich foods." Calcium, riboflavin (Vitamin B2), and protein are the key nutrients needed to build the basic structure and strength of bones and teeth, assist in the production of energy needs, and help in the growth and maintenance of every living cell. If you are not a milk drinker, other foods in the milk group (Table 13.1) will supply the calcium, riboflavin, and protein you need.

## Meat and Beans Group

"Go lean with protein." Key nutrients in this group are iron, protein, niacin, thiamin, zinc, and B12 (Table 13.2).

### Table 13.1 Nutrient-Density Ratings of Milk Group

| Rating: | Food Choices in Ranked Order for Calcium |
|---|---|
| ★ ★ ★ ★ ★ | nonfat plain yogurt, nonfat milk<br>nonfat cream cheese<br>nonfat fruit yogurt<br>low fat milk (1%)<br>buttermilk<br>lowfat cheese<br>reduced-fat milk (2%) |
| ★ ★ ★ ★ | part-skim ricotta cheese<br>whole milk<br>regular fat cheese<br>lowfat chocolate milk (1%)<br>lowfat fruit yogurt<br>nonfat frozen yogurt |
| ★ ★ | pudding<br>custard<br>lowfat frozen yogurt<br>light ice cream |
| ★ | milkshake<br>cottage cheese<br>ice cream<br>nonfat sour cream |

Even though this group is sometimes called simply the "meat group," plant foods, when eaten together, can supply the needed protein, niacin, iron, and thiamin and are considered alternatives to eating meat. (In fact, a separate eating plan for those who choose to eat only alternatives to meat is included under the web-link, *Tips and Resources* of *MyPyramid*.)

Some of the plant food combinations that complement each other (allowing the amino acids to combine to form balanced protein) are dried beans and whole wheat, dried beans and corn or rice, and peanuts and wheat.

One serving is equal to 2 to 3 ounces of cooked lean meat, fish, or poultry, or the protein equivalent.

### Table 13.2 Nutrient-Density Ratings of Meat and Beans Group

| Rating: | Food Choices in Ranked Order for Iron and Protein |
|---|---|
| ★ ★ ★ ★ | fish, shellfish<br>poultry (light meat, skinless)<br>turkey ham<br>beef (round and sirloin)<br>pork (tenderloin)<br>veal (leg and shoulder)<br>lentils |
| ★ ★ ★ | beef (rib, chuck, flank and ground)<br>ham (lean)<br>tofu<br>veal and lamb (leg and loin)<br>poultry (dark meat with skin)<br>pork (loin chop, and rib)<br>Canadian bacon<br>poultry sausage<br>dried beans and peas<br>eggs |
| ★ ★ | hot dogs<br>pork sausage<br>chicken nuggets<br>fish sticks<br>nuts and seeds |
| ★ | peanut butter<br>bologna |

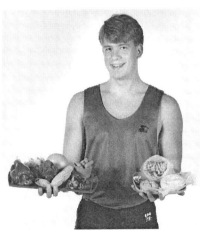

**Figure 13.3** Nutrient-Dense Foods versus Calorie-Dense Foods

## Table 13.3 Nutrient-Density Ratings for Vegetables Group

| Rating: | Food Choices in Ranked Order for Folic Acid and Vitamins A and C* |
|---|---|
| ★ | red and green bell peppers |
| ★ | mustard greens |
| ★ | bok choy |
| ★ | spinach |
| | leaf lettuce |
| | broccoli |
| | carrots |
| | cauliflower |
| ★ | cabbage |
| ★ | chard |
| ★ | asparagus |
| ★ | kale |
| | vegetable juice |
| | Brussels sprouts |
| | salsa |
| | iceberg lettuce |
| | sweet potato |
| | tomato |
| | snow peas |
| | zucchini |
| | okra |
| | winter squash |
| | green beans |
| ★ | beets |
| ★ | cucumber |
| | celery |
| | jicama |
| | artichoke |
| | peas |
| | mushrooms |
| ★ | eggplant |
| | corn |
| | avocado |
| | potato |

*Based on 100-calorie portions

## Table 13.4 Nutrient-Density Ratings for Fruits Group

| Rating: | Food Choices in Ranked Order for Folic Acid, Vitamins A and C |
|---|---|
| ★ | papaya |
| ★ | strawberries |
| ★ | kiwi |
| ★ | orange, grapefruit |
| ★ | orange juice |
| | cantaloupe |
| | mandarin oranges |
| | mango |
| ★ | honeydew |
| ★ | raspberries |
| ★ | apricots |
| ★ | rhubarb |
| | pineapple |
| | watermelon |
| | pineapple juice |
| | blueberries |
| ★ | peach |
| ★ | banana |
| | plum |
| | cherries |
| | frozen fruit |
| | juice bar |
| | canned fruit |
| ★ | pear |
| | apple |
| | dried fruit |
| | grapes |
| | raisins |

## Table 13.5 Nutrient-Density Ratings for Grains Group

| Rating: | Food Choices in Ranked Order for Fiber and Complex Carbohydrate |
|---|---|
| ★ | barley |
| ★ | bulgur |
| ★ | bran or whole-grain cereals |
| ★ | popcorn (air-popped or lite microwave) |
| | whole-grain breads |
| | oatmeal |
| | whole-grain pasta |
| | corn or whole-wheat tortilla |
| ★ | brown rice |
| ★ | bran muffin |
| ★ | whole-grain crackers |
| ★ | soft pretzel |
| | English muffin |
| | enriched pasta |
| | popcorn (oil-popped) |
| ★ | flour tortilla |
| ★ | bagel |
| | enriched breads, |
| | enriched rice |
| | pancakes |
| | waffles |
| | graham crackers |
| | saltines |
| | sweetened cereal |
| | dry pretzels |
| ★ | cornbread |
| | fruit or nut bread |
| | biscuit |
| | stuffing |
| | croissant |

Visually, a 2- to 3-ounce portion fills the palm of an average hand and is the width of the little finger. All excess fat should be removed from any meat you eat. You should remove the skin from poultry and eat only the meat, eliminating unnecessary calories.

## Vegetables Group

"Vary your veggies." Key nutrients derived from the Vegetables group are folic acid, Vitamins A and C—which are catalysts or action starters—and fiber (Table 13.3). Their most important functions are:

- forming and maintaining skin and body linings

- cementing substances to promote strength in cells and hastening healing of injuries

- functioning in all visual processes

- aiding in the use of iron

**Sources of Vitamin A** Remembering two simple colors—orange and green—will remind you that foods of these colors provide Vitamin A. You should eat dark green, leafy, and orange vegetables (such as carrots, sweet potatoes, and greens) regularly. Because Vitamin A is stored in the fat tissue of the body, an overdose through supplementation in pill form can be harmful and even fatal. (The same is true for the other fat-soluble vitamins—D, E, and K.)

**Sources of Vitamin C** Daily servings of vegetables such as broccoli, bell peppers, and spinach are recommended for supplying the needed catalyst Vitamin C. Vitamin C is water-soluble, which means that if you take in too much, the excess is excreted through the urine. If you decide to take Vitamin C supplement pills in massive doses, your body will react by increasing the level it needs. If you then stop taking Vitamin C supplements suddenly, your body will react as if it were deficient! Supplementation is costly and unnecessary for well people who eat properly.

## Fruits Group

"Focus on fruits." Key ingredients in the Fruits group are folic acid, Vitamins A and C, and fiber (Table 13.4). Thus, the Fruits group is similar in nutrients to the Vegetables group.

## Grains Group

"Make half your grains whole." Your number-one daily need is energy to perform every function from sleeping to aerobics. Although the Grains group assists with the growth and maintenance of cells and with the elimination process (fiber provides bulk to your waste for easy removal), the major function is to provide energy.

If you do not use this carbohydrate food for the expenditure of energy, for growth and repair, or eliminate it, you wear it as body fat—future energy. It's like constantly carrying around extra gasoline for your car. If you are an active person, such as a varsity or endurance athlete, you will need an abundance of this energy food.

Key nutrients in the Grains group are fiber, complex carbohydrate, thiamin, iron, and niacin (Table 13.5).

## *MyPyramid* Program Flexibility

At each calorie level, individuals who eat nutrient-dense foods may be able to meet their recommended nutrient intake without consuming their full calorie allotment. The remaining calories ~ *the discretionary calorie allowance* ~ allow individuals flexibility to consume some foods and beverages that may contain added fats, added sugars, and alcohol.[11]

## Discretionary Foods

"Know the limits on fats, sugars and salt (sodium)." The foods classified as extras or Discretionary foods provide little or no nutrition and are often high in sugar, salt, fat, and calories. Among them are:

bacon
bouillon
butter
cakes
candy
coffee
condiments
cookies
snack crackers
cream
regular-fat cream cheese
doughnuts
French fries
fruit-flavored drinks
gelatin dessert
gravy
honey
jam
jelly
margarine
mayonnaise
nondairy creamer
olives
onion rings
pickles
pies

potato chips
salad dressings
sauces
seasonings
sherbet
soft drinks
sour cream
sugar
tea
tortilla chips
vegetable oils.[12]

Recommendations to follow when including oils, solid fats, and sugars have been assigned to each of the [12] *MyPyramid* eating plans. For oils, allowances are listed in *teaspoons,* and when adding the limited extras of solid fats and sugars, it is listed in *extra calorie* allowances per day.[13]

## Alternative/Vegetarian Diets

Viable options are available and you can make good choices in every dimension of the lifetime fitness program you're designing for yourself. Your eating plan is no exception. The *MyPyramid* Food System also provides an alternative eating plan you also might choose to consider if you are a vegetarian.[14]

To understand this acceptable alternative to eating, according to the food plans mentioned previously, ask yourself the following three questions. More detailed questions to ask yourself pertaining to each point are provided at the end of this chapter on Exercise 13.1, Considerations for Vegetarian Meal Planning:

1. What group(s) are you choosing to eat in an alternative way (meat and beans group, milk group, meat and beans and milk groups, discretionary fats/oils/sweets) and the reason for each choice?

2. Do you understand the required nutrients (provided in each group) that you have to consider and replace with other forms of alternative food choices (that likewise can provide those required nutrients)?

3. Does this choice of eating plan fulfill your needs regarding the six total wellness dimensions of your life?

Once you've assessed all of your needs regarding this complex topic you can proceed with considering an alternative eating plan.

Some research findings to consider are as follows:

- A high animal-based diet is more likely to lead to heart disease, cancer, high blood pressure, diabetes, stroke, and obesity.[15]
- A plant-based diet is higher in vitamins and fiber and lower in cholesterol and other animal fats that may reduce or even reverse the risk of the aforementioned health risks.[16,17]
- A well-planned vegetarian eating regimen can generally meet all of the nutrient requirements for energy, growth, and repair of tissues.[18,19]
- If strict vegan diets (described in Exercise 13.1) are adopted or if you are in a special-needs group (pregnant, lactating, infant, child, or adolescent), you *must* consult with a registered dietitian or a licensed nutritionist. This certified professional is qualified to answer your questions about alternative food choices and is able to design an alternative eating plan for your own special needs.

A variety of menu-planning approaches can provide vegetarians with adequate nutrition. The text accompanying the *MyPyramid Vegetarian Diets* is useful. In addition, the following guidelines can help vegetarians plan healthful diets.

- Choose a variety of foods, including whole grains, vegetables, fruits, legumes, nuts, seeds and, if desired, dairy products and eggs.
- Vegetarians who choose not to use milk, yogurt, or cheese need to select other food sources rich in calcium. For a list of calcium-rich foods, see Figure 1, 1997 American Dietetics Association Position Paper on Vegetarian Diets.[20]
- Choose whole, unrefined foods often, and minimize your intake of highly sweetened, fatty, and heavily refined foods.
- Choose a variety of fruits and vegetables.
- If you eat animal foods such as dairy products and eggs, choose lower-fat versions of these foods. Limit cheeses and other high-fat dairy foods and eggs in the diet because of their saturated fat content and because their frequent use displaces plant foods in some vegetarian diets.
- If you are a vegan include a regular source of Vitamin B12 in your diet along with a source of Vitamin D if sun exposure is limited.

## Fluid Replacement Pyramid

Water is the best fluid for hydrating the body, especially when exercising for up to 60 to 90 continuous minutes.[21] In general, adults need 1 milliliter of water for every calorie expended. This formula converts into *6–8 cups per day*. To keep your body cool, more is required in warm weather and during exercise (see Figure 13.4a, Fluid Replacement Pyramid).

Some fluid replacement pointers are:[22,23]

- Adequate fluid intake hydrates the body and, in turn, enhances all performance and reduces the possibility of a heat stress illness.
- Fluids should be consumed on a regular basis, not just when you get thirsty. Thirst usually reflects

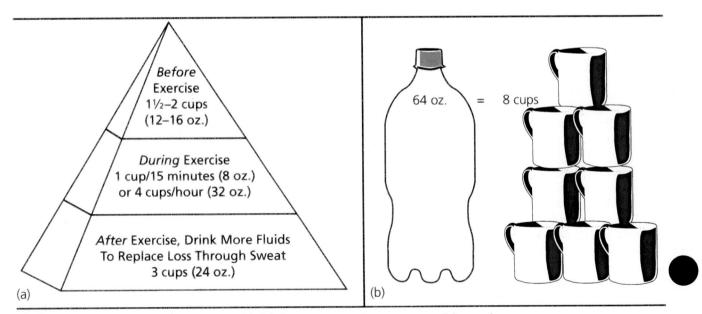

(a)

*Before* Exercise
1½–2 cups (12–16 oz.)

*During* Exercise
1 cup/15 minutes (8 oz.) or 4 cups/hour (32 oz.)

*After* Exercise, Drink More Fluids To Replace Loss Through Sweat
3 cups (24 oz.)

(b)

64 oz. = 8 cups

**Figure 13.4** Fluid Replacement Pyramid: (a) for your exercise program; (b) per day

dehydration and a loss of important fluids and electrolytes.

- When exercising for longer endurance periods (more than 90 continuous minutes), sports drinks may be considered a viable option to assist in replacement of important fluids and electrolytes.

- The visual key to check if you are adequately hydrating yourself is clear, light-colored urine.

As an action plan for fluid replacement:

- Measure 64 oz. (8 cups) of water (Figure 13.4b), and be sure to consume it throughout that day. This can be easily accomplished by refilling a sports squeeze bottle continually with this measured-out amount and taking it with you.

- Drink water as your choice beverage for snacks, breaks, and mealtimes.

- Cooling alternatives: If you'd prefer a hydrating change to water, choose fluids with no caffeine or alcohol and little sugar or sodium. Consider any of these three alternatives:

  — Mix 100% juice with plain or sparkling water.

  — Mix unsweetened, decaffeinated iced tea with orange juice or lemonade.[24]

  — Squeeze a wedge of lemon, lime, or orange into unflavored carbonated water, or add a mint sprig.

## Monitoring Your Food/Beverage Intake

Do you eat *a wide variety of foods in moderation,* as shown in the USDA *MyPyramid* Food System (Figures 13.1 and 13.2), or in the *Pyramid Plus* Starred Nutrient Density Tables 13.1–13.5 ranking the best choices, or in the *MyPyramid* Vegetarian Diets guidelines? After you have accessed your customized eating plan from the *MyPyramid* web site (it'll look similar to Figure 13.2), think about what you

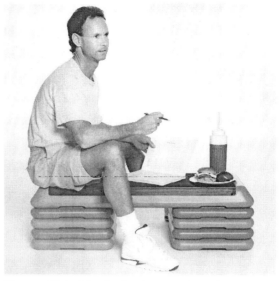

**Figure 13.5** Monitoring Your Eating Plan

have consumed today, and record all of the foods and beverages you ate and drank (Figure 13.5).

Two options are available for you to monitor and record your eating plan:

1. http://www.mypyramidtracker.gov/ This option allows for the long-term tracking of your eating and physical activity.

2. Exercise 13.2, Food and Beverage Intake for 1-3 Days. This option provides a simple method of monitoring and recording for just 1-3 days, using the charts in the textbook (you are encouraged to record longer in your Fitness Journal, especially if you are on a weight loss program). It includes observing one's eating patterns (regarding variety, volume, and nutrient density), and also includes monitoring one's emotional eating patterns, a key to weight management. This second option identifies:

- today's date

- nutrient density starred ratings

- appropriate food group for each item

- cups and ounces of food consumed

- with whom, where, why

- duration of time taken to eat

- other activity engaged in while eating

- Chapter 14 will request an additional entry, rating how "empty" or "full" you feel, before/during/ after consumption

For listing a combination food, think about what foods went into it and identify those foods with the appropriate food group. For example, the cheese on a pizza would be recorded in the Milk group, the tomatoes and any other vegetables in the Vegetables group, and the crust in the Grains group. The ingredients in a combination food may not always count as a full serving from the food group. Think in terms of the quantity consumed, along with its nutrient category. (Consult the web site's information on how to count mixed dishes when recording food entries.[25])

If you're finding it's helpful, continue monitoring your intake for a few days in your Fitness Journal, recording the same categories of entries. (Chapter 14 will have you consider monitoring and recording your intake for 60 days, if you are choosing to follow the weight loss program presented there.) How does it measure up to the standards established for a balanced diet with special

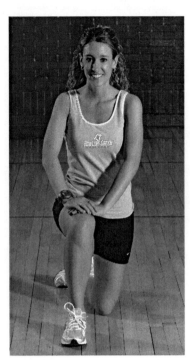

**Figure 13.6** Nutrition and the Athlete

attention to selecting nutrient-dense foods? If your diet lacks variety, moderation, or foods from one of the food groups, you might not be getting all the nutrients and energy you need.

It's easy to improve your diet if you take it one step, one choice at a time. Start by choosing one challenge to work on (see Goal-Setting Challenge at the end of the chapter), come up with a solution, and spend 1 week trying to correct it. After mastering it, choose a second eating challenge, and then continue until you have a well-managed eating plan.

## Nutrition and the Athlete

The food groups already presented form the foundation of the diet recommended for young athletes (Figure 13.6). Any of the plans presented serves as the nucleus for meals both in and out of athletic seasons. There is a vast leeway in the choice of foods within each of the food groups. Basic nutritional needs of athletes and non-athletes do not differ much except in terms of calories.[26]

Total caloric needs vary with individual metabolism and physical activity. An intake of 2000 calories a day should be the bare minimum allowed for an athlete involved in a vigorous training program. The number of calories a young male athlete expends in serious training might be as high as 4000 to 6000 calories per day. Calorie intake that exceeds expenditure for basal body functions, for physical activity, and for growth of lean body mass, however, will still form body fat, so pay attention to your training diet.

---

### Basic nutritional needs of athletes and nonathletes do not differ except in terms of calories.

---

A pregame meal should:

- Support blood sugar levels to avoid hunger sensations
- Leave the stomach and upper bowel empty at the time of competition (feeling sense is comfortable, light, and can breathe easily)
- Provide maximum hydration
- Minimize stomach upset; promote maximum performance
- Provide a psychological edge by including foods the athlete likes and believes will help him or her win

*Carbohydrates* in the diet will support blood sugar and provide glycogen stores to maintain these levels. Glycogen, the storage form of carbohydrate, is the quickest and most efficient source of energy.

High-carbohydrate foods include:

apples
applesauce
bagels
baked potatoes
baking powder biscuits
bananas
boiled potatoes
bread (white, whole wheat)
cheese pizza
egg noodles

graham crackers
hard rolls
macaroni and cheese
mashed potatoes
oatmeal
oranges and orange juice
orange sherbet
pancakes (enriched)
pears
spaghetti
sponge cake
sweet potatoes
waffles

Carbohydrates are digested more rapidly than protein and fat. A breakfast of toast and jam, cereal with low-fat milk, and fruit or juice will leave the stomach much sooner than a meal of eggs with steak, sausage, or bacon.

Optimum hydration is important to athletes, especially those involved in endurance events, such as long-distance swimming and running. The immediate pregame diet should consist of two to three glasses of a beverage, with no fewer than eight full glasses every 24 hours.

Whole milk is not recommended because of its high fat content. Caffeine also should be avoided because it may increase nervous tension and agitation before the contest. Noncarbonated fruit drinks are generally good choices.

*Energy gels* (highly concentrated carbohydrates) claim to quickly replace glycogen. Leading health/fitness professionals have stated:

While gels may give endurance athletes an extra boost, most athletes can ensure they have adequate glycogen stores by eating foods rich in carbohydrates before and following exercise.[27]

Energy gels are best suited to endurance athletes who participate in aerobic exercise for more than $1\frac{1}{2}$ to 2 hours . . . and they must have access to water to take them.[28]

Athletes should avoid concentrated sources of simple sugar such as glucose tablets and undiluted honey, as they can cause gas and discomfort. Also, bulky foods high in fiber or cellulose are not good choices before an event. And, athletes should avoid heavily salted foods on the day of competition, because these can cause water retention, which decreases athletic performance.

The athlete should eat the pregame meal 3 to 4 hours before the contest. For a highly demanding sport, a 1000-calorie meal is ideal. A 500-calorie meal suffices for a sport that requires lower energy.

Athletes must be prepared physically to meet the special demands on their bodies. The starting block is sound nutrition knowledge coupled with practice. If you sacrifice physical excellence to an inefficient or harmful diet, reduced strength and endurance and a poor performance will be the result.

## Dietary Guidelines for Americans, 2005  USDA

The *Dietary Guidelines* is an official document produced by the U.S. Government that provides the foundation and supporting research for all of the nutrition advice we follow. Its designers and contributors are a panel of professionals with credentials specializing in the field of nutrition. The document, in its entirety, is 80 pages in length and provides much insight into all aspects of the science of human nutrition.

The following is a listing of the ten chapters within the *Dietary Guidelines*, followed briefly by the Key Recommendations being promoted. Further considerations on these key recommendations follow several entries, and all Key Recommendations for Special Populations have been omitted here; they can be found in their entirety on the U.S. Government's web site, http://www.healthierus.gov/dietaryguidelines.

## CHAPTERS:

### 1 EXECUTIVE SUMMARY[29]

The *Dietary Guidelines for Americans [Dietary Guidelines]* provides science-based advice to promote health and to reduce risk for major chronic diseases through diet and physical activity. Major causes of morbidity and mortality in the United States are related to poor diet and a sedentary lifestyle. Some specific diseases linked to poor diet and physical inactivity include cardiovascular disease, type 2 diabetes, hypertension, osteoporosis, and certain cancers. Furthermore, poor diet and physical inactivity, resulting in an energy imbalance (more calories consumed than expended), are the most important factors contributing to the increase in overweight and obesity in this country. Combined with physical activity, following a diet that does not provide excess calories according to the recommendations in this document should enhance the health of most individuals.[30] The following is a listing of the *Dietary Guidelines* by chapter.

### 2 ADEQUATE NUTRIENTS WITHIN CALORIE NEEDS

#### Key Recommendations

- Consume a variety of nutrient-dense foods and beverages within and among the basic food groups while choosing foods that limit the intake of saturated and *trans* fats, cholesterol, added sugars, salt, and alcohol.
- Meet recommended intakes within energy needs by adopting a balanced eating pattern, such as the USDA Food Guide or the DASH (Dietary Approaches to Stop Hypertension) Eating Plan.[31]

### 3 WEIGHT MANAGEMENT

#### Key Recommendations

- To maintain body weight in a healthy range, balance calories from foods and beverages with calories expended (see Table 13.6).

## Table 13.6  Calories Should Be in Proportion to Activity[32]

Estimated calorie needs for different age groups and activity levels:
- **Sedentary:** Includes only light physical activity associated with day-to-day life.
- **Moderately active:** Includes walking 1.5 to 3 miles a day at 3 to 4 mph or the equivalent in another activity.
- **Active:** Includes physical activity equivalent to walking more than 3 miles a day at 3 to 4 mph.

**Calories needed:** ■ = Female   □ = Male

| Ages | Sedentary | | Moderately active | | Active | |
|---|---|---|---|---|---|---|
| 2-3 | 1000 | 1000 | 1000–1400 | 1000–1400 | 1000–1400 | 1000–1400 |
| 4-8 | 1200 | 1400 | 1400–1600 | 1400–1600 | 1400–1800 | 1600–2000 |
| 9-13 | 1600 | 1800 | 1600–2000 | 1800–2200 | 1800–2200 | 2000–2600 |
| 14-18 | 1800 | 2200 | 2000 | 2400–2800 | 2400 | 2800–3200 |
| 19-30 | 2000 | 2400 | 2000–2200 | 2600–2800 | 2400 | 3000 |
| 31-50 | 1800 | 2200 | 2000 | 2400–2600 | 2200 | 2800–3000 |
| 51 plus | 1600 | 2000 | 1800 | 2200–2400 | 2000–2200 | 2400–2800 |

Source: Dietary Guidelines for Americans, 2005

- To prevent gradual weight gain over time, make small decreases in food and beverage calories and increase physical activity.

Consider this: If you eat 100 more food calories a day than you burn, you'll gain about 1 pound in a month. That's about 10 pounds in a year. The bottom line is that to lose weight, it's important to reduce calories and increase physical activity.

## 4 PHYSICAL ACTIVITY

### Key Recommendations

- Engage in regular physical activity and reduce sedentary activities to promote health, psychological well-being, and a healthy body weight.

- To reduce the risk of chronic disease in adulthood: Engage in at least 30 minutes of moderate-intensity physical activity, above usual activity, at work or home on most days of the week.

- For most people, greater health benefits can be obtained by engaging in physical activity of more vigorous intensity or longer duration.

- To help manage body weight and prevent gradual, unhealthy body weight gain in adulthood: Engage in approximately 60 minutes of moderate- to vigorous-intensity activity on most days of the week while not exceeding caloric intake requirements.

- To sustain weight loss in adulthood: Participate in at least 60 to 90 minutes of daily moderate-intensity physical activity while not exceeding caloric intake requirements. Some people may need to consult with a healthcare provider before participating in this level of activity.

- Achieve physical fitness by including cardiovascular conditioning, stretching exercises for flexibility, and resistance exercises or calisthenics for muscle strength and endurance.

## 5 FOOD GROUPS TO ENCOURAGE

### Key Recommendations

- Consume a sufficient amount of fruits and vegetables while staying within energy needs. Two cups of fruit and 2 $\frac{1}{2}$ cups of vegetables per day are recommended for a reference 2000-calorie intake, with higher or lower amounts depending on the calorie level.

- Choose a variety of fruits and vegetables each day. In particular, select from all five vegetable subgroups (dark green, orange, legumes, starchy vegetables, and other vegetables) several times a week.

- Consume 3 or more ounce-equivalents of whole-grain products per day, with the rest of the recommended grains coming from enriched or whole-grain products. In general, at least half the grains should come from whole grains.

- Consume 3 cups per day of fat-free or low-fat milk or equivalent milk products.

## 6 FATS

### Key Recommendations

- Consume less than 10% of calories from saturated fatty acids and less than 300 mg/day of cholesterol, and keep *trans* fatty acid consumption as low as possible.

- Keep total fat intake between 20 to 35% of calories, with most fats coming from sources of polyunsaturated and monounsaturated fatty acids, such as fish, nuts, and vegetable oils.

- When selecting and preparing meat, poultry, dry beans, and milk or milk products, make choices that are lean, low-fat, or fat-free.

- Limit intake of fats and oils high in saturated and/or *trans* fatty acids, and choose products low in such fats and oils.

Consider this: If you have a high blood cholesterol level, you have a greater chance of incurring a heart attack. A population such as that in the United States, with diets high in saturated fats and cholesterol, tends to have high blood cholesterol levels.

*Cholesterol* is a necessary constituent of body tissues. When the circulating amount in the blood is higher than 200 milligrams (mg) (mild risk) or higher than 240 mg (high risk), it can cause early atherosclerosis. Atherosclerosis is a process of fatty build-up

## Table 13.7 Blood Lipid Profile

| | | | | Near or | Borderline | |
|---|---|---|---|---|---|---|
| **Type** | **Low** | **Desirable** | **Optimal** | **Above Optimal** | **High** | **High** |
| Total Cholesterol | | <200 | | | 200–239 | >240 |
| HDL | <35 | 35–59 | >60 | | | |
| LDL | | | <100 | 100–129 | 130–159 | 160–189 |

Listed in milligrams / deciliter or mg/dl

Adapted from the AMA, 2001, *Journal of the AMA*, 285 (19), 2486-97.

in the walls of the blood vessels, eventually leading to narrowing of the arteries and poor circulation. Cholesterol is one of the three major risk factors for coronary heart disease (CHD). (The other two are high blood pressure and cigarette smoking.)

*High-density lipoproteins (HDL),* the "good cholesterol," coat the inside of artery walls, providing a protective layer of grease to prevent fatty deposits from building up. They also serve as scavengers by actually helping dissolve fatty deposits when they do occur. A high amount in the blood indicates protection and decrease in the risk for heart attack. Certain people genetically have higher amounts. HDL also can be increased by weight loss and by regular aerobic exercise. A very low level in the blood indicates a serious risk for heart attack.

*Triglycerides* (another type of fat) are diet-related and usually are not involved in the atherosclerotic process. High values occur in certain fat metabolism disorders and in diabetes.

*Low-density lipoproteins (LDL)* are related to dietary habits. LDLs form dangerous deposits on the walls of blood vessels, are the primary culprits in clogged arteries and atherosclerosis, and place a person at high risk for heart attack. If cholesterol and HDL values are borderline, LDL values may decide the risk.

*Risk ratio* is a calculated value (total cholesterol divided by your HDL value) that most experts use to predict an individual's risk of heart attack. Having a high HDL cholesterol value and a low LDL cholesterol value reduces the risk.

Cholesterol is measured by a simple blood test that shows milligrams (mg) of total cholesterol (HDL, LDL, and VLDL, very low-density lipoproteins) per deciliter (dl) of blood. If your blood lipid values are tested and indicate increased risk for heart disease (see Table 13.7), you may benefit from improving your diet and increasing your exercise.

Experts differ in their recommendations for healthy Americans. For the U.S. population as a whole, however,

reducing the intake of total fat, saturated fat, and cholesterol is sensible.

- Limit use of animal fats, hard margarines, and partially hydrogenated shortenings.
- Choose lean meats, fish, skinless poultry, dried beans, and peas as your protein sources.
- Choose fat-free or low-fat dairy products.
- Use egg yolks and whole eggs in moderation (use egg whites and egg substitutes freely).
- Limit breaded and deep-fried foods, and foods with creamy sauces.
- Trim fats from meats.
- Broil, bake, and boil rather than fry.
- Read food labels carefully to determine amounts and types of fat and cholesterol in foods.
- Consume 300 mg/day or less of cholesterol.
- Limit fat to 30% or less of total daily calories. To determine the percentage of calories in a product that come from fat: 1 gram of fat equals 9 calories. Multiply the grams of fat in a serving times 9. The result equals the number of calories from fat in a serving. Divide the fat calories by the total calories in a serving to determine the percentage.

For example, if a chili label reads:

> 1 cup serving = 200 calories
> Fat, 10g • Carbohydrate, 5g • Sodium, 980mg
> 1 cup of chili has 10 grams of fat
> 10g fat x 9 calories/gram of fat = 90 calories from fat in 1 cup
> 90 fat calories / 200 total calories = 45% of the calories in 1 cup of chili comes from fat.[33]

## 7 CARBOHYDRATES

### Key Recommendations

- Choose fiber-rich fruits (Figure 13.7), vegetables, and whole grains often.
- Choose and prepare foods and beverages with little added sugars

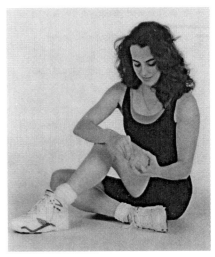

**Figure 13.7** Choose Fiber-rich Fruits Often

or caloric sweeteners, such as amounts suggested by the USDA Food Guide and the DASH Eating Plan.

- Reduce the incidence of dental caries by practicing good oral hygiene and consuming sugar- and starch-containing foods and beverages less frequently.

Consider this: To determine how many teaspoons of sugar a product contains:

> *Note:* 1 teaspoon = 5 grams of sugar
> Divide the grams of sugar in a serving, by 5.
> For example, if a cereal box label reads:
> 1 cup serving = 140 calories
> Carbohydrates/starch, 10g
> • Sucrose, 15g • Fiber, 1gm
> 1 cup of cereal contains 15 grams of sucrose (sugar)
> 15 grams of sucrose ÷ 5 grams of sugar per teaspoon =
> 3 teaspoons of simple sugar in 1 cup of cereal.

Products are healthier when the amount of sucrose (simple sugar) is low.[34]

## 8 SODIUM AND POTASSIUM

### Key Recommendations

- Consume less than 2300 mg (approximately 1 tsp. of salt) of sodium per day.

- Choose and prepare foods with little salt. At the same time, consume potassium-rich foods, such as fruits and vegetables.

Consider this: The major hazard posed by excessive sodium is its effect on blood pressure. In populations where high-sodium intake is common, high blood pressure is also common. In populations with low-sodium intake, high blood pressure is rare. Establish preventive measures, such as the following:

- Use herbs, spices, and fruits to flavor foods.

- Add little or no salt at the table.

- Limit salty foods.

- Read the Nutrition Facts label to compare and help identify foods lower in sodium.

- Use sparingly condiments such as soy sauce, ketchup, mustard, pickles, and olives.

## 9 ALCOHOLIC BEVERAGES

### Key Recommendations

- Those who choose to drink alcoholic beverages should do so sensibly and in moderation—defined as the consumption of **up to one drink per day for women** and **up to two drinks per day for men**.

- Alcoholic beverages should not be consumed by some individuals, including those who cannot restrict their alcohol intake, women of childbearing age who may become pregnant, pregnant and lactating women, children and adolescents, individuals taking medications that can interact with alcohol, and those with specific medical conditions.

- Alcoholic beverages should be avoided by individuals engaging in activities that require attention, skill, or coordination, such as driving or operating machinery.

Consider this: Alcoholic beverages tend to be high in calories and low in other nutrients. Heavy drinkers may lose their appetite for foods that contain essential nutrients. Vitamin and mineral deficiencies occur commonly in heavy drinkers because of poor nutrient intake and because alcohol alters absorption and use of some essential nutrients.

One or two drinks daily seem to cause no harm in adults, but even moderate drinkers should remember that alcohol is a high-calorie, low-nutrient food. If you wish to achieve or maintain your recommended weight, alcohol intake must be well monitored. Drinking alcohol with meals slows its absorption. Pregnant women should not use alcohol. If you drink, do not drive. Research indicates that women have higher blood alcohol levels than men after having one drink. This is because women have less activity of an enzyme that helps to metabolize alcohol in the body. Thus, women are more vulnerable to the acute and chronic complications of alcoholism.

*Count a drink as:*

- 12 fluid ounces of regular or light beer

- 5 fluid ounces of table wine

- 3 1/2 fluid ounces of dessert wine

- 7 fluid ounces of light wine

- 3 1/2 fluid ounces of gin, rum, or whiskey (80 proof)

- 1 mixed drink[35]

## 10 FOOD SAFETY

### Key Recommendations

- To avoid microbial food-borne illness:

  - Clean hands, food contact surfaces, and fruits and vegetables. Meat and poultry should not be washed or rinsed.

  - Separate raw, cooked, and ready-to-eat foods while shopping, preparing, or storing foods.

  - Cook foods to a safe temperature to kill microorganisms.

  - Chill (refrigerate) perishable food promptly and defrost foods properly.

  - Avoid raw (unpasteurized) milk or any products made from unpasteurized milk, raw or partially cooked eggs or foods containing raw eggs, raw or undercooked meat and poultry, unpasteurized juices, and raw sprouts.

## *Nutrition Facts Label*

The federal government establishes the requirements for labels on commercially sold food products. The benefit of a standardized label makes it relevant to today's health concerns. It is a label you can understand, and one that can help you plan healthy meals and snacks.

What we eat actually can raise or lower our risks for acquiring certain diseases. For this reason, the Food and Drug Administration allows claims linking a nutrient, or food, to the risk of a disease or health-related condition. Only seven health messages are allowed because these are the only ones supported by scientific evidence (e.g., "low fat" and "a link between fruits and vegetables and a lower risk of cancer"). These claims must meet strict requirements enforced by the federal government, so when you see them, you can trust what they say. (Foods without the claims, however, are not necessarily less nutritious.)

The package must feature a nutrition panel called "Nutrition Facts" (see Figure 13.8). Almost all packaged foods will have to carry this nutrition information. It includes ingredient labeling on the labels of all foods with more than one ingredient. Try these tips:

- Keep these low: saturated fats, *trans* fats, cholesterol, and sodium.

- Get enough of these: potassium, fiber, vitamins A and C, calcium, and iron.

- Use the % Daily Value (DV) column when possible.

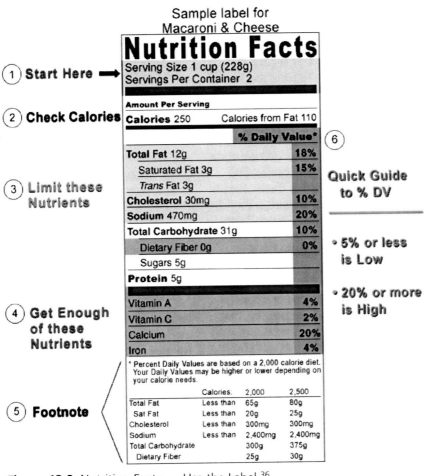

**Figure 13.8** Nutrition Facts. . . Use the Label.[36]

- **Check Servings and Calories.** The *serving size* is the basis for measuring a food's nutrient content and is the first place to consult on the Nutrition Facts panel. Look at the serving size and how many servings you are actually consuming. The serving sizes are close to the amounts people eat. If you choose to eat more, or less, than the serving size given on the label, adjust the amounts of nutrients accordingly. If you double the servings you eat, you double the calories and nutrients, including the % DVs.

- **Make Your Calories Count.** Look at the calories on the label and compare them with what nutrients you are also getting to decide whether the food is worth eating. When one serving of a single food item has over 400 calories per serving, it is high in calories.

- **% Daily Value.** The amount of certain nutrients in a food is expressed in two ways:

1. Amount by weight per serving.
2. As a percentage of the Daily Value (a unique nutritional reference tool). By using the Percent Daily Values, you can determine easily whether a given food contributes little (has a low percentage) or a lot (has a high percentage) of a specific nutrient. Five percent DV or less is low, 20% DV or more is high. You also can compare different foods with no need to do any calculations. The goal is to choose a variety of foods that, together, give you close to 100% of each nutrient for a day, or average about 100% a day over several days. The Percent Daily Values listed

on the nutrition panel are based on consuming 2000 calories a day. If you eat more or less calories a day, you'll have to adjust the values accordingly.

- **Don't Sugarcoat It.** Since sugars contribute calories with few, if any, nutrients, look for foods and beverages low in added sugars. Read the ingredient list and make sure that added sugars are not one of the first few ingredients. Some names for added sugars (caloric sweeteners) include sucrose, glucose, high fructose corn syrup, corn syrup, maple syrup, and fructose.

- **Know Your Fats.** Look for foods low in saturated fats, *trans* fats, and cholesterol to help reduce the risk of heart disease (5% DV or less is low, 20% DV or more is high). Most of the fats you eat should be polyunsaturated and monounsaturated fats. Keep total fat intake between 20% to 35% of calories.

- **Reduce Sodium (salt), Increase Potassium.** Research shows that eating less than 2300 milligrams of sodium (about 1 tsp. of salt) per day may reduce the risk of high blood pressure. Most of the sodium people eat *comes from processed foods,* not from the saltshaker. Also look for foods high in potassium, which counteracts some of sodium's effects on blood pressure.

## Major Changes Set for Food Labels

Beginning January 1, 2006 there are a host of changes on the horizon for food labels. The Food and Drug Administration

- now requires that food packages and some supplements list the amount of *trans* fat on the label;

- requires labeling for the eight allergen groups: tree nuts, milk, eggs, fish, crustacean shellfish, peanuts, soybeans, and wheat;

- is expected to define the term "whole grain" for labels in 2006;

■ is considering giving calories more prominence on the label (increasing type size of calorie list), and specifying nutrition information for an entire package, not just for "servings".[37]

These changes are just a beginning. Food labeling is actively in transition, so keep up with the latest research as it becomes available and the resulting FDA requirements.

# Disordered Eating

Research from the National Institute of Mental Health (NIMH)[38] reveals that in the United States, more than 90% of the individuals affected with serious or life-threatening disordered eating (anorexia nervosa, bulimia nervosa, and binge-eating disorder) are adolescent and young adult women, who go on strict diets to achieve an "ideal" figure. (Less than 10% of the afflicted are men and older women.) Such stringent dieting can play a key role in triggering their disordered eating.

*Anorexia nervosa* is a dangerous condition in which individuals intentionally starve themselves (literally to death, without intervention). The chief manifestation is extreme weight loss—at least 15% below an individual's normal body weight. Afflicted people suffer terribly from hunger pains, but they think they are overweight even when they are bone-thin, because they are terrified of gaining any weight. Food and weight become obsessions. They often develop strange rituals. For instance, they might collect recipes and prepare gourmet feasts for family and friends but not partake in the meals themselves. They might adhere to strict exercise routines to keep weight off. Anorexic women may cease to menstruate, and men with anorexia often become impotent.

*Bulimia nervosa* is a destructive pattern characterized by excessive overeating, followed by purging (vomiting) to control the weight. Typical behaviors include abusing laxatives and diuretics, taking enemas, exercising excessively, or a combination of these behaviors. Because individuals with bulimia tend to binge and purge in secret (from once or twice a week to several times a day) and maintain a normal or above normal body weight, they often successfully hide their problem from others for years. Dieting heavily between episodes is common. Eventually, half of those with anorexia develop bulimia. Many people with bulimia are ashamed of these unusual habits, and as a consequence, they do not seek help until they reach their 30s and 40s. By this time, their eating pattern is deeply ingrained and is difficult to change.

*Binge-eating disorder* is an illness that resembles bulimia but differs in that it does not include purging. The individuals eat large quantities of food and do not stop until they are uncomfortably full. As a consequence, they are obese and have a history of weight fluctuations. This disordered eating occurs more frequently in women than men and afflicts 30% of the people participating in medically supervised weight-control programs.

## Causes of Disordered Eating

Individuals with disordered eating are characterized by:

■ low self-esteem

■ feelings of helplessness

■ fear of becoming fat

■ using the disorder as a way of handling stress and anxieties

Disordered eating seems to run in families and have both genetic and environmental contributing factors. Anorexia and bulimia are found most often in Caucasians and in professions that emphasize thinness (such as modeling, gymnastics, and wrestling).

The consequences of disordered eating can be severe, and one in 10 cases of anorexia leads to death from starvation, cardiac arrest, other medical complications, or suicide. Increasing awareness of the dangers of disordered eating has led many of those afflicted to seek help. NIMH-supported research has found that people with disordered eating who get early treatment have a better chance of full recovery than those who wait years before getting help. (For instance, group therapy, in which individuals share experiences, is especially effective with individuals with bulimia.)

The key for help in all categories is to change abnormal thoughts and behaviors. Chapters 2, 12, and 14 provide many helpful suggestions. Treatment can save the life of someone who exhibits disordered eating.[39]

# Problems and Solutions

Below is a list of seven problem-eating behaviors that indicate the need for help, followed by 26 solutions—your ABC's of eating!

### Problem-Eating Behaviors

■ overeating when stimulated by seeing a certain restaurant, establishment (like the movies), or when attending specific occasions

■ binge-eating certain foods and beverages or when very hungry or when feeling certain emotions (such as anger, depression, boredom, anxiety, frustration, loneliness)

■ choosing food portions that are too large or too high-calorie

■ eating too fast, everything on the plate even when no longer hungry, leftovers because it is "a sin to waste food," while watching TV, reading, or doing other passive activities, throughout the day, or when not hungry

■ overeating when stimulated by the sight, smell, nearness of food, in social situations, or at the persuasion of family and friends

■ eating as a reward

■ skipping meals (usually breakfast and/or lunch), but overeating at dinner or later in the day.

## Solutions

**A =** Ask family and friends not to give food as a present or reward.

**B =** Before eating anything, ask yourself if you really need or want it.

**C =** Chew each bite thoroughly before swallowing; enjoy textures.

**D =** Drink a glass of water before eating, and "doggy bag" leftovers when done.

**E =** Eat foods high in fiber; they require more chewing.

**F =** Find nonfood ways to reward yourself.

**G =** Give away the meal's leftover foods to guests, or freeze them immediately.

**H =** Hunger is the best cue to eat; don't eat unless you feel hungry!

**I =** Ice water is necessary and filling; hydrate yourself daily using the replacement pyramid (see Figure 13.4).

**J =** Journaling your food and beverage intake can be fun!

**K =** Keep available lower-calorie foods, such as fruits and vegetables, for snacks and keep them visible and ready to eat.

**L =** Leave the table after eating a meal, stay and talk while sipping a glass of ice water, and learn to say *no* gracefully.

**M =** Moderation in all food.

**N =** Never put food on the fork until you have chewed, swallowed, and savored the last forkful of food.

**O =** Ordering is the key behavior to learn when eating out. Decide your meal beforehand by "future picturing" what you need and want and, most important, how you choose to feel when you are done eating (aim for a "5"on the control dial, Figure 14.5).

**P =** Put down the utensils between bites, and enjoy conversing with others.

**Q =** Quotes encouraging positive eating choices are great refrigerator decorations. What's your favorite quote?

**R =** Read labels and learn about the nutrient and caloric values of foods. Avoid foods that are high in calories and low in nutrients.

**S =** "Seconds" are indicators of overeating. Size up your entire meal the first time it is served, and stop eating when you are full, comfortable, feel light, and can breathe easy ( a "5" on the control panel with large dial, Figure 14.5).

**T =** Television mute buttons are great devices to use when food commercials air. When the sound is gone, close your eyes and relax for several minutes until your show returns.

**U =** Use small plates so small portions appear larger.

**V =** Votive candlelight is soothing to the digestion. Light a candle to calm your desire to overeat.

**W =** Write out all of the scenarios that happened prior to overeating, to analyze the "trigger(s)" and behavior chain involved with pain and subsequent pleasure linking to reduce stress.

**X =** "Xtra" food stays on the stove. Don't serve food family style when overeaters are present.

**Y =** Yoga, tai chi, and relaxation using guided imagery are great substitutes for inappropriate eating, as are reading a good book, physical activity, and all of your positive stress relievers that are not associated with consuming food and beverages.

**Z =** "Zero-starred" foods and those with few stars in Tables 13.1 through 13.5 that are tempting can be avoided by simply not buying them!

## A Caveat

Better or best nutrition choices can be made by following the various guidelines mentioned in this chapter. If you know little about human physiology—how your vital processes work—an abundance of scientifically based, easy-to-read literature explains how to balance the needed nutrients. Select guidelines developed by well-established medical and fitness sources, such as those referred to in this chapter, rather than those from your favorite movie and television stars or supermarket trade magazines.

## Goal-Setting Challenge

✔ You can set many possible small goals regarding nutrition. Begin by reviewing the chapter subtitles and listing topics or points that require your attention. Prioritize this list in order of your needs. Enjoy the challenge of balancing your intake (eating) with your expenditure (exercise). Or, if a course goal is to lose fat weight or gain lean weight, *imbalancing* might be your goal.

✔ Write a Nutrition Goal for Chapter 13 in your Fitness Journal, following the guidelines in Exercise 2.3, Fitness Course Goals, at the end of Chapter 2. Consider what phase(s) of your program requires attention—Eating *nutrient-dense* foods? Monitoring the *amount and serving sizes* you eat? Consuming enough *fluids*, before/during/after exercise? We all have areas in which we can improve when it comes to nutritionally fueling ourselves.

# Exercise 13.1    Considerations for Vegetarian Meal Planning

**1** Identify the group(s) you're choosing to eat in an alternative way (meat and beans group; milk group; meat and beans and milk groups; discretionary fats/oils/sweets) and the reason for each choice:

I am alternatively eating the:
\_\_\_\_ Milk Group \_\_\_\_ Both Meat and Beans and Milk Group
\_\_\_\_ Meat and Beans Group \_\_\_\_ Fats, Oils, and Sweets

**My reasons for this choice:** _____

_____

Here are six eating style definitions,* including each plan's name and the main food choices. Check (✔) the plan you're choosing to eat:

\_\_\_\_ *Animal/Meat-Based Diet:* beef, pork, chicken, turkey, fish, eggs, and dairy products

\_\_\_\_ *Plant-Based Diet:* fruits, vegetables, grains, legumes, seeds, and nuts

\_\_\_\_ *Vegetarian Diet:* plant-based diet that may include seafood, fish, eggs, or dairy products

\_\_\_\_ *Lacto-Ovo Vegetarian Diet:* plant-based diet plus eggs and dairy products

\_\_\_\_ *Lacto-Vegetarian Diet:* plant-based diet plus dairy products

\_\_\_\_ *Vegan (VEE-gun) Diet:* plant-based diet only (excludes all animal foods, meat, poultry, fish, eggs, and dairy products)

*Source: Tammy Kime-Sheets, author of original teaching tool entitled, *How To Eat Without the Meat*, in section "Cut the Animal Fat," p. 2, distributed to clients at Nutritional Wellness seminars and workshops in greater Toledo, Ohio area, 1996–1998.

**2** Do you understand *what the required nutrients and their functions are* (provided in each food group), that have to be considered and replaced by other forms of alternative food choices (that, likewise, can provide those required nutrients)?

\_\_\_\_ Yes.   If your answer is \_\_\_\_ No:

Especially consider your needs for all of the following essential nutrients and the functions each performs to keep you healthy: amino acids (ensuring adequate nitrogen retention), calcium, iron, linolenic acid, Vitamin $B_{12}$, Vitamin D, zinc. Identify *naturally occurring foods* (not *manufactured* pills/potions/products) that you enjoy eating and drinking and an accompanying serving size you'll eat that provides each nutrient in your new plan.

| Nutrient | Foods I Enjoy That Provide This | A Serving Size Equals |
|---|---|---|
| Essential amino acids | _____ | _____ |
| Calcium | _____ | _____ |
| Iron | _____ | _____ |
| Linolenic acid | _____ | _____ |
| Vitamin $B_{12}$ | _____ | _____ |
| Vitamin D | _____ | _____ |
| Zinc | _____ | _____ |

This information is fully detailed on the Internet website of The *Vegetarian Resource Group* at http://www.vrg.org/ and can provide you with valuable assistance in your meal planning for vegetarian eating.

**3** Does this new choice of eating plan fulfill *your* physical, social, emotional, spiritual, intellectual, and talent expression needs?

Answer these questions:

**Physical:** Will my food and beverage choices provide for all of my needs regarding basal metabolism, growth, repair, and energy? _____

(We usually find out the answer to this question when the *lack* shows up and we don't have enough nutrients present to provide needed energy/proper growth/ability to repair in a timely fashion/or when illness and disease take over.)

Do I eat a variety of food *colors* (*resembling a rainbow*) and *crunches** that provides naturally for these four needs? \_\_\_\_

**Social:** Can I *easily* eat with my plan around family and friends, and *enjoy* all of my choices in their presence? \_\_\_\_

**Emotional:** Does my eating plan \_\_\_\_ *predominantly* include \_\_\_\_ *occasionally* include \_\_\_\_ *never* include "comfort" food I may choose to eat? (Comfort food is usually characterized as having a soft, mushy texture, and white, creamy, beige, or brown in color.) Are my eating choices primarily focused \_\_\_\_ *toward* promoting my best health or  \_\_\_\_ *away from* experiencing illness and disease?

**Spiritual/Philosophical:** Does the eating plan I'm choosing to follow include a belief that "nature" can supply all the essential nutrients (from naturally existing sources), or must I rely on self-prescribed supplementation using *manufactured* pills, potions, and products to obtain all of the necessary nutrients I need to stay healthy?

\_\_\_\_ All from nature.

\_\_\_\_ Inadequate, so I must self-supplement to have all of the required nutrients I need.

**Intellectual:** Would my combined choices fulfill the eating guidelines established by the federal government, the American Dietetics Association, a local registered dietitian or licensed nutritionist, and/or my family physician?

\_\_\_\_ Yes, from any of these sources.

\_\_\_\_ No, not from any of these sources. The source for guidelines I choose to follow is:

_____

**Talent Expression:** If I am an athlete, is my eating plan providing all of the nutrients I need to stay well, grow, and repair, in addition to the increased energy and fluid replacement needs I have?

\_\_\_\_ Yes      \_\_\_\_ No

(Athletes in training must adjust to their increased energy needs by eating significantly more calories of the carbohydrate foods and replace the loss of fluids by consuming more water or other appropriate fluids.)

*Source: Tammy Kime-Sheets, *How To Eat Without The Meat*, in section "Lifestyle Profile of Nutrition Choice, You Are How You Eat," 1996–1998.

## Exercise 13.2 Monitoring Your Food and Beverage Intake For 1 to 3 Days

**Directions:** Record your food and beverage intake for 1 to 3 days. It will require just a moment's reflection as you identify the points listed. Afterwards, ask yourself: "How do my choices measure up to the standards established for a balanced diet, with special attention to selecting nutrient-dense foods?" Identify:

- Today's date.
- Nutrient-density starred ratings (4/3/2/1/0) before each food/beverage entry.
- Appropriate food group for each item.

Then:

- Comment regarding the social and emotional aspects of your eating patterns.
- Practice the feeling sense and rate 0–10 how "empty" or "full" you feel before and after your meals or snacks (see Figure 14.5 for more information).
- Set a goal to improve one aspect of your diet or eating actions that require the most attention:

➡ **GOAL:** _____

### Food and Beverage Intake Diary — For 1 Day

| Date: | *Nutrient Density | Name of Food | Food Groups: Mi/Me/VF/G/DF | How Much | With Whom | | | Where | Eating Dial | | Why | | | | | | | How Long (Number of Minutes) | Other Activity While Eating |
|---|---|---|---|---|---|---|---|---|---|---|---|---|---|---|---|---|---|---|---|
| | | | | | Alone | Family | Friends | | Before | After | Worried | Bored | Depressed | Tired | Social | Hungry | Other: | | |
| BREAKFAST | | | | | | | | | | | | | | | | | | | |
| SNACK | | | | | | | | | | | | | | | | | | | |
| LUNCH | | | | | | | | | | | | | | | | | | | |
| SNACK | | | | | | | | | | | | | | | | | | | |
| DINNER | | | | | | | | | | | | | | | | | | | |
| SNACK | | | | | | | | | | | | | | | | | | | |

**Food and Beverage Intake Diary — For 1 Day**

| Date: | *Nutrient Density | Name of Food | Food Groups: Mi/Me/V/F/G/DF | How Much | With Whom | | | Where | Eating Dial | | Why | | | | | | | How Long (Number of Minutes) | Other Activity While Eating |
|---|---|---|---|---|---|---|---|---|---|---|---|---|---|---|---|---|---|---|---|
| | | | | | Alone | Family | Friends | | Before | After | Worried | Bored | Depressed | Tired | Social | Hungry | Other: | | |
| BREAKFAST | | | | | | | | | | | | | | | | | | | |
| SNACK | | | | | | | | | | | | | | | | | | | |
| LUNCH | | | | | | | | | | | | | | | | | | | |
| SNACK | | | | | | | | | | | | | | | | | | | |
| DINNER | | | | | | | | | | | | | | | | | | | |
| SNACK | | | | | | | | | | | | | | | | | | | |

**Food and Beverage Intake Diary — For 1 Day**

| Date: | *Nutrient Density | Name of Food | Food Groups: Mi/Me/V/F/G/DF | How Much | With Whom | | | Where | Eating Dial | | Why | | | | | | | How Long (Number of Minutes) | Other Activity While Eating |
|---|---|---|---|---|---|---|---|---|---|---|---|---|---|---|---|---|---|---|---|
| | | | | | Alone | Family | Friends | | Before | After | Worried | Bored | Depressed | Tired | Social | Hungry | Other: | | |
| BREAKFAST | | | | | | | | | | | | | | | | | | | |
| SNACK | | | | | | | | | | | | | | | | | | | |
| LUNCH | | | | | | | | | | | | | | | | | | | |
| SNACK | | | | | | | | | | | | | | | | | | | |
| DINNER | | | | | | | | | | | | | | | | | | | |
| SNACK | | | | | | | | | | | | | | | | | | | |

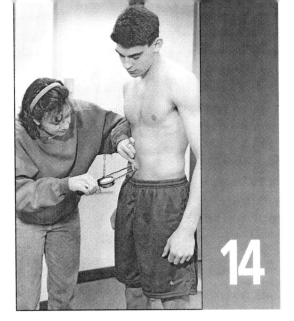

# Weight Management

## 14

Your body is composed of two types of weight: lean weight (also called lean body mass or fat-free mass) and fat weight (fat mass). Lean weight is composed primarily of bones, muscles, internal organs, and body fluids. Your lean weight begins to weigh less after maturity when you stop growing every year. Fat weight is stored energy and protection for present and future use. The amount of each type of weight you carry is important to know so you can understand what is best for the health of your heart and lungs (cardiovascular and respiratory systems).

## Body Composition

Body fat can be classified as either essential fat or storage fat. *Essential fat* is needed for normal physiological functions. Without it, your health begins to deteriorate. This essential fat constitutes about 3% of the total fat in men and 10 to 12% in women. The percentage is higher in women because it includes gender-related fat such as that found in the breast tissue, the uterus, and other gender-related areas.

*Storage fat* is the fat stored in adipose tissue, mostly beneath the skin (subcutaneous fat) and around major organs in the body. This fat serves three basic functions:

1. As an insulator to retain body heat
2. As energy substrate for metabolism
3. As padding against physical trauma to the body

The amount of storage fat does not differ between men and women except that men tend to store fat around the waist and women more so around the hips and thighs.[1]

Each person can "wear" a certain percentage of fat to maintain ideal cardiovascular and respiratory efficiency and minimize the risk factors associated with heart disease. Perhaps you are wearing less than a recommended percentage of fat. This doesn't matter unless you are malnourishing yourself or you wish to look heavier cosmetically. A number of people don't wear the recommended percentages. For example, endurance athletes such as marathon runners and Olympic gymnasts carry much less fat. They burn it off and don't carry the excess. They usually eat right to provide the necessary nutrients and energy and thus display a firm, trim, toned look, yet they stay well.

In contrast are individuals who have anorexia nervosa (see Chapter 13). They, too, carry less than the recommended percentage of body fat, but they do this by also eliminating their lean weight. They desire a trim look but go about it in a way that is against all physiological principles of proper weight loss. To them, weight loss means dropping pounds to be slim at all cost, no matter what kind of weight it is, fat or lean. This is an extremely detrimental way to lose weight. The concept of healthy slimness and unhealthy slimness is presented later in the chapter.

## Determining Your Recommended Weight

A recommended weight cannot be determined just by looking at someone. Therefore, an assessment determining an individual's body composition must be done. This includes calculating, as precisely as possible, body fat percentage in relation to lean weight mass. Knowing these values enables an estimation of an individual's "best" or recommended weight.

Two methods for determining your recommended weight (and the accompanying health risks from not maintaining that weight) are the following

1. *Skinfold Thickness.* Skinfold thickness initially is measured by a well-trained fitness professional using precision laboratory instruments. Then the person being measured uses the number values received to figure individual results. The formula to figure skinfold thickness is provided in this chapter (see Exercise 14.1, Tables 14.1–14.4, Goal Setting Challenge, and Exercise 14.2).

2. *Body Mass Index (BMI).* A person can easily calculate BMI, using Exercise 14.3, Calculating Adult BMI. (see page 166). A requirement to start this calculation is having a recent and accurate measurement of your weight (in pounds) and your height (in inches).

The BMI calculation procedure and all the necessary accompanying research (health risks related to the index value you are assigned), procedures to follow (properly measuring your height and weight to provide accuracy in your results), and suggestions to consider (eating and exercising to attain your recommended weight) are provided on several professionally rated sites,[2] listed on page 182, *Websites*. Before beginning, review each site, including any your instructor may add to this list.

Each of these methods approach the topic of determining one's recommended weight from a different perspective, and both have advantages and disadvantages. Therefore, it is suggested that students become aware of how both methods are calculated to obtain a recommended weight.

## Measuring Skinfold Thickness

The skinfold thickness measurement technique can determine whether an individual is at recommended weight, or is underweight, overweight (overfat), or obese, and then quantify exactly by how much. Specific goals then can be set to obtain or maintain the recommended weight. Because of the relative accuracy, availability of equipment, and ease of use in a fitness class setting, measuring skinfold thickness is currently the most frequently used technique with this population. It also is considered a more accurate method for certain populations to use than is the Body Mass Index (BMI) calculation.

Assessment of body composition using skinfold thickness is based on the principle that approximately half of the body's fatty tissue is deposited directly beneath the skin. If this tissue is estimated validly and reliably, it can produce a good indication of percent body fat.

This test is done with the aid of a precision instrument called a *skinfold caliper*. Three specific sites must be measured with the calipers and then added together to reflect the total percentage of fat. These measurements may vary slightly on the same person when they are taken by different professionals. Therefore, pre- and post-measurements preferably should be taken by the same technician.

Using the three-site skinfold testing, the procedure for assessing percent body fat follows:

1. Specific anatomical sites are tested. For men, these are the chest, abdomen, and thigh (Figure 14.1). For women, the suprailium, thigh, and triceps areas are tested (Figure 14.2). All measurements should be taken on the right side of the body with the person standing. The proper anatomical landmarks for skinfolds are:

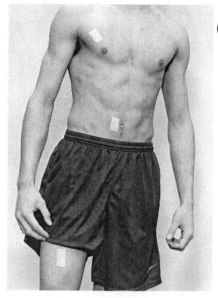

**Figure 14.1** Anatomical Sites for Skinfold Testing of Men

**Men**

| | |
|---|---|
| **Chest:** | A diagonal fold halfway between the shoulder crease and the nipple. |
| **Abdomen:** | A vertical fold taken about 1 inch to the right of the umbilicus. |
| **Thigh:** | A vertical fold on the front of the right thigh, midway between the knee and hip. (Weight-bear on left foot.) |

**Women**

| | |
|---|---|
| **Suprailium:** | A diagonal fold above the crest of the ilium (on the side of the hip) (a). |
| **Thigh:** | A vertical fold on the front of the right thigh, midway between the knee and hip (a). (Weight-bear on left foot.) |
| **Triceps:** | A vertical fold on the back of the upper arm, halfway between the shoulder and the elbow (b). |

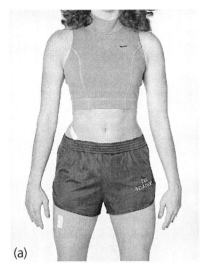

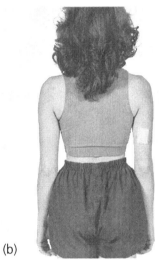

**Figure 14.2** Anatomical Sites for Skinfold Testing of Women

2. The technician conducts the measurements by grasping a thickness of skin in the key locations just mentioned, with a thumb and forefinger, and pulling the fold slightly away from the muscular tissue. The calipers are held perpendicular to the fold, and the measurement is taken ½" below the finger hold. Each site is measured three times, and the values are read to the nearest .1–.5 mm. The average of the two closest readings is recorded as your final value. The readings are taken in close succession to avoid excessive compression of the skinfold. Releasing and regrabbing the skinfold is required between readings.

3. When doing pre- and post-assessments, the measurement should be conducted at the same time of day. The best time is early in the morning to avoid hydration changes resulting from activity or exercise.

## Determining Your Percent Body Fat

Record your findings in Exercise 14.1. The percent fat is obtained by adding all three skinfold measurements, then looking up the respective values on Table 14.1 for women, Table 14.2 for men under age 40, and Table 14.3 for men over 40.

---

### Exercise 14.1 Calculating Your Percent Body Fat

Record your three skinfold readings, add them together, and enter the total value.

_____

_____

_____

―――――――

_____ Total of 3 skinfold readings

Using Tables 14.1, 14.2, or 14.3, determine your current percent body fat, according to your age and gender, and record it here:

_____ . _____ **%**

---

## Determining Your Classification

After finding out your percent body fat on Table 14.1, 14.2, or 14.3, you can determine your current body composition *classification* according to Table 14.4. In this table you will find the "health fitness" label and the "high physical fitness" label for percent fat standards. For example, the recommended health fitness fat percentage for a 20-year-old female is 28% or less. The health fitness standard is established at the point where there seems to be no detriment to health in terms of percent body fat. A high physical fitness range for this same woman is between 18% and 23%.

The high physical fitness standard does not mean that you cannot be somewhat below this number. As mentioned earlier, many highly trained athletes' measurements are below the percentages set. *The 3% essential fat for men and 12% for women are the lower limits for people to maintain good health.* Below these percentages, normal physiologic functions can be seriously impaired.

In addition, some experts point out that a little storage fat (over the essential fat) is better than none at all. As a result, the health and high fitness standards for percent fat in Table 14.4 are set higher than the minimum essential fat requirements, at a point conducive to optimal health and well-being. Also, because lean tissue decreases with age, one extra percentage point is allowed for every additional decade of life.

---

**Therefore, my current classification from Table 14.4 is:**

―――――――――――

---

## Table 14.1 Percent Fat Estimates for Women Calculated from Skinfold Thickness

| Sum of 3 Skinfolds | | | | Age to the Last Year | | | | |
|---|---|---|---|---|---|---|---|---|
| | Under 22 | 23 to 27 | 28 to 32 | 33 to 37 | 38 to 42 | 43 to 47 | 48 to 52 | 53 to 57 | Over 58 |
| 23–25 | 9.7 | 9.9 | 10.2 | 10.4 | 10.7 | 10.9 | 11.2 | 11.4 | 11.7 |
| 26–28 | 11.0 | 11.2 | 11.5 | 11.7 | 12.0 | 12.3 | 12.5 | 12.7 | 13.0 |
| 29–31 | 12.3 | 12.5 | 12.8 | 13.0 | 13.3 | 13.5 | 13.8 | 14.0 | 14.3 |
| 32–34 | 13.6 | 13.8 | 14.0 | 14.3 | 14.5 | 14.8 | 15.0 | 15.3 | 15.5 |
| 35–37 | 14.8 | 15.0 | 15.3 | 15.5 | 15.8 | 16.0 | 16.3 | 16.5 | 16.8 |
| 38–40 | 16.0 | 16.3 | 16.5 | 16.7 | 17.0 | 17.2 | 17.5 | 17.7 | 18.0 |
| 41–43 | 17.2 | 17.4 | 17.7 | 17.9 | 18.2 | 18.4 | 18.7 | 18.9 | 19.2 |
| 44–46 | 18.3 | 18.6 | 18.8 | 19.1 | 19.3 | 19.6 | 19.8 | 20.1 | 20.3 |
| 47–49 | 19.5 | 19.7 | 20.0 | 20.2 | 20.5 | 20.7 | 21.0 | 21.2 | 21.5 |
| 50–52 | 20.6 | 20.8 | 21.1 | 21.3 | 21.6 | 21.8 | 22.1 | 22.3 | 22.6 |
| 53–55 | 21.7 | 21.9 | 22.1 | 22.4 | 22.6 | 22.9 | 23.1 | 23.4 | 23.6 |
| 56–58 | 22.7 | 23.0 | 23.2 | 23.4 | 23.7 | 23.9 | 24.2 | 24.4 | 24.7 |
| 59–61 | 23.7 | 24.0 | 24.2 | 24.5 | 24.7 | 25.0 | 25.2 | 25.5 | 25.7 |
| 62–64 | 24.7 | 25.0 | 25.2 | 25.5 | 25.7 | 26.0 | 26.2 | 26.4 | 26.7 |
| 65–67 | 25.7 | 25.9 | 26.2 | 26.4 | 26.7 | 26.9 | 27.2 | 27.4 | 27.7 |
| 68–70 | 26.6 | 26.9 | 27.1 | 27.4 | 27.6 | 27.9 | 28.1 | 28.4 | 28.6 |
| 71–73 | 27.5 | 27.8 | 28.0 | 28.3 | 28.5 | 28.8 | 29.0 | 29.3 | 29.5 |
| 74–76 | 28.4 | 28.7 | 28.9 | 29.2 | 29.4 | 29.7 | 29.9 | 30.2 | 30.4 |
| 77–79 | 29.3 | 29.5 | 29.8 | 30.0 | 30.3 | 30.5 | 30.8 | 31.0 | 31.3 |
| 80–82 | 30.1 | 30.4 | 30.6 | 30.9 | 31.1 | 31.4 | 31.6 | 31.9 | 32.1 |
| 83–85 | 30.9 | 31.2 | 31.4 | 31.7 | 31.9 | 32.2 | 32.4 | 32.7 | 32.9 |
| 86–88 | 31.7 | 32.0 | 32.2 | 32.5 | 32.7 | 32.9 | 33.2 | 33.4 | 33.7 |
| 89–91 | 32.5 | 32.7 | 33.0 | 33.2 | 33.5 | 33.7 | 33.9 | 34.2 | 34.4 |
| 92–94 | 33.2 | 33.4 | 33.7 | 33.9 | 34.2 | 34.4 | 34.7 | 34.9 | 35.2 |
| 95–97 | 33.9 | 34.1 | 34.4 | 34.6 | 34.9 | 35.1 | 35.4 | 35.6 | 35.9 |
| 98–100 | 34.6 | 34.8 | 35.1 | 35.3 | 35.5 | 35.8 | 36.0 | 36.3 | 36.5 |
| 101–103 | 35.2 | 35.4 | 35.7 | 35.9 | 36.2 | 36.4 | 36.7 | 36.9 | 37.2 |
| 104–106 | 35.8 | 36.1 | 36.3 | 36.6 | 36.8 | 37.1 | 37.3 | 37.5 | 37.8 |
| 107–109 | 36.4 | 36.7 | 36.9 | 37.1 | 37.4 | 37.6 | 37.9 | 38.1 | 38.4 |
| 110–112 | 37.0 | 37.2 | 37.5 | 37.7 | 38.0 | 38.2 | 38.5 | 38.7 | 38.9 |
| 113–115 | 37.5 | 37.8 | 38.0 | 38.2 | 38.5 | 38.7 | 39.0 | 39.2 | 39.5 |
| 116–118 | 38.0 | 38.3 | 38.5 | 38.8 | 39.0 | 39.3 | 39.5 | 39.7 | 40.0 |
| 119–121 | 38.5 | 38.7 | 39.0 | 39.2 | 39.5 | 39.7 | 40.0 | 40.2 | 40.5 |
| 122–124 | 39.0 | 39.2 | 39.4 | 39.7 | 39.9 | 40.2 | 40.4 | 40.7 | 40.9 |
| 125–127 | 39.4 | 39.6 | 39.9 | 40.1 | 40.4 | 40.6 | 40.9 | 41.1 | 41.4 |
| 128–130 | 39.8 | 40.0 | 40.3 | 40.5 | 40.8 | 41.0 | 41.3 | 41.5 | 41.8 |

NOTE: Body density is calculated based on the generalized equation for predicting body density of women developed by A. S. Jackson, M. L. Pollock, and A. Ward and published in *Medicine and Science in Sports and Exercise* 12 (1980): 175–182. Percent body fat is determined from the calculated body density using the Siri formula. Hoeger and Hoeger, *Principles and Labs for Fitness and Wellness*, Wadsworth, Cengage Learning, 2002, reproduced with permission.

## Table 14.2 Percent Fat Estimates for Men under 40 Calculated from Skinfold Thickness

| Sum of 3 Skinfolds | | | | Age to the Last Year | | | |
|---|---|---|---|---|---|---|---|
| | Under 19 | 20 to 22 | 23 to 25 | 26 to 28 | 29 to 31 | 32 to 34 | 35 to 37 | 38 to 40 |
| 8–10 | .9 | 1.3 | 1.6 | 2.0 | 2.3 | 2.7 | 3.0 | 3.3 |
| 11–13 | 1.9 | 2.3 | 2.6 | 3.0 | 3.3 | 3.7 | 4.0 | 4.3 |
| 14–16 | 2.9 | 3.3 | 3.6 | 3.9 | 4.3 | 4.6 | 5.0 | 5.3 |
| 17–19 | 3.9 | 4.2 | 4.6 | 4.9 | 5.3 | 5.6 | 6.0 | 6.3 |
| 20–22 | 4.8 | 5.2 | 5.5 | 5.9 | 6.2 | 6.6 | 6.9 | 7.3 |
| 23–25 | 5.8 | 6.2 | 6.5 | 6.8 | 7.2 | 7.5 | 7.9 | 8.2 |
| 26–28 | 6.8 | 7.1 | 7.5 | 7.8 | 8.1 | 8.5 | 8.8 | 9.2 |
| 29–31 | 7.7 | 8.0 | 8.4 | 8.7 | 9.1 | 9.4 | 9.8 | 10.1 |
| 32–34 | 8.6 | 9.0 | 9.3 | 9.7 | 10.0 | 10.4 | 10.7 | 11.1 |
| 35–37 | 9.5 | 9.9 | 10.2 | 10.6 | 10.9 | 11.3 | 11.6 | 12.0 |
| 38–40 | 10.5 | 10.8 | 11.2 | 11.5 | 11.8 | 12.2 | 12.5 | 12.9 |
| 41–43 | 11.4 | 11.7 | 12.1 | 12.4 | 12.7 | 13.1 | 13.4 | 13.8 |
| 44–46 | 12.2 | 12.6 | 12.9 | 13.3 | 13.6 | 14.0 | 14.3 | 14.7 |
| 47–49 | 13.1 | 13.5 | 13.8 | 14.2 | 14.5 | 14.9 | 15.2 | 15.5 |
| 50–52 | 14.0 | 14.3 | 14.7 | 15.0 | 15.4 | 15.7 | 16.1 | 16.4 |
| 53–55 | 14.8 | 15.2 | 15.5 | 15.9 | 16.2 | 16.6 | 16.9 | 17.3 |
| 56–58 | 15.7 | 16.0 | 16.4 | 16.7 | 17.1 | 17.4 | 17.8 | 18.1 |
| 59–61 | 16.5 | 16.9 | 17.2 | 17.6 | 17.9 | 18.3 | 18.6 | 19.0 |
| 62–64 | 17.4 | 17.7 | 18.1 | 18.4 | 18.8 | 19.1 | 19.4 | 19.8 |
| 65–67 | 18.2 | 18.5 | 18.9 | 19.2 | 19.6 | 19.9 | 20.3 | 20.6 |
| 68–70 | 19.0 | 19.3 | 19.7 | 20.0 | 20.4 | 20.7 | 21.1 | 21.4 |
| 71–73 | 19.8 | 20.1 | 20.5 | 20.8 | 21.2 | 21.5 | 21.9 | 22.2 |
| 74–76 | 20.6 | 20.9 | 21.3 | 21.6 | 22.0 | 22.2 | 22.7 | 23.0 |
| 77–79 | 21.4 | 21.7 | 22.1 | 22.4 | 22.8 | 23.1 | 23.4 | 23.8 |
| 80–82 | 22.1 | 22.5 | 22.8 | 23.2 | 23.5 | 23.9 | 24.2 | 24.6 |
| 83–85 | 22.9 | 23.2 | 23.6 | 23.9 | 24.3 | 24.6 | 25.0 | 25.3 |
| 86–88 | 23.6 | 24.0 | 24.3 | 24.7 | 25.0 | 25.4 | 25.7 | 26.1 |
| 89–91 | 24.4 | 24.7 | 25.1 | 25.4 | 25.8 | 26.1 | 26.5 | 26.8 |
| 92–94 | 25.1 | 25.5 | 25.8 | 26.2 | 26.5 | 26.9 | 27.2 | 27.5 |
| 95–97 | 25.8 | 26.2 | 26.5 | 26.9 | 27.2 | 27.6 | 27.9 | 28.3 |
| 98–100 | 26.6 | 26.9 | 27.3 | 27.6 | 27.9 | 28.3 | 28.6 | 29.0 |
| 101–103 | 27.3 | 27.6 | 28.0 | 28.3 | 28.6 | 29.0 | 29.3 | 29.7 |
| 104–106 | 27.9 | 28.3 | 28.6 | 29.0 | 29.3 | 29.7 | 30.0 | 30.4 |
| 107–109 | 28.6 | 29.0 | 29.3 | 29.7 | 30.0 | 30.4 | 30.7 | 31.1 |
| 110–112 | 29.3 | 29.6 | 30.0 | 30.3 | 30.7 | 31.0 | 31.4 | 31.7 |
| 113–115 | 30.0 | 30.3 | 30.7 | 31.0 | 31.3 | 31.7 | 32.0 | 32.4 |
| 116–118 | 30.6 | 31.0 | 31.3 | 31.6 | 32.0 | 32.3 | 32.7 | 33.0 |
| 119–121 | 31.3 | 31.6 | 32.0 | 32.3 | 32.6 | 33.0 | 33.3 | 33.7 |
| 122–124 | 31.9 | 32.2 | 32.6 | 32.9 | 33.3 | 33.6 | 34.0 | 34.3 |
| 125–127 | 32.5 | 32.9 | 33.2 | 33.5 | 33.9 | 34.2 | 34.6 | 34.9 |
| 128–130 | 33.1 | 33.5 | 33.8 | 34.2 | 34.5 | 34.9 | 35.2 | 35.5 |

NOTE: Body density is calculated based on the generalized equation for predicting body density of men developed by A. S. Jackson and M. L. Pollock and published in the *British Journal of Nutrition* 40 (1978): 497–504. Percent body fat is determined from the calculated body density using the Siri formula. Hoeger and Hoeger, *Principles and Labs for Fitness and Wellness*, Wadsworth, Cengage Learning, 2002, reproduced with permission.

## Table 14.3    Percent Fat Estimates for Men Over 40 Calculated from Skinfold Thickness

| Sum of 3 Skin-folds | Age to the Last Year | | | | | | | |
|---|---|---|---|---|---|---|---|---|
| | 41 to 43 | 44 to 46 | 47 to 49 | 50 to 52 | 53 to 55 | 56 to 58 | 59 to 61 | Over 62 |
| 8–10 | 3.7 | 4.0 | 4.4 | 4.7 | 5.1 | 5.4 | 5.8 | 6.1 |
| 11–13 | 4.7 | 5.0 | 5.4 | 5.7 | 6.1 | 6.4 | 6.8 | 7.1 |
| 14–16 | 5.7 | 6.0 | 6.4 | 6.7 | 7.1 | 7.4 | 7.8 | 8.1 |
| 17–19 | 6.7 | 7.0 | 7.4 | 7.7 | 8.1 | 8.4 | 8.7 | 9.1 |
| 20–22 | 7.6 | 8.0 | 8.3 | 8.7 | 9.0 | 9.4 | 9.7 | 10.1 |
| 23–25 | 8.6 | 8.9 | 9.3 | 9.6 | 10.0 | 10.3 | 10.7 | 11.0 |
| 26–28 | 9.5 | 9.9 | 10.2 | 10.6 | 10.9 | 11.3 | 11.6 | 12.0 |
| 29–31 | 10.5 | 10.8 | 11.2 | 11.5 | 11.9 | 12.2 | 12.6 | 12.9 |
| 32–34 | 11.4 | 11.8 | 12.1 | 12.4 | 12.8 | 13.1 | 13.5 | 13.8 |
| 35–37 | 12.3 | 12.7 | 13.0 | 13.4 | 13.7 | 14.1 | 14.4 | 14.8 |
| 38–40 | 13.2 | 13.6 | 13.9 | 14.3 | 14.6 | 15.0 | 15.3 | 15.7 |
| 41–43 | 14.1 | 14.5 | 14.8 | 15.2 | 15.5 | 15.9 | 16.2 | 16.6 |
| 44–46 | 15.0 | 15.4 | 15.7 | 16.1 | 16.4 | 16.8 | 17.1 | 17.5 |
| 47–49 | 15.9 | 16.2 | 16.6 | 16.9 | 17.3 | 17.6 | 18.0 | 18.3 |
| 50–52 | 16.8 | 17.1 | 17.5 | 17.8 | 18.2 | 18.5 | 18.8 | 19.2 |
| 53–55 | 17.6 | 18.0 | 18.3 | 18.7 | 19.0 | 19.4 | 19.7 | 20.1 |
| 56–58 | 18.5 | 18.8 | 19.2 | 19.5 | 19.9 | 20.2 | 20.6 | 20.9 |
| 59–61 | 19.3 | 19.7 | 20.0 | 20.4 | 20.7 | 21.0 | 21.4 | 21.7 |
| 62–64 | 20.1 | 20.5 | 20.8 | 21.2 | 21.5 | 21.9 | 22.2 | 22.6 |
| 65–67 | 21.0 | 21.3 | 21.7 | 22.0 | 22.4 | 22.7 | 23.0 | 23.4 |
| 68–70 | 21.8 | 22.1 | 22.5 | 22.8 | 23.2 | 23.5 | 23.9 | 24.2 |
| 71–73 | 22.6 | 22.9 | 23.3 | 23.6 | 24.0 | 24.3 | 24.7 | 25.0 |
| 74–76 | 23.4 | 23.7 | 24.1 | 24.4 | 24.8 | 25.1 | 25.4 | 25.8 |
| 77–79 | 24.1 | 24.5 | 24.8 | 25.2 | 25.5 | 25.9 | 26.2 | 26.6 |
| 80–82 | 24.9 | 25.3 | 25.6 | 26.0 | 26.3 | 26.6 | 27.0 | 27.3 |
| 83–85 | 25.7 | 26.0 | 26.4 | 26.7 | 27.1 | 27.4 | 27.8 | 28.1 |
| 86–88 | 26.4 | 26.8 | 27.1 | 27.5 | 27.8 | 28.2 | 28.5 | 28.9 |
| 89–91 | 27.2 | 27.5 | 27.9 | 28.2 | 28.6 | 28.9 | 29.2 | 29.6 |
| 92–94 | 27.9 | 28.2 | 28.6 | 28.9 | 29.3 | 29.6 | 30.0 | 30.3 |
| 95–97 | 28.6 | 29.0 | 29.3 | 29.7 | 30.0 | 30.4 | 30.7 | 31.1 |
| 98–100 | 29.3 | 29.7 | 30.0 | 30.4 | 30.7 | 31.1 | 31.4 | 31.8 |
| 101–103 | 30.0 | 30.4 | 30.7 | 31.1 | 31.4 | 31.8 | 32.1 | 32.5 |
| 104–106 | 30.7 | 31.1 | 31.4 | 31.8 | 32.1 | 32.5 | 32.8 | 33.2 |
| 107–109 | 31.4 | 31.8 | 32.1 | 32.4 | 32.8 | 33.1 | 33.5 | 33.8 |
| 110–112 | 32.1 | 32.4 | 32.8 | 33.1 | 33.5 | 33.8 | 34.2 | 34.5 |
| 113–115 | 32.7 | 33.1 | 33.4 | 33.8 | 34.1 | 34.5 | 34.8 | 35.2 |
| 116–118 | 33.4 | 33.7 | 34.1 | 34.4 | 34.8 | 35.1 | 35.5 | 35.8 |
| 119–121 | 34.0 | 34.4 | 34.7 | 35.1 | 35.4 | 35.8 | 36.1 | 36.5 |
| 122–124 | 34.7 | 35.0 | 35.4 | 35.7 | 36.1 | 36.4 | 36.7 | 37.1 |
| 125–127 | 35.3 | 35.6 | 36.0 | 36.3 | 36.7 | 37.0 | 37.4 | 37.7 |
| 128–130 | 35.9 | 36.2 | 36.6 | 36.9 | 37.3 | 37.6 | 38.0 | 38.5 |

NOTE: Body density is calculated based on the generalized equation for predicting body density of men developed by A. S. Jackson and M. L. Pollock and published in the *British Journal of Nutrition* 40 (1978): 497–504. Percent body fat is determined from the calculated body density using the Siri formula. Hoeger and Hoeger, *Principles and Labs for Fitness and Wellness*, Wadsworth, Cengage Learning, 2002, reproduced with permission.

## *Table 14.4    Body Composition Classification According to Percent Body Fat*

| MEN | | | | | |
|---|---|---|---|---|---|
| **Age** | **Excellent** | **Good** | **Moderate** | **Overweight** | **Obese** |
| ≤19 | 12.0 | 12.1–17.0 | 17.1–22.0 | 22.1–27.0 | ≥27.1 |
| 20–29 | 13.0 | 13.1–18.0 | 18.1–23.0 | 23.1–28.0 | ≥28.1 |
| 30–39 | 14.0 | 14.1–19.0 | 19.1–24.0 | 24.1–29.0 | ≥29.1 |
| 40–49 | 15.0 | 15.1–20.0 | 20.1–25.0 | 25.1–30.0 | ≥30.1 |
| ≥50 | 16.0 | 16.1–21.5 | 21.1–26.0 | 26.1–31.0 | ≥31.1 |

| WOMEN | | | | | |
|---|---|---|---|---|---|
| **Age** | **Excellent** | **Good** | **Moderate** | **Overweight** | **Obese** |
| ≤19 | 17.0 | 17.1–22.0 | 22.1–27.0 | 27.1–32.0 | ≥32.1 |
| 20–29 | 18.0 | 18.1–23.0 | 23.1–28.0 | 28.1–33.0 | ≥33.1 |
| 30–39 | 19.0 | 19.1–24.0 | 24.1–29.0 | 29.1–34.0 | ≥34.1 |
| 40–49 | 20.0 | 20.1–25.0 | 25.1–30.0 | 30.1–35.0 | ≥35.1 |
| ≥50 | 21.0 | 21.1–26.5 | 26.1–31.0 | 31.1–36.0 | ≥36.1 |

▨ "High physical fitness" standard

▨ "Health fitness" standard

Source: *Principles & Labs for Physical Fitness & Wellness* by Werner W. K. Hoeger (Englewood, CO: Morton Publishing Company, 1994), p. 62.

To continue calculating your recommended body weight, first complete the Goal-Setting Challenge shown here. Then, place the percentage you chose on page 165, in Step 3 of Exercise 14.2 and complete the figuring of this exercise now.

---

### *Goal-Setting Challenge*

 Your recommended body weight is computed based on your choosing a "health" or a "high fitness" fat percentage for your respective age and gender. Your selection of a *desired/recommended fat percentage* should be based on:

- your current percent body fat; and
- your personal health-fitness goals and objectives.

Select your desired/*recommended* body *fat percentage* (RFP) from Table 14.4 based on your goals and the "health" or "high fitness" standards given. Express this percentage in decimal form:

● _____% (RFP) Goal    Place this percentage (decimal) on Step 3, Exercise 14.2.

## Exercise 14.2

### Determining Your
### Recommended Body Weight

### Calculate Here:

1. **Fat Weight:** Multiply your total body weight in pounds (BW) by the current percent fat (%F) you're carrying (see Tables 14.1, 14.2, and 14.3), expressing this percentage in decimal form. (BW × .____ %F). This is your *fat weight* (FW), the actual number of pounds of fat you now carry.

$$\underline{\quad} \times .\underline{\quad} = \underline{\quad}$$
(BW  ×  %F  =  FW)

2. **Lean Weight:** Subtract your fat weight (FW) from your total body weight (BW − FW). This is your current *lean weight* (LW).

$$\underline{\quad} - \underline{\quad} = \underline{\quad}$$
(BW  −  FW  =  LW)

3. Place your desired/*recommended fat percentage* (RFP) that you selected here (see Goal Setting Challenge in the chapter), expressing this percentage in decimal form.

$$.\underline{\qquad} \% \ (RFP)$$

4. **Recommended Weight:** To calculate your recommended weight, use the following formula: LW ÷ (1.0 − .RFP) = RW (Recommended Weight).

$$\underline{\quad} \div (1.0 - .\underline{\quad}) = \underline{\quad}$$
LW          RFP          RW

**GOAL:**  Subtract your recommended body weight from your current body weight (BW − RW). This tells you exactly how many pounds you'll goal-set to lose or gain. (Note: Positive numbers = weight to *lose*. Negative numbers = weight to *gain*.)

$$\underline{\quad} - RW = \underline{\qquad}$$
BW          Actual pounds
I'm setting a goal
to lose/gain.

---

*Example:* A 19-year-old female who weighs 136 pounds and is 25% fat would like to know what her recommended weight should be, with a "desired"/recommended fat percentage of 17%, which is the "high physical fitness" standard.

Gender:  female
Age:     19
BW:      136
%F:      25% (.25 in decimal form)
RFP:     17% (.17 in decimal form)

- FW = BW × %F
  FW = 136 × .25 = 34 lbs.
- LW = BW − FW
  LW = 136 − 34 = 102 lbs.
- RFP: 17% (.17 in decimal form)
- RW = LW ÷ (1.0 − .RFP)
  RW = 102 ÷ (1.0 − .17)
  RW = 102 ÷ (.83) = 122.9 lbs.*

*Recommended Body Weight

**Goal-Set Timeframe
to Lose/Gain Weight:**

$$\underline{\qquad\qquad} /pounds$$
1 week

$$\underline{\qquad\qquad} /pounds$$
1 month

$$\underline{\qquad\qquad} /pounds$$
3 month

$$\underline{\qquad\qquad} /pounds$$
6 month

$$\underline{\qquad\qquad} /pounds$$
1 year

**GOAL:**  To reach her recommended body weight, she'll set a goal to lose 13.1 pounds of fat weight (subtracting *recommended body weight from current weight (136 − 122.9 = 13.1).

## Determining Your Recommended Weight by Calculating Body Mass Index

### Exercise 14.3 Calculating Adult BMI[3]

**Directions:** Locate your height (listed in feet and inches) in the left-most column. Read across the row for that height, to your weight (listed in pounds). Follow the column of your weight up to the top row, which lists the BMI. Note: BMI of 18.5–24.9 is *healthy* weight range; BMI of 25–29.9 is *overweight* range; BMI of 30 and above is *obese* range.

| BMI➡ ⬇Height | 19 | 20 | 21 | 22 | 23 | 24 | 25 | 26 | 27 | 28 | 29 | 30 | 31 | 32 | 33 | 34 | 35 |
|---|---|---|---|---|---|---|---|---|---|---|---|---|---|---|---|---|---|
| | | | | | | | Weight in Pounds | | | | | | | | | | |
| 4'10" | 91 | 96 | 100 | 105 | 110 | 115 | 119 | 124 | 129 | 134 | 138 | 143 | 148 | 153 | 158 | 162 | 167 |
| 4'11" | 94 | 99 | 104 | 109 | 114 | 119 | 124 | 128 | 133 | 138 | 143 | 148 | 153 | 158 | 163 | 168 | 173 |
| 5' | 97 | 102 | 107 | 112 | 118 | 123 | 128 | 133 | 138 | 143 | 148 | 153 | 158 | 163 | 168 | 174 | 179 |
| 5'1" | 100 | 106 | 111 | 116 | 122 | 127 | 132 | 137 | 143 | 148 | 153 | 158 | 164 | 169 | 174 | 180 | 185 |
| 5'2" | 104 | 109 | 115 | 120 | 126 | 131 | 136 | 142 | 147 | 153 | 158 | 164 | 169 | 175 | 180 | 186 | 191 |
| 5'3" | 107 | 113 | 118 | 124 | 130 | 135 | 141 | 146 | 152 | 158 | 163 | 169 | 175 | 180 | 186 | 191 | 197 |
| 5'4" | 110 | 116 | 122 | 128 | 134 | 140 | 145 | 151 | 157 | 163 | 169 | 174 | 180 | 186 | 192 | 197 | 204 |
| 5'5" | 114 | 120 | 126 | 132 | 138 | 144 | 150 | 156 | 162 | 168 | 174 | 180 | 186 | 192 | 198 | 204 | 210 |
| 5'6" | 118 | 124 | 130 | 136 | 142 | 148 | 155 | 161 | 167 | 173 | 179 | 186 | 192 | 198 | 204 | 210 | 216 |
| 5'7" | 121 | 127 | 134 | 140 | 146 | 153 | 159 | 166 | 172 | 178 | 185 | 191 | 198 | 204 | 211 | 217 | 223 |
| 5'8" | 125 | 131 | 138 | 144 | 151 | 158 | 164 | 171 | 177 | 184 | 190 | 197 | 203 | 210 | 216 | 223 | 230 |
| 5'9" | 128 | 135 | 142 | 149 | 155 | 162 | 169 | 176 | 182 | 189 | 196 | 203 | 209 | 216 | 223 | 230 | 236 |
| 5'10" | 132 | 139 | 146 | 153 | 160 | 167 | 174 | 181 | 188 | 195 | 202 | 209 | 216 | 222 | 229 | 236 | 243 |
| 5'11" | 136 | 143 | 150 | 157 | 165 | 172 | 179 | 186 | 193 | 200 | 208 | 215 | 222 | 229 | 236 | 243 | 250 |
| 6' | 140 | 147 | 154 | 162 | 169 | 177 | 184 | 191 | 199 | 206 | 213 | 221 | 228 | 235 | 242 | 250 | 258 |
| 6'1" | 144 | 151 | 159 | 166 | 174 | 182 | 189 | 197 | 204 | 212 | 219 | 227 | 235 | 242 | 250 | 257 | 265 |
| 6'2" | 148 | 155 | 163 | 171 | 179 | 186 | 194 | 202 | 210 | 218 | 225 | 233 | 241 | 249 | 256 | 264 | 272 |
| 6'3" | 152 | 160 | 168 | 176 | 184 | 192 | 200 | 208 | 216 | 224 | 232 | 240 | 248 | 256 | 264 | 272 | 279 |
| | Healthy Weight | | | | | | Overweight | | | | | | Obese | | | | |

Source: Evidence Report of Clinical Guidelines on the Identification, Evaluation, and Treatment of Overweight and Obesity in Adults, 1998. NIH/National Heart, Lung, and Blood Institute (NHLBI).

## Achieving a Healthy Slimness

We seem to admit readily that a primary goal in taking fitness courses is to appear healthy and slim. We desire this goal because we can see directly when our body looks nice, lean, and toned; likewise, we can see directly when it looks out of shape and flabby. Many individuals, therefore, focus initially on a form of fitness or being in shape that they can readily see.

Your outer appearance, however, is not the entire, or even major, focus of a quality fitness program. You can live without well-toned muscles or a trim figure, but you can't live very long without a strong heart and lungs. Looking attractive and feeling good about your appearance are good ancillary goals (Figure 14.3). The key word, however, is *healthy* slimness.

To review your current understanding of healthy slimness, turn to Exercise 14.4, Establishing a Weight Wellness Mindset, at the end of the chapter. Be honest with yourself. How do you picture, feel, and talk to yourself about weight management, eating/drinking, and exercising? This survey will help you formulate a starting point to begin a weight management mental training program.

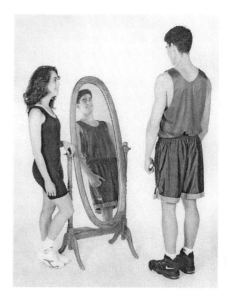

**Figure 14.3** Outer Appearance, a Secondary Goal

## Goals of Weight Management

Weight management means controlling the amount of body fat in relation to the amount of lean tissue. Weight management includes:

1. *Weight maintenance* (keeping the same ratio of fat to amount of lean you're currently carrying).

2. *Weight gain* (almost always in terms of lean weight gain, not fat weight gain).

3. *Weight loss* (always in terms of loss of body fat).

## Weight Maintenance

Weight maintenance is the goal when your current body composition of fat to lean tissue is ideal for your best cardiovascular and respiratory health and you are pleased with how you look. You have enough strength to function well in your daily life of work and recreation, whatever that may encompass. To remain at this constant weight, your energy must be in balance:

calories in (eating) =
calories out (exercise).

Calculate the calories for your weight maintenance on Exercise 14.5. Because "calories out" declines with aging (your metabolism slows down and you are less active), a decline in "calories in" (eating less) must accompany the aging processes.

## Weight Gain

Weight gain almost always refers to gaining *lean* tissue, or thickening muscle fiber. When you want to look better aesthetically or to increase your strength for a sport or for daily needs, weight training is the type of activity in which to engage. If you are overfat, to *gain lean weight and lose extra body fat* simultaneously will require you to eat less while providing *more exercise* through weight training. Only if you are at recommended

---

## Exercise 14.5
## Calculating Weight Maintenance

1. Record your present weight, in pounds.

2. Record your lifestyle. Number values are:
   12 = sedentary
   15 = active physically
   18 = pregnant/nursing
   20 = varsity athlete or physical laborer

3. Multiply (1) × (2).

This is your weight maintenance number, or the number of calories per day you need to eat to *stay* at your current weight.

_____ (1) weight

× _____ (2) lifestyle
_____

_____ Calories for Weight Maintenance

Source: *The Aerobic Way*, by Kenneth H. Cooper (New York: Evans & Co. 1977), p. 142.

---

weight or underfat weight should you accompany this weight-gain program with an increase in caloric intake.[4]

Weight gain, then, means increasing muscle mass, or thickening of muscle fibers. You do not gain more muscle cells; you thicken what you presently have.

Here are four points from the research professionals that will encourage you to consider a *lean weight gain* program, either by itself, or in conjunction with a fat weight loss program:

1. "Strength training to gain lean weight has many benefits, but the one that is the most underappreciated is its impact on metabolism. Under proper conditions (adequate calorie intake and proper exercise program design), strength training will develop muscle. *Your muscle is the primary control of your metabolism. The more muscle you have, the more fat you will burn.*"[5]

2. A widely respected strength training researcher states, "People need to understand the importance of replacing muscle and increasing their metabolism as at least one part of the process of maintaining and reaching a healthy body weight. In addition to endurance exercise and proper nutrition, I promote strength training due to its metabolic benefit. Research from Tufts University indicates that if you replace about three pounds of muscle, you will increase your metabolic rate by about 7% which reverses about 14 years of the aging process."[6]

3. "An underlying reason people struggle with weight management is a drop in lean body mass as they age. This decrease in lean body mass is directly correlated with a five percent drop in metabolic rate for each decade a person lives. We can reverse the loss of lean body mass and in conjunction reverse the drop

in our metabolism through strength training. The additional lean body mass created through strength training creates a solid foundation of weight management."[7]

4. "If men and women who want to get in shape cut back calories too far and overemphasize cardiovascular exercise, their body will have no choice but to burn muscle as fuel. Since their body will cannibalize their own muscle tissue, lean body mass will drop, metabolic rate will drop, fat loss will plateau, and they will not reach their long term fitness goal . . . That's the science of it."[8]

## Weight Loss

Weight loss refers to purposefully losing *fat weight*, never lean weight. The weight loss, of course, can be both lean and fat, depending on how you go about losing the weight. Before you spend your money on any unique new weight-reduction plan, claim, product, device, or book, call your local Better Business Bureau. If you completely understand the principles of weight loss, you will be able to determine a product's or a program's worth before you spend time, money, and energy on it. Weight-loss principles are as follows.

1. *Fat weight is the only kind of weight to lose.* If a product or program claims to "get rid of excess body fluids," beware! Body fluids are not fat. Unnatural water retention, *edema*, is a condition to be monitored and treated by a doctor, not by self-prescribed procedures or products.

2. *If water weight (fluid) is lost by sweating during exercise, it should and will return in 24 hours* to maintain the body's chemical balance. The energy-producing (metabolic) processes perform best when all of the necessary components are present. Dropping water weight is not effective weight loss. It is part of the fat-free weight and is vital to continuous

well-being. You can understand, then, why weighing yourself after a strenuous exercise session will produce inaccurate results.

3. *Fat is metabolized more readily and efficiently by performing moderate-intensity exercise for a long time.* If you are able to work continuously at a moderate intensity (lower end of your training zone) for more than 30 minutes, you will tap into the most physiologically sound way to metabolize (burn off) unwanted body fat. You need to exercise for *more than 30 minutes at a time, to make significant changes in the fat content of the body.*

To maximize metabolic efficiency, increase one, two, or all three of the aerobic exercise criteria: *frequency*, *intensity*, and *time duration*. Refer to Chapter 1 to determine what the safe maximum levels of each criterion are for you to use.

Wearing rubber suits, transparent plastic wrap around body parts, or heavy, long-sleeved sweats, pantyhose, or tights on hot days inhibits the free flow of sweat and does not allow it to perform its function of cooling. In hot and humid settings, wear as little as possible when performing fitness exercises. You cannot metabolize (burn up) fat faster by wearing more clothes.

4. *Fat burns off your body in a general way.* You can't "spot-reduce." Spot-reducing is perhaps the most prevalent misconception concerning fat-weight loss. Many unscrupulous people are defrauding unsuspecting overfat Americans out of millions of dollars every year.

By your genetic constitution, your body will use up its stored energy (fat) any way it is programmed to do. You cannot do 50 leg lifts a day and hope to reduce the fat deposits in the area. You will shape up (thicken) the muscle fiber in the area, and toned muscles contain more of the enzymes involved in breaking down fat, but you do not burn off the fat there or at any spe-

cific location. As energy is needed, it is withdrawn first from the immediate sources, and when this is used up, randomly from more permanent storage. It then is converted to an immediate usable form. Thus, at first you may lose weight in places you don't necessarily wish to, such as your face or chest/breast area. With perseverance, however, you'll burn off the fat in problem areas, too.

5. *Loss of fat weight is accomplished most readily through a combined program of monitoring your food intake carefully and exercising aerobically.* When you monitor food intake (and eat less) and exercise (expend more calories or energy), you lose almost 100% fat. This is the only kind of weight you want to lose. Exercise speeds weight loss by burning calories while you're working out, and also by revitalizing your metabolism so you continue to burn calories more readily for the next few hours.

Losing fat weight by simply eating less food is difficult. If you avoid exercise and severely restrict your food intake only, the weight loss is not just fat. According to the way in which you have "dieted," your weight loss is approximately one-half to two-thirds fat loss and *one-third to one-half lean weight loss.* If your lifestyle and habits of eating and exercising don't change after you stop dieting and you gain back your lost weight, what you gain back is all fat. You are worse off because you lost both fat and lean tissue and regained only fat.

Over a lifetime of "yo-yo" crash dieting, the entire body composition changes to your detriment. You can lose fat weight in many ways but the only way to *keep* fat weight off is by following a regular exercise program.[9]

6. *Weight can be both gained and lost through an endurance exercise program.* You will be burning off fat for energy and building up muscle simultaneously. Therefore,

if you do not see a change on the scale immediately, don't be disappointed.

7. *A light exercise program tends to increase appetite, and a strenuous exercise program decreases appetite.* After an endurance (aerobic) hour, the desire for food diminishes greatly. You will have time to carefully select or prepare what you know is good for you rather than ravenously grab that easy, high-calorie food (see Chapter 13) sitting around.

8. *Eating less food is easier than exercising it off.* In most high-intensity fitness sessions, you will burn only about 300 calories. If you are seriously interested in losing extra fat weight, think twice about rewarding yourself with high-calorie treats afterward. Instead, replenish your water loss with noncaloric, yet quite filling, ice water.

9. *Low calorie dieting does not work for the long term* because it drops a person's metabolism like a rock! You want to counteract this result by properly "fueling your furnace." Remember, the bigger the furnace (the more lean weight you develop), the more calories you'll burn, and the easier and more efficient becomes your fat weight loss.

10. *There is no such thing as a constipated endurance aerobic exerciser or athlete.* Regular, rhythmic stimulation of the entire digestion and elimination processes is one of the side benefits of aerobic exercise.

11. *The body's energy balance determines whether a person gains or loses body fat.* Proper weight loss is the result of *taking in less caloric energy and expending more.*

12. Stress and your waistline: stress may be making you fat![10] There's growing evidence that chronic stress can make you thick

around the middle. Here are five key points that are interesting researchers:

- Basically, people gain weight because they consume more calories than they burn.
- Research is now suggesting that gaining belly fat may be the body's *coping mechanism* for turning off the stress response. As one accumulates more belly fat, stress hormone levels went down; the higher the belly fat, the lower the stress hormones.[11]
- Stress plays a role in weight gain. Research shows that "night-eating syndrome" (a problem that causes sufferers to binge eat) is linked to high stress hormones.[12]
- The stress-fat link does suggest that many of the nation's dieters are missing out on a key component of weight management, if they aren't also trying to manage their stress.[13]
- Exercise is an obvious way to manage stress, but even less strenuous options—like yoga, meditation or massage—may be useful in a weight-loss program. "One of the things people miss is that exercise not only burns calories, but it changes the way you respond to stress, which may be one of the reasons why exercise is important, and under appreciated. Stress management might be the one weight loss strategy that society hasn't really addressed."[14]

## *Weight-Loss Strategies*

The challenge involved in losing weight may involve the need for any of the following: (a) gaining a better self-image, (b) instituting a naturally slender eating strategy, (c) learning effective ways to become motivated and make decisions, (d) resolving a

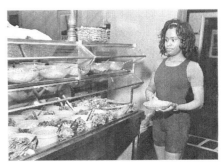

**Figure 14.4** Creating Future-Tense Pictures, Self-Talk, and Feelings

phobic response to childhood abuse, (e) learning better social skills, or (f) learning better coping skills.[15]

## ◆ "Naturally Slender" Eating

Naturally slender and overweight individuals differ in their mental images and self-talk concerning food. Overweight people usually construct *present-tense* pictures and self-talk. They see, smell, hear, or experience food, and state internally, "Boy, am I hungry!" The result is that they eat immediately. They focus only on the moment as they eat.

Naturally thin people usually do not have this present-tense strategy. Instead they create *future-tense* pictures, self-talk, and feelings. They experience how they'll feel over time[16]. Naturally slender people, as they approach a restaurant food bar (see Figure 14.4) or order from a menu, *determine ahead of time how they choose to feel when they are all finished eating.* This proactive, plan-ahead approach can be the difference between being naturally slender or being overweight for a lifetime.

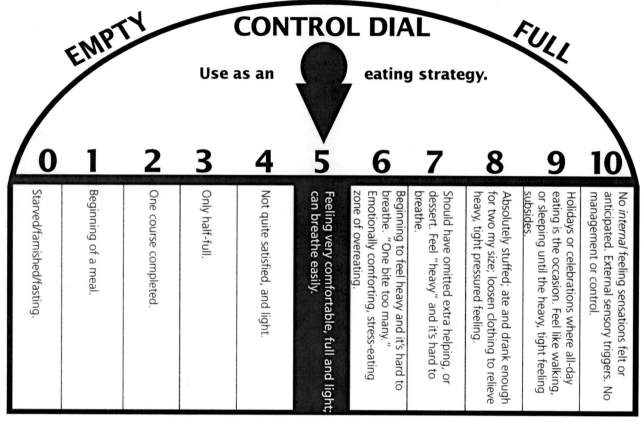

**Figure 14.5** Control Panel for Eating Strategy

## ◆ Control Panel with One Large Dial

A control panel, such as the one introduced in Chapter 12, can be used as an eating strategy (Figure 14.5) to reflect how "empty" or "full" you feel:

— before you eat;

— during the meal;

— when you're done eating.

First, you have to "go inside" where your hunger cues are. Predetermine how empty or full you are. Give that feeling a number from 0 to 10 and an accompanying label.

Then, when selecting and eating food, adjust your control panel to how you feel currently, how you choose to feel while eating, and how you choose to feel when you're done eating and drinking. Add this feeling sense to the three days of monitoring your eating and beverage intake, at the end of Chapter 13, in Exercise 13.2. This is also key information to record in your Fitness Journal.

### Caloric Expenditure

Every moment of every day, no matter what activity you engage in, from sleeping to aerobic exercise, you are using up calories. Caloric energy expenditure is influenced most by how physically active you are all day. The body's basic needs are more or less fixed, but the amount of physical exertion is a personal decision.

How physically active your life is depends on your choices of profession and recreational activities. It depends upon a multitude of day-to-day choices: whether to walk to the local store or drive the car; use the stairs or elevator; rake the leaves or hire someone to do it; go out for a bicycle ride after dinner or watch a TV show. How physically active your life is depends as much on attitude as it does on opportunity.[17]

### Caloric Expenditures for Various Activities

How many calories you burn per minute during any activity depends upon two criteria:

1. *Intensity* (high-, medium-, or low-level work or exercise)

2. *Body weight*

The higher the intensity, the more calories you burn per minute. For example, you expend more energy and calories running a mile than you do walking that mile. The more you weigh, the more calories per minute you will burn (just as full-size cars burn more fuel per mile than small, compact models).

## Caloric Intake Needed to Gain Lean Weight

Adequate muscle is a long-term key component to a healthy metabolism that burns fat. It also keeps us looking "toned" and protects us from injury. You'll notice you will "tone up" before you "bulk up."[18]

To add 1 pound of body muscle requires 2500 calories. (This includes about 600 calories for the muscle and the extra energy needed for exercise to develop the muscle.) Thus, the daily caloric excess, over your maintenance number just figured, is 360.[19] You must be at or below your recommended weight to go on an excess calorie-eating program to gain muscle. You want to use your excess body fat first for your energy requirements.

*To gain 1 pound of muscle:*

2500 calories equivalent to 1 pound of muscle

÷ 7 days in a week

= 360 daily excess calories to eat over your maintenance intake number

Taking in more than 1000 calories per day over the number needed to maintain weight, however, is likely to result in weight gain as body fat even if you are exercising strenuously on a regular basis.[20]

Since your nutrition is at least 50% responsible for a toned "ripped" look, start with a firm foundation—eat lean protein, complex carbohydrates, and fibrous vegetables to build muscle mass.

## Caloric Intake Needed to Lose Body Fat

To lose more than 2 to 3 pounds of body fat per week is physiologically impossible.[21] Weight loss greater than this is in the form of water and lean body tissue. To drop unwanted extra body fat systematically, you need to drop 3500 calories a week. This translates into 500 per day, to lose one pound of body fat per week, or 250 per day to lose one-half pound per week.

*To lose 1 pound fat:*

3500 calories

÷ 7 days per week

= 500 calories a day fewer than your maintenance number

If you desire to drop more pounds per week but the total caloric intake would be less than 1200, you need to reestablish your goal to lose only 1 pound per week. You never want to eat fewer than 1200 calories per day. A daily diet of fewer than 1200 calories is likely to be deficient in needed nutrients for you to grow, repair, stay well, and have energy to perform daily tasks and leisure. Sometimes, on a one-to-one basis, a doctor will have a patient eat fewer than 1200 calories per day but will provide extensive guidelines and supplementation. This should be done only under the strict supervision of a doctor.

"An ideal program is one that assists you to lose 3 to 5 lbs. of fat and gain 2 to 3 lbs. of lean weight (muscle) the first month. On the bathroom scales, it will reflect 1 to 2 lbs. a month weight loss. *This* is the right way to do it!"[22] It means that your metabolism will actually *be higher after the month.*[23] Fad diets cannot do this for you. It requires eating a balanced diet of wholesome foods along with moderate amounts of proper exercise.

## Successful Weight Loss Accomplished In Record Time!

Throughout this *Fourth Edition,* you have been given great ideas to consider and powerful educational tools to implement into your journey toward total fitness. Here now are *"10 Rules for Successful Weight Loss Accomplished in Record Time!"* to begin using *daily,* and continue *for just* 10 *to* 15 *weeks.* At the conclusion of this time, if you like these new patterns and are enjoying the results you're getting, continue on with them as long as they continue to serve you. Some of these ideas are new; others have been presented in earlier chapters of this text. Many of these ideas have been recently published in other noted authors' works, with great success reported from their clients.[24] Make the commitment to yourself to begin using all 10 rules, today! Of course, moderation in healthy eating, combined with your weight-loss specific *exercise* program,* are additional catalysts that boost the success of these 10 easy rules.

*Includes exercising for 60-90 minutes, continuously, using moderate intensity, low/no impact movement, 4–7 days per week.

### 1. Establish a Time to Stop Eating. Determine a *time of day* to complete all hunger-cued eating and drinking beverages. Commit not to eat and drink anything after this hour. [This 'beverage drinking' does *not* include plain water.] Select one of these times: 7:00 p.m./7:30 p.m./ 8:00 p.m.—and at this time each day you'll stop eating all food and drinking beverages. Make it a cut-off time that is at least 2 hours, or more, before your regular bedtime.

**2. Begin at the Starting Gate: Eat a Great Breakfast!** Establish the routine of eating a nutritional and filling breakfast each morning. This provides your system with that initial boost of energy *to get your metabolism moving each day, burning those calories!* Each morning, consider eating breakfasts that provide only nutrient dense foods, selecting at least one favorite food from each of the five food groups. Remember to include lean protein (chicken, fish) sources because proteins support your metabolism and help you retain muscle during a weight loss program.[25] Early morning fuel provides the jumpstart your metabolism requires, after awakening from 6-8 hours of sleep, when your metabolism and calorie burning was also at rest. When you've stopped eating at your designated evening cut-off time, you'll be *ready* to eat and 'break the fast' when you arise!

Then, a great eating plan to consider for the remainder of your day if your goal is fat weight loss and lean weight gain consists of all of the following points:

- six meals per day; we get a metabolic boost every time we eat;

- include lean protein at each meal; there is a positive thermogenic (heat producing) effect from proteins;

- minimum of refined sugars ("empty calories");

- include a vegetable or fruit each meal (a good source of fiber, vitamins, minerals as well as helping to minimize any acidity created by protein intake).

- a starchy carbohydrate or piece of fruit each meal (allows for an increase carbohydrate intake, so that you have sufficient energy to train hard);

- guard against eating too few calories. A diet that is too low in calories *slows your metabolism* and ends up making it harder to reach your twin goals of losing fat weight and gaining lean weight.[26]

**3. Journal Your Daily Progress.** Monitor and record your food/beverage consumption for 60-70 days. See Chapter 13 for an easy-to-use food/beverage monitoring chart. After the 1-3 days of monitoring in the text, have your Instructor review your monitoring before you continue for 60-70 days, to be sure you're on track. Next, record all of the columns and headings* into a pocket-sized journal. Write your entries as you consume nourishment during the day. Research has proven that if you monitor food/beverage intake by daily journalizing all consumption, it can be another key to successful weight loss in record time. [27] And, if you choose to continue to monitor and journal after the recommended 10-15 weeks, especially over holidays, you'll ensure continued weight loss, instead of the classic '500% holiday weight gain.'[28]

*Note: Consider journalizing these four practical ideas, all of which have already been presented in this textbook, earlier in this chapter, or in Chapter 13. *They are also the basic tools to teach small children how to eat healthfully:*

1. Understand and mention when recording your self-talk, how the nutrients you are consuming are working for your body (milk provides strong bones and teeth, to enable me to perform my fitness moves and smile doing them).

2. Stay connected to your body signals of hunger, and eat accordingly: '0' empty on the dial -to-'4' almost full; '5' full and satisfied; '6'overate -to-'10' stuffed.

3. Separate hunger from other feelings like boredom, sadness, or anxiety. Know your hunger cues and how they feel.

4. Develop the skill to make smart decisions around food. Manage the desire to make your 'tongue happy' with cravings, to making rational and realistic choices considering what each choice will mean for you[29] (right amount = proper energy, growth and devel-

opment; too much = extra body fat stored and risk factors increase; too little = lack of energy, lack of growth and development).

**4. Eat to Satisfy Only Physical Hunger Cues.** All other cues are considered emotional or comfort eating. Eating food or consuming beverages in order to suppress a negatively experienced life event from the past, or to fill a void left by a great loss, never fills *that* kind of 'emptiness.' Wait to eat until you *feel physically empty* and in need of nourishment (those stomach-growling, empty tank sensations). Your eating and drinking is completed at a meal when you then register "5" on the Control Panel with One Large Dial— Used as an Eating Strategy, provided earlier in this Chapter.

**5. Continuously Hydrate with Plain Water.** Drink 64 ounces of plain water every day. To regulate this routine, fill a 64-ounce plastic bottle with your day's supply, then pour it into an 8- or 16- ounce plastic bottle and carry this with you. Replenish the small bottle from your main container. Or, consider drinking a half-cup of water every waking hour. Begin with lesser amounts and work up to the recommended amount, if it is difficult to consume this volume in the beginning.

**6. Eliminate Alcohol for 60 days.** Alcohol slows down metabolism, when you are purposefully trying to *speed it up* on a daily basis! It consists of calories that provide energy and very few nutrients. If this energy is not expended it is, of course, stored as body fat. Many times it is regularly consumed for emotional comfort after the 'stop eating/drinking' hour you've selected (in Rule #1), so it is no longer a viable choice anyway. And, it negatively affects your judgment and decision-making ability. At a time when you have made a commitment to achieve weight loss in record time, you don't need cloudy judgment and decision making to take over, when you're in eating and drinking environments that regularly pressure you to participate in over consumption in order to socially 'fit in.' Instead, abstain from alcohol use and enjoy the role of 'designated driver'!

### 7. Speak Positive Self-Talk—Reframe Your Negative Talk.

Listen to yourself talking internally, and when you hear the negatives pop up concerning these 10 rules, *reframe* the thoughts immediately into being positive, nurturing, staying the course, and keeping the goal of successful weight loss in record time! Correcting negative, disabling thoughts ("How can I *ever* give up alcohol and my *beloved* midnight snack?") immediately into making confident statements like, "I really *enjoy* the new disciplined eating pattern I am following, which stops all of my eating and drinking beverages after 7:30 p.m.!", provides the internal support you need.

### 8. Consider Your Eating Environment.

Choose to sit, relax to your favorite soothing music and candlelight, and provide at least 20 minutes of quiet time to eat your meal, savoring each bite, every time you eat. In this way, you can be purposeful and conscious about *what* and *how much* you eat, *feeling* and *listening to* the internalized Control Panel with One Large Dial within your head. Hearing, "I am at the '3' and that reflects I am still hungry" or, "I have reached the '5' and that reflects I am now registering *'full'* and need to immediately stop eating food and drinking beverages" can be very powerful to experience at mealtime. When you control your eating environment, it helps to slow down the eating process and makes following these 10 rules a fun and an enjoyable experience.

### 9. Replace Emotional Eating with Another Type of Comfort or Passion.

Exercise! Read! Volunteer! Consider this: How do I enjoy releasing my stress? What activity am I *passionate* about doing? What are my talents, hobbies, collections? How do I express my talents when I volunteer? As you either get moving and exercise, or divert your mind and emotions to engaging in your favorite stress outlets, you'll be replacing the emotional feelings of loneliness, boredom, depression, and anger that trigger emotional eating, and begin focusing now on emotionally fulfilling activities that help you express your giftedness. This helps everyone! It can provide personal gain for you in a number of ways, and help is always well received by others when their needs are being met.

### 10. Enjoy Relaxation: Morning, Noon or Night.

When you awaken in the morning, take the first 3 minutes of your day to first, feel your pulse for a full minute, noting if it is continuing to lower on a regular basis. Then talk to yourself with your favorite phrase, to awaken your body to an alert status ("It is so great to be *alive* today!"). Finally, review your day as to what's on your mental calendar's 'to-do' list. At mid-day when a 10-minute break becomes available, practice imagery that focuses on your new emerging figure/physique, how you are now committed to these 10 rules and how you're choosing to look. Get very clear mental pictures and feelings about the *results* you are choosing and the positive choices you are making during each day, to enable those images and feelings to happen. At the end of your day after you have gotten into bed, select one of the numerous relaxation techniques presented here in Chapter 12 and enjoy putting a peaceful closure to the day. Conclude with a new imaging technique that you've now created that specifically clarifies your using all ten of these rules for eating your meals and snacks, and drinking water. These rules all become programmed patterns into your mental makeup *when you regularly repeat them*, either by your daily actions and choices, or by imaging the new patterns while in a deeply relaxed state. With these images on your mind as you drop off each night, even while you're sleeping, your mind can remain focused on achieving your weight-loss goal, in record time!

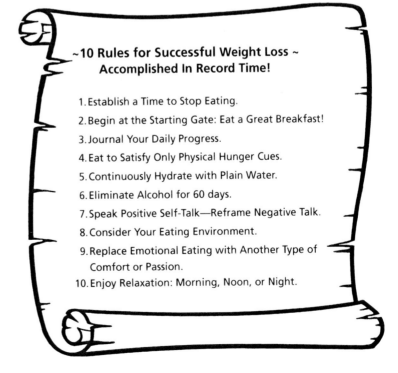

~ 10 Rules for Successful Weight Loss ~
**Accomplished In Record Time!**

1. Establish a Time to Stop Eating.
2. Begin at the Starting Gate: Eat a Great Breakfast!
3. Journal Your Daily Progress.
4. Eat to Satisfy Only Physical Hunger Cues.
5. Continuously Hydrate with Plain Water.
6. Eliminate Alcohol for 60 days.
7. Speak Positive Self-Talk—Reframe Negative Talk.
8. Consider Your Eating Environment.
9. Replace Emotional Eating with Another Type of Comfort or Passion.
10. Enjoy Relaxation: Morning, Noon, or Night.

## In Short—

To maintain a specific weight, caloric input must equal caloric output. To gain or lose weight requires an imbalance of energy in your eating and exercising lifestyle habits. Weight management involves:

- Assessing your weight

- Getting involved in programs that can assist you in weight management

- Reviewing your time priorities and setting short- and long-range goals to achieve or maintain your recommended weight

Educating yourself about how to manage your weight will help you understand how the human body works and how it does not work physiologically. Then you can be alert to all of the false notions, especially regarding weight loss, that are rampant today. Equipped with accurate information, you can develop a program that will work for you for a lifetime!

---

### Goal-Setting Challenge

  Set a goal to become more aware of your thinking and actions regarding your body composition or self-image—what may be taking up a lot of your mental energy at present. Convert your wishes into small, continual, conscious choices. Write a weight management goal for Chapter 14, first following the four steps presented in Chapter 2, Exercise 2.3, then recording it in your Fitness Journal.

## *Exercise 14.4* *Establishing a Weight-Wellness Mindset*[30]

Change can be exciting! If you are ready to improve your body composition and establish a healthy slimness, change must *begin* at the internal motivational sensory level (see Chapter 2). Assess how you have thought about weight management, eating, and exercising. Is it the "diet-thinking" mentality that is basically *pain*-motivated? Or is it the pleasure-based weight-wellness mindset? Reflect on the following challenges and check where your mindset is now, by *circling the bullet(s)* that reflect your thinking in each challenge category. Set goals to reframe your thinking and actions to a more positive mindset.

### "Diet" Thinking versus "Weight-Wellness" Mindset

| "Diet" Thinking | Challenge | Weight-Wellness Mindset |
|---|---|---|
| ■ Any weight loss as measured on scales that society/others think I should lose<br><br>■ Achieve body image determined by society | GOAL | ■ Personal self-confidence in my ability to continually make the best choices from available food options<br>■ Wellness/balance is my choice of lifestyle |
| ■ Any *rapid* weight loss is acceptable — fat weight OR lean weight | PROGRESS/ PROCESS | ■ Gradual lifestyle changes for the better; awareness of all choices and options |
| ■ Overall: negative<br>■ Perfectionistic<br>■ Many limitations and restrictions<br>■ Feel self-conscious when eating in front of others | ATTITUDE | ■ Overall: positive<br>■ Flexible; can flow with available options<br>■ Many possibilities/choices available<br>■ Can socially eat and quietly monitor eating |
| ■ Only after achieving weight loss | SELF ACCEPTANCE/ WORTH | ■ Beginning now, and increasing with each moment, as more distinctions are made |
| ■ It's "work"; a painful necessity<br>■ Stop exercising during stressful times<br>■ Confusion: some say I should, some say I shouldn't<br>■ Forget to exercise<br>■ If you miss one day of exercise, you feel disgusted with yourself<br>■ Start exercising to look good for an event | EXERCISE | ■ I enjoy moving as a pleasurable necessity<br>■ It's energizing, fun, and a positive outlet for stress<br>■ Have specific exercise goals and track them in a Fitness Journal<br>■ Understand that it's a required part of the energy formula for proper weight loss/gain |
| ■ Slow-moving | SPEED OF MOVEMENT | ■ Fast-moving |
| ■ Negative: food is the enemy; I must deprive myself and use my willpower against desires<br>■ Select only "diet" labels<br>■ Count calories in all foods | FOOD | ■ Food is the friend<br>■ Celebrate! Enjoy, taste, savor each bite<br>■ Creativity of choices and color variety<br>■ Count servings and choose just enough |
| ■ Fast (as if this were "the last supper"!)<br>■ Very slow (methodical; avoidance; deceptive) | SPEED OF EATING | ■ Savoring-paced. |
| ■ All-or-nothing approach: "I can eat it all"/ "I can't have any of *that*!" | SELF-TALK | ■ "I enjoy having it if and when I really choose it; moderation is my guideline." |
| ■ Limited "diet" dictates<br>■ No choices | CHOICE | ■ I am in charge and I decide what and when to eat—freedom |
| ■ External<br>■ Blame others or the environment frequently; "victim"<br>■ Go on and off "diets" frequently | CONTROL | ■ Internal<br>■ Take ownership/ "victor"; have learned to eat anything |

| "Diet" Thinking | Challenge | Weight-Wellness Mindset |
|---|---|---|
| ■ Weigh self once or more a day | SCALES | ■ Scales are used to determine starting point, landmarks of time (end of a class) or to monitor/control fat weight gain |
| ■ Entree is 2/3 meat; 1/3 other foods | "THE AMERICAN PLATE" | ■ 2/3 breads/grains, vegetables and fruits with meat as a *side* dish |
| ■ Brown, white, soft, mushy | "COMFORT FOODS" ARE | ■ Colorful/rainbow of colors; crunchy, fresh |
| ■ The "discretionary" foods with no stars | "SNACKS" ARE | ■ Complex carbohydrates, low in fat/salt, with 3 or 4 nutrient density stars |
| ■ Drink lots to suppress my appetite<br>■ Eliminate it by wearing rubber suits during exercise because it's extra weight | WATER | ■ Needed to maintain or replenish lost fluids for vital functions |
| ■ "Moments on the lips, forever on the hips" | EATING A SUGARED FOOD | ■ Gives me energy! |
| ■ Don't wait for, or experience, internal cues<br>■ Use "appetite" or *mental* cues such as the external sensory cues of sight/sound/smell/taste/touch to eat.<br>■ Use distress to trigger eating response (boredom, anxiety, social acceptance, etc.) | CUES TO EAT | ■ Physical cues<br>■ I am in tune with my body's internal cues for physical hunger such as: empty tank (stomach contracts); headachy; shaky; "too light"; ready for fuel! Or can acknowledge feeling of fullness and not eat<br>■ Consider nonfood response to stress, such as walking, writing, sports, friends |
| ■ Reactionary<br>■ Satisfy now | WILL POWER | ■ Proactive: *plan for* various results I choose<br>■ Patience, can wait |
| ■ *Comfort*, for now<br>■ Emotionally feel better immediately<br>■ Enjoy the "full and heavy" feeling before they stop eating ("6-plus" on the dial). Or "very empty and very light" ("0–2" on the dial) | FEELING SENSE | ■ Nurturing for growth and the future<br>■ Know what "satisfied, comfortable, full, yet light" feels like ("5" on dial); know how much to select, and when to stop eating |
| ■ Needed protection from: neglect; physical or sexual abuse; low self-image; poor social or coping skills | BODY FAT VIEWED AS | ■ Stored energy<br>■ Necessary protection of my vital organs; required storage for my fat-soluble vitamins |
| ■ Have a self-prescribed best way(s) to achieve weight loss<br>■ Follow movie stars' diets | WEIGHT-LOSS PRESCRIPTION | ■ Follow guidelines and programs from certified fitness professionals |
| ■ Avoiding pain: moving-away-from reasons<br>■ Present tense in terms of picturing/self-talking/feeling<br>■ "See food" diet: see food and am "hungry" | MOTIVATION DERIVED FROM | ■ Gaining pleasure: moving-toward reasons<br>■ Future pictures, talk, and feelings<br>■ "That'll: sit well; give me gas; make me feel just right and satisfied; feel too full" |
| ■ Focused on "diet" they're following; label claims, amounts, and caloric value of food before, during, and after eating | CONVERSATION | ■ New people, surroundings, and ideas<br>■ Sensory stimuli experience at this moment—aesthetics, aromas, colors, crunches, tastes |
| ■ Only when goal weight is achieved | SUCCESS DEFINED | ■ Recommended lean-to-fat ratio best health is assessed, understood, and worked on through daily living choices in *all* 6 dimensions of life |

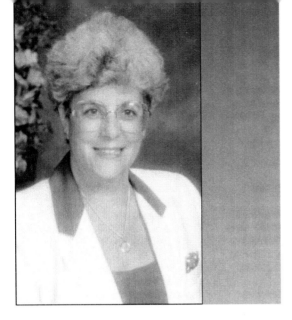

# *Notes*

**Karen S. Mazzeo, M.Ed.**
**Educator • Author • Consultant**

## CHAPTER 1

1. Dr. Steven Blair, President and CEO, Cooper Institute, Dallas, TX, in President's Lecture Series address, BGSU, Bowling Green, OH, January 12, 2005.
2. Terry W. Parsons, "Positive Lifestyle Strategies," lecture quoting Kenneth Cooper's research to Anchor Fitness Course, September 18, 1990.
3. Kenneth H. Cooper, "Run Dick, Run Jane," (Provo, UT: Brigham Young University, 1971) (Film).
4. Blair.
5. Kenneth H. Cooper, *The Aerobics Way* (New York: M. Evans and Company, 1977), p. 10.
6. National Vital Statistics Div., National Center for Health Statistics, Rockville, MD, 1994.
7. Blair.
8. American College of Sports Medicine 1990: Position Stand, "The Recommended Quality and Quantity of Exercise for Developing and Maintaining Cardiorespiratory and Muscular Fitness in Healthy Adults," *Medical Science Sports Exercise, 22*(2), (1990), pp. 265–274.
9. American College of Sports Medicine (ACSM) position stand on, "Physical Activity and Bone Health," *MSSE,* November, 2004. www.acsm.org
10. St. Julian's Fitness Inc., Tom and Shane St. Julian, Owners, 1096 North Main Street, Bowling Green, OH 43402 (419) 354-5060.
11. Blair.
12. Bonnie Berger, Ph.D., "Coping With Stress: Effectiveness of Exercise and Other Techniques," *Quest,* American Academy of Kinesology and Physical Education, 1994, 46, p.105.
13. Berger.
14. Berger.
15. Berger, p.106.
16. Polar®F11™ Heart Rate Monitor, http://www.polarusa.com/Products/

fseries/f//.asp?cat=consumer, (800) 290-6330. Polar Electro, Inc., Sylvia Hom, Marketing Director, Business to Business, 1111 Marcus Ave., Lake Success, NY 11042 (516) 364-0400 Fax: (516) 364-5454.
17. Unpublished research data by Karen S. Mazzeo collected on students enrolled in aerobic dance courses, 1984–1986.
18. G. A. V. Borg, "Psychophysical Bases of Perceived Exertion," *Medicine and Science in Sport and Exercise* 14 (1982).
19. Charlotte A. Williams, "THR Versus RPE: The Debate Over Monitoring Exercise Intensity," *IDEA Today,* April 1991, p. 42.
20. Williams.
21. Andrea Petersen, "The Baby Boomer Tune-up," *The Wall Street Journal,* Tuesday, March 8, 2005, D1.

## CHAPTER 2

1. Bernie Rabin, Ed.D, educational and clinical psychologist, guest speaker for Karen S. Mazzeo's Tension Management and Health Methods courses, Bowling Green State University, 1978–1988.
2. Shad Helmstetter, *What To Say When You Talk to Yourself* (New York: Pocket Books/ Simon & Schuster, 1986), p. 98.
3. Karen S. Mazzeo, *Stress*Time* Life Management* Principles, Methods, and Assessment Techniques* (Bowling Green, OH: Mazzeo Reprographics, 2001) p. 42.
4. Anthony Robbins, *Unlimited Power* (New York: Fawcett/ Columbine 1986), pp. 125–148.
5. Connirae Andreas et al., *Heart of the Mind* (Moab, UT: Real People Press, 1989), pp. 254–255.
6. Robert Dilts et al., *Neuro-Linguistic Programming: The Study of the Structure of Subjective Experience* (Cupertino, CA: Meta Publications, 1980).
7. David Gordeon et al., *The Neuro-Linguistic Programming Home Study Guide* (San Rafael, CA: FuturePace).

## CHAPTER 3

1. Lenore Zohman et al., *The Cardiologists' Guide to Fitness and Health Through Exercise* (New York: Simon and Schuster, 1979), p. 81.
2. Zohman.
3. American College of Obstetricians and Gynecologists, *Safety Guidelines for Women Who Exercise* (ACOG Home Exercise Programs No. 2, Washington DC: ACOG, 1986), p. 6.
4. Douglas H. Richie, Jr. "How to Choose Shoes," *IDEA Today,* April 1991, p. 67.
5. Richie.
6. ACOG, p. 5.
7. ACOG, pp. 4–5.
8. Orthotic for sports shoe prescribed and dispensed by Dr. Charles Marlowe, podiatrist to Karen S. Mazzeo, Summer 1983.
9. *Therapeutic Foot Massage,* Hydropedes™ Glycerin Filled Insoles with Cambrelle®, 300 East Grace St., Barstow, CA 92311 www.hydropedes.com (760) 256-4404 M-F 8-5 pm PST.
10. *Therapeutic Foot Massage,* Hydropedes™.
11. ACOG, p. 5.
12. Committee on Nutritional Misinformation, Food and Nutrition Board, National Research Council, National Academy of Sciences, "Water Deprivation and Performance of Athletics," distributed by Nutritional Education and Training Program, Bowling Green State University, 1981.
13. American Alliance for Health, Physical Education, and Recreation, *Nutrition for Athletes. A Handbook for Coaches* (Washington, DC: AAHPERD, 1971), p. 42.
14. AAHPERD, *Nutrition for Sport Success* (Reston, VA: AAHPERD), 1984, p. 2.
15. American College of Sports Medicine, *Encyclopedia of Sports Sciences and Medicine* (New York: Macmillan, 1971), p. 215.
16. ACSM, p. 216.
17. ACSM.

18. Doug Jackson, CSRS, ACE, *Personal Fitness Advantage Newsletter*, "Fitness Question and Answer; Round Two—My Turn", www.personalfitnessadvantage. com, November 22, 2004, p.2.
19. Interview with Jane Steinberg, athletic trainer of intercollegiate sports, Bowling Green State University, Bowling Green, Ohio, spring 1982.
20. ACOG, p. 6.
21. Steinberg.
22. *Harvard Medical School Health Letter*, *11* (5), p. 4.

## CHAPTER 5

1. Kenneth H. Cooper, *Running Without Fear* (New York: M. Evans and Company, 1985), p. 128.
2. Cooper, p. 192.
3. Cooper, p. 197.
4. Cooper, *The Aerobics Program for Total Well Being* (New York: M. Evans and Company, 1982), pp. 141–142. Dr. Kenneth Cooper, in correspondence with *Fitness* author Karen S. Mazzeo, dated December 1, 2000, stated that the three 1982 copyrighted Cooper Fitness Tests presented in this text are still valid fitness testing instruments and should be used exactly as published.
5. Lenore R. Zohman et al., *The Cardiologists' Guide to Fitness and Health Through Exercise* (New York: Simon and Schuster, 1979), p. 87.

## CHAPTER 6

1. Candace Copeland-Brooks, *Moves . . . and More!* (San Diego: IDEA, Inc., 1990) (videotape).
2. Copeland, *The Low-Impact Challenge for the Fitness Professional* (Newark, NJ: PPI Entertainment Group/Parade Video, 1991) (videotape).
3. Julie Moo-Bradley and Jerrie Moo-Thurman, *Aerobics Choreography in Action: The High-Low Impact Advantage.* (San Diego: IDEA, Inc. 1990) (videotape).
4. Lynne Brick, *Total Body Workout* (Philadelphia: Creative Instructors Aerobics, 1991) (videotape).
5. Amy Jones, "Point-Counterpoint: Sequencing a Dance-Exercise Class," *Dance Exercise Today*, May/June 1985.
6. American College of Obstetricians and Gynecologists, *Safety Guidelines for Women Who Exercise* (ACOG Home Exercise Programs) (Washington, DC: ACOG, 1986).
7. James L. Hesson, *Weight Training for Life* (Englewood, CO: Morton Publishing, 1985).
8. SPRI Products, 1554 Barclay Blvd., Buffalo Grove, IL 60089, *Pumping Rubber* (instructions for product use), 1988, 1-800-222-7774).

9. John Patrick O'Shea, *Scientific Principles and Methods of Strength Fitness*, 2d ed. (Reading, MA: Addison-Wesley, 1976).
10. Len Kravitz et al., "Static & PNF Stretches," *IDEA Today*, March 1990.

## CHAPTER 7

1. Ken Alan, "A Choreography Primer," *IDEA Today*, January 1989.
2. Lorna Francis et al., "Moderate-Impact Aerobics," *IDEA Today*, September 1989.
3. Lorna Francis et al., "Injury Prevention. Low-Impact Aerobics: 'Do's and Don'ts'." *Dance Exercise Today*, Nov./Dec. 1986.
4. Alan.
5. Francis, "Moderate-Impact Aerobics."
6. Francis, "Injury Prevention."
7. Francis, "Moderate-Impact Aerobics." Also, *Aerobics Choreography* (San Diego: IDEA, Association for Fitness Professionals, 1990).
8. Candace Copeland, *The Low-Impact Challenge for the Fitness Professional* (Newark, NJ: PPI Entertainment Group/ Parade Video, 1991) (videotape).
9. Francis, "Moderate-Impact Aerobics."
10. Copeland, 1991.
11. Francis, "Moderate-Impact Aerobics," 1989.
12. Francis.
13. Francis.
14. "Research: Caloric Expenditure in LIA vs HIA" from study, 'The Metabolic Cost of Instructor's Low Impact and High Impact Aerobic Dance Sequences,' *IDEA Today*, January 1991, p. 8.
15. "Tempo and Ground Reaction Forces for LIA and HIA," from study, 'Comparison of Forces in High and Low Impact Aerobic Dance at Various Tempos,' *IDEA Today*, May 1991, p. 9.
16. IDEA, *Aerobics Choreography* (San Diego: IDEA: Association for Fitness Professionals, 1989).
17. Doug Jackson, CSRS, ACE, *Personal Fitness Advantage Newsletter*, "Optimizing Your Cardio Training for Fitness and Fat Loss", www.personalfitnessadvantage. com, February 18, 2005, p. 2.
18. Jackson.
19. Jackson, pp. 2-3.
20. Jackson, p. 3.
21. Jackson, p. 3-4.
22. Jackson, p. 4.
23. Karen S. Mazzeo et al., *Aerobic Dance—A Way to Fitness*, 2d ed. (Englewood, CO: Morton Publishing, 1987), p. 112.
24. Mazzeo, 113.
25. Lauren M.Mangili et al., *Step Training Plus,* 2d ed. (Englewood, CO: Morton Publishing, 1999) p.80.
26. Mangili.
27. B. Bellinger, et al. "Energy Expenditure of a Non Contact Boxing Training Session Compared with Submaximal Treadmill

Running," *Medicine & Science in Sport & Exercise*, 29:12 (1997), 1653– 1656.
28. E. Rodriguiez, "Putting the Punch in Your Boxing Classes," *IDEA Health & Fitness Source*, June 1998, pp. 23–28.

## CHAPTER 8

1. Joan Price, "Stepping Basics," *IDEA Today*, Nov./Dec. 1990, p. 57.
2. Len Kravitz and Rich Deivert, "The Safe Way to Step," *IDEA Today*, April 1991, pp. 47–50.
3. Sports Step, Inc. videotape accompanying The Step, *Introduction to Step Training*, Atlanta 1989.
4. Lynne Brick and David Essel, *Pump N' Step* [videotape], 1991.
5. Lorna Francis, Peter Francis, and Gin Miller, *Step-Reebok. The First Aerobic Training Workout with Muscle. Instructor Training Manual.* (Reebok International, Ltd., 1990).
6. Francis, p. 6.
7. M. S. Olson, et al., "Cardiorespiratory Responses to 'Aerobic' Bench Stepping Exercise in Females," *Medicine and Science in Sports and Exercise* (abstract), *23*: 4 (April 1991), S27.
8. D. L. Blessing, et al., "The Energy Cost of Bench Stepping With and Without One and Two Pound Hand-Held Weights," *Medicine and Science in Sports and Exercise* (abstract), *23*: 4 (April 1991), S28.
9. F. Goss, et al., "Energy Cost of Bench Stepping and Pumping Light Handweights in Trained Subjects," *Research Quarterly for Exercise and Sport*, *60*: 4 (1989), pp. 369–372.
10. L. Calarco, et al., "The Metabolic Cost of Six Common Movement Patterns of Bench Step Aerobic Dance," *Medicine and Science in Sports and Exercise* (abstract), *23*: 4 (April 1991), S140.
11. Ralph La Forge, "What the Latest Research Has to Say About STEP Exercise," *IDEA Today*, September, 1991, pp. 31–35.
12. D. Stanforth et al., "The Effect of Bench Height and Rate of Stepping on the Metabolic Cost of Bench Stepping," *Medicine and Science in Sport and Exercise* (abstract), 23:4 (April 1991), S143.
13. American College of Sports Medicine, "Position Statement on the Recommended Quantity and Quality of Exercise for Developing and Maintaining Cardio-respiratory and Muscular Fitness in Healthy Adults," *Medicine and Science in Sports and Exercise*, 22(1990), pp. 265–274.
14. M.S. Olson, et al., "The Physiological Effects of Bench/ Step Exercise," *Sports Medicine*, 3 (1996), pp. 164–175.
15. S. Woodby-Brown, K. Berg, and R. W. Latin, "Oxygen Cost of Aerobic Bench

Stepping at Three Heights," *Journal of Strength & Conditioning Research, 7,* 163–167.

16. Calcarco et al.

17. K. Greenlaw, et al., "The Energy Cost of Traditional Versus Power Bench Step Exercise at Heights of Four, Six, and Eight Inches," *Medicine and Science in Sport and Exercise, 27,* 5 (June 1995, supplement), abstract #1343.

18. M. Scharff-Olsen, et al., "Psyiological Responses of Males and Females to Bench Step at Two Different Rates," Sports Medicine, 3 (1996): 164–175.

19. Scharff-Olsen.

20. Kravitz.

21. Step Reebok, 1997 Revised Guidelines for Step Reebok, "Guidelines for Step Height and Music Speed", Reebok University, 1997.

22. M. Groupe-Kennedy, "Managing Step Intensity," *ACE Certified News,* 2:5 (1997), p. 9.

23. Deborah Kern, Ph.D., "The Power of Music. How to make the best musical selections for your mind-body classes", IDEA Health & Fitness Source, April 2000, p.48.

24. Step Reebok Guidelines, ACE Chapter 9, p. 277.

25. Kravitz, p. 48.

26. Francis, p. 23.

27. Francis, pp. 23–25.

28. Francis.

29. Francis.

30. Francis.

31. Francis.

32. Karen S. Mazzeo and Lauren M. Mangili, *Instructor's Manual for Step Training Plus* (Englewood, CO: Morton Publishing, 1993) p. 33. (Adapted for this textbook).

33. Mazzeo.

## CHAPTER 9

1. Kenneth H. Cooper, *The Aerobics Program for Total Well-Being* (New York: M. Evans and Company, 1982), p. 129.

2. Cooper, p. 144.

3. American Institute for Cancer Research NEWSLETTER, "Walk Your Way to Good Health", Spring 2003, Issue 79, p.5.

4. American Institute for Cancer Research NEWSLETTER, "Pedometers Make Americans Move", Fall 2002, Issue 77, p. 4.

5. Ruth Carver, President and CEO Walk4Life, Inc.™, 12137 Rhea Drive, Unit B, Plainfield, IL 60544, (888) 422-1806, www.walk4life.com, provided research (April, 2005) conducted by various institutions and professionals who reported their results in the March 2005 issue of the official journal of ACSM, and *Medicine and Science in Sports and Exercise,* Vol. 37, No. 3. The Walk4Life™ promotional pieces provided were

entitled, "Pedometers 101", "New Study Confirms Walk4Life Pedometer 'Activity Time' Feature a More Accurate Way of Assessing Student Activity Levels" and "Frequently Asked Questions and Answers About Pedometers."

6. Carver.

7. Carver.

8. AIC, "Pedometers Make America Move."

9. Robert P. Pangrazi, Arizona State University, "Questions You Always Wanted to Ask About Pedometers," presentation and handout given to attendees at the Walk4Life™ presentation, AAHPERD National Convention, Chicago, IL, April 13, 2005, p.1, 2.

10. Carver.

11. Walk4Life, Inc™ DUO 2-Function Digital Pedometer, information brochure included with product purchase.

12. Pangrazi, p. 2.

13. Pangrazi, p. 3.

14. Pangrazi.

15. Pangrazi.

16. Pangrazi.

17. Carver.

18. Carver.

19. Level I Walking Only Program was written by Dr. Richard W. Bowers, ACSM-certified program director, Fitwell Program, Student Recreation Center, Bowling Green State University, Bowling Green, Ohio, 1990.

20. Steven N. Blair, *Exercise and Health: Sports Science Exchange* (Gatorade Sports Science Institute, November 1990) (Vol. 3, #29).

21. Top-notch fitness facilities like St. Julian's Fitness, 1096 North Main St., Bowling Green, OH 43402 (419) 354-5060, Tom and Shane St. Julian owners, provide Elliptical Trainers for their clients' use.

22. ACSM Development of Product Recommendations Committee, American College of Sports Medicine Elliptical Trainer Brochure 0180GNBR "Selecting and Effectively Using an Elliptical Trainer."

23. ACSM.

## CHAPTER 10

1. Doug Jackson, CSRS, ACE, *Personal Fitness Advantage Newsletter*, "Prevent or Slow Osteoporosis with the SAID Principle," p. 2, www.personalfitnessadvantage.com, April 28, 2005, p. 2.

2. Jackson.

3. James L. Hesson, *Weight Training for Life* (Englewood, CO: Morton Publishing, 2000), p. 4.

4. American College of Obstetricians and Gynecologists, Safety Guidelines for Women Who Exercise (ACOG Home Exercise Programs) (Washington, DC: ACOG, 1986), p. 6.

5. Hesson, pp. 23, 25.

6. Hesson, p. 23.

7. Steven J. Fleck et al., *Designing Resistance Training Programs,* 2d ed. (Champaign, IL: Human Kinetics,1997), p. 19.

8. American College of Sports Medicine: Position Stand, "The Recommended Quality and Quantity of Exercise for Developing and Maintaining Cardio-Respiratory and Muscular Fitness in Healthy Adults," *Medicine and Science in Sports and Exercise 22:* 2 (1990), pp. 265–274.

9. Doug Jackson, CSRS, ACE, *Personal Fitness Advantage Newsletter,* "Solutions For Your Fitness Lifestyle," www.personalfitnessadvantage.com, May 2003, Vol. 1, Issue 3, p. 4.

10. Doug Jackson, CSRS, ACE, *Personal Fitness Advantage Newsletter,* "Don't Miss This Interview with Women's Fitness Expert Kelli Calabrese", www.personalfitnessadvantage.com, March 19, 2005, p. 3.

11. Doug Jackson, CSRS, ACE, *Personal Fitness Advantage Newsletter,* "Getting Lean: My Interview with Body Transformation Specialist Billy Hofacker," www.personalfitnessadvantage.com, November 15, 2004, p.3 quoting a linked article that can be found at http://www.msnbc.msn.com/id/6391058.

12. Fleck, p. 8.

13. Jackson, p 2.

14. Fleck, p. 8.

15. Doug Jackson, CSRS, ACE, *Personal Fitness Advantage Newsletter*, "Don't Miss This: Building Stability with Jonathan Ross", www.personalfitnessadvantage.com, April 4, 2005, p. 4.

16. Sports Step, Inc. Videotape accompanying *The Step, Introduction to Step Training* (Atlanta: Sports Step, 1989).

17. SPRI Products, Inc., *Pumping Rubber* (instructions for product use) (Buffalo Grove, IL, 1988).

18. SPRI.

19. SPRI.

20. SPRI.

21. Jackson, pp. 2-3.

22. Jackson, p. 4.

23. American College of Sports Medicine: Position Stand: pp. 265–274.

24. James L. Hesson, *Weight Training for Life* (Englewood, CO: 1985), pp. 164–165.

25. Doug Jackson, CSRS, ACE, *Personal Fitness Advantage Newsletter,* "Getting Lean: My Interview with Body Transformation Specialist Billy Hofacker," www.personalfitnessadvantage.com, November 15, 2004, pp. 1-2, quoting a linked article that can be found at http://www.msnbc.msn.com/id/6391058.

26. SPRI.

27. Lynn Brick and David Eassel, *Pump N' Step* (1991) (videotape).
28. SPRI Products, Inc. and Brick Bodies, *Step Strength* (Buffalo Grove, IL: SPRI Products).
29. Program developed by Doug Jackson, M.Ed., CSCS, ACE, Expert Fellow of the National Board of Fitness Examiners, Certified Personal Trainer and Managing Partner, Fitness 21 Express™, 1474 Coral Ridge Drive, Coral Springs, FL 33071 (954)755-9121 www.personalfitnessadvantage.com .
30. James L. Hesson, *Weight Training for Life, 5th Edition* (Englewood, CO: Morton Publishing, 2000) p. 88.
31. Howley and Franks, *Health Fitness Instructor's Handbook* (Champaign, IL: Human Kinetics, 2003) p. 257.
32. Hesson, p. 96.
33. B.J. Cardinal and M. Kosma, "Don't Forget Muscular Fitness!" *Physical Activity Today*, a publication of the Research Consortium of AAHPERD, Vol. 10, No.3, p.1.
34. John Patrick O'Shea, *Scientific Principles and Methods of Strength Fitness*, 2nd ed. (Reading, MA: Addison-Wesley, 1976), p. 89.

## CHAPTER 11

1. Kirpal Singh Mahal, professor Tusculum College, Greeneville, TN and invited guest speaker to the AAHPERD National Convention and Exposition, April 14, 2005, in presentation entitled, "YOGA: Brighten Your Present and Future by Practicing Yoga," and handout of information, "Breath Rhythm During The Salutation to the Sun".
2. Andre van Lysebeth, *YOGA Self-Taught* (Boston, MA: Weiser Books, 1999), p. 243.
3. van Lysebeth, p. 243.
4. Len Kravitz et al., "Static & PNF Stretches," *IDEA Today*, March 1990.
5. Kravitz et al.
6. Kravitz et al.
7. Kravitz et al.

## CHAPTER 12

1. Roman Carek, Director of the Counseling and Career Development Center, Bowling Green State University, Bowling Green, Ohio, from his stress management presentation in the LIFE Seminar Workshop Series, held at the Student Recreation Center of BGSU, 1982.
2. John S. J. Power, *Why Am I Afraid to Tell You Who I Am?* (Allen, TX: Tabor Publishing, 1969), p. 56.
3. Hans Selye, *Stress Without Distress* (Toronto: McClelland and Stewart Limited, 1974), p. 141.
4. The Kerr House, International Health Resort and Spa, Laurie Hostetler, Owner/Director, 17777 Beaver St., Grand Rapids, OH 43522, (419) 832-

1733, info@thekerrhouse.com www.thekerrhouse.com.
5. Harbor Employee Assistance, *Healthy Alternatives Newsletter*, "Stressed Out?" (Toledo, OH) 2005. www.harbor.org.
6. Former Special Agents of the Federal Bureau of Investigation, *The Grapevine*, Family Assistance News, May 2005, p.4.
7. Technique by Dr. Bernie Rabin, psychologist and lecturer to Karen Mazzeo's Personal Wellness, Health Methods, and Stress Management classes 1980–1988, Bowling Green State University, Bowling Green, Ohio.
8. Developed by Karen S. Mazzeo, M.Ed., for Tension Management courses at Bowling Green State University, Bowling Green, Ohio, 1998. Creativity inspired from two techniques: "Riding Through a Rainbow," by Don E. Gibbons, and "Recycling Emotions," by Richard Bolstad and Margot Hambett.
9. Developed by Karen S. Mazzeo, M.Ed., for Tension Management courses at Bowling Green State University, Bowling Green, Ohio, 1985.
10. Mazzeo.

## CHAPTER 13

1. Nutrition Education Services, "*Pyramid Plus, A Star-Studded Guide to Food Choices for Better Health*" (Portland, Oregon Dairy Council, 1999).
2. Judy Tillapaugh, "Cross-Training in the Kitchen," *IDEA Today*, October, 1991, p. 21.
3. American Institute for Cancer Research, *Newsletter*, "Water Down Your Summer Thirst," 60 (Summer 1998), p. 5.
4. Gatorade Company (division of Quaker Oats Company) "Fluid Pyramid" pamphlet (1-800-884-2867).
5. Nanci Hellmich, "U.S. diet guide stresses exercise", *USA Today*, Thursday, January 13, 2005, Section A, p.1.
6. U.S. Department of Agriculture, *Dietary Guidelines for Americans 2005* and *MyPyramid ~ Steps to a Healthier You* (Washington, D.C.) www.MyPyramid.gov.
7. Margo Wootan, Director of the Center for Science in the Public Interest, Washington, D.C. quoted in *The Wall Street Journal*, "The Food Pyramid Gets Personalized", Wednesday, April 20, 2005, Sect.D, pp. 1-2.
8. Tim Radak, Director of Nutrition, Physicians Committee for Responsible Medicine, Washington, D.C., quoted in *The Wall Street Journal*, "The Food Pyramid Gets Personalized", Wednesday, April 20, 2005, Section D, p 2.
9. Nutrition Education Services.
10. Nutrition Education Services.
11. U.S. Department of Agriculture, http://www.health.gov/dietaryguidelines/dga2005/document/html/executivesummary.htm , p. 2.

12. Nutrition Education Services.
13. U.S. Department of Agriculture, http://www.MyPyramid.gov/mypyramid/index.aspx. It is then listed on the individualized eating plan you're given.
14. U.S. Department of Agriculture, http://www.MyPyramid.gov/tips_resources/vegetarian_diets.html .
15. Tammy Kime-Sheets, author of original teaching tool entitled, "How to Eat Without the Meat," in the section, 'Cut the Animal Fat,' p. 2, distributed to clients at Nutrition Wellness seminars and workshops in the greater Toledo, Ohio area, 1998.
16. Kime-Sheets, p. 2.
17. Vegetarian Resource Group, http://www.vrg.org/nutrition/adapaper.htm ,pp.1-3.
18. Kime-Sheets.
19. Vegetarian Resource Group.
20. American Dietetics Association, http://www.eatright.org
21. American Institute for Cancer Research,*Newsletter*, p. 5.
22. American Institute for Cancer Research.
23. Tammy Kime-Sheets, *W.I.C. Wellness News . . . You Can Use!* "W.A.T.E.R. = Water A 'Treat' Everyone Requires;" "Water-The Perfect Drink!" "Water Replacement Plan" (Fulton/Henry County, OH: W.I.C.), August 1997.
24. American Institute for Cancer Research.
25. U.S. Department of Agriculture, http://www.MyPyramid.gov/tips resources/mixed food information print.html .
26. Jan Lewis, "Nutrition Notes: Nutrition and the Athlete" Workshop Series, Nutrition Education and Training Program, Bowling Green State University, Bowling Green, OH, 1981.
27. Mayo Clinic Diet and Nutrition Resource Center, http://www.mayo.ivi.com/mayo/commonhtm/dietpage.htm Mayo Health O@sis section, "Energy gels- At the competitive edge," p. 2.
28. Mayo Clinic Diet and Nutrition Resource Center.
29. U. S. Department of Agriculture, http://www.health.gov/dietaryguidelines/dga2005/document/html/executivesummary.htm , p.1.
30. U. S. Department Agriculture.
31. U.S. Department of Agriculture, http://www.healthierus.gov/dietaryguidelines/index.html .
32. Nanci Hellmich, "New, healthier plate is full," *USA Today*, Wednesday, January 19, 2003, Section D, p. 7.
33. Lucy M. Williams, lecture and literature, "Shopping Tips for Low Fat, Low Salt, Low Cholesterol Diets," delivered to Karen S. Mazzeo's Anchor Fitness-Personal Excellence class, February, 1991.
34. Williams.
35. U. S. Department of Agriculture, Human Nutrition Information Service, *Home & Garden Bulletin No. 253*-8, p. 2, July

1993 (Washington, DC: Government Printing Office).

36. U.S. Department of Agriculture, http://www.cfsan.fda.gov/~dms/foodlab.html .

37. Jane Zhang, "Major Changes Set For Food Labels," *The Wall street Journal*, Wednesday, December 28, 2005, p. D1 and D4.

38. Lee Hoffman, *Eating Disorders, Decade of the Brain* (NIH Publication No. 94-3477) (Washington, DC: National Institute of Mental Health, Office of Scientific Information, 1994).

39. Hoffman.

## CHAPTER 14

1. Werner W. K. Hoeger, *Principles & Labs for Physical Fitness & Wellness* (Englewood, CO: Morton Publishing, 1994), pp. 49–64.

2. Tufts University Nutrition Navigator, http://navigator.tufts.edu/profess.html. About the Ratings section, pp. 1–2, and Health Professionals section. 3. http://www.health.gov/dietaryguidelines/dga2005/document/html/chapter3.htm.

4. Jan Lewis, *Nutrition Notes. Dietary Guidelines 2*, Bowling Green State University, Bowling Green, OH, 1981.

5. Doug Jackson, CSRS, ACE, *Personal Fitness Advantage Newsletter*, "3 Keys to Staying in Shape through the Holidays," www.personalfitnessadvantage.com, December 9, 2004, p. 1.

6. Doug Jackson, CSRS, ACE, *Personal Fitness Advantage Newsletter*, "Doug's Two Cents on New Federal Health Recommendations," www.personalfitnessadvantage.com January 21, 2005, p. 2.

7. Jackson.

8. Jackson, p. 3.

9. Dr. Steven Blair, keynote speaker at American Alliance for Health, Physical Education, Recreation, & Dance National Convention, Indianapolis, 1992.

10. Tara Parker-Pope, "Stress and Your Waistline: Gaining Belly Fat May Be Body's Way of Coping," *The Wall Street Journal*, Health Journal, Tuesday, July 19, 2005, p.D2.

11. Parker-Pope.

12. Parker-Pope.

13. Parker-Pope.

14. Parker-Pope, quoting Carol Shively, a pathology professor at Wake Forrest University School of Medicine.

15. Connirae Andreas and Steven A. Andreas, *Heart of the Mind* (Moab, UT: Real People Press, 1989), p. 251.

16. Andreas, p. 125.

17. Lewis, p. 6.

18. Doug Jackson, CSRS, ACE, *Personal Fitness Advantage Newsletter*, "Solutions For Your Fitness Lifestyle ", www.personalfitnessadvantage.com, May 2003, Vol.1,Issue 3, p. 4.

19. Lewis, p. 4.

20. Lewis.

21. Lewis.

22. Jackson, p. 5.

23. Jackson.

24. Bob Greene, *Bob Greene's Total Body Makeover* (New York, NY: Simon and Schuster, 2005), pp. 142–165.

25. Jackson.

26. Doug Jackson, CSRS, ACE, *Personal Fitness Advantage Newsletter*, "3 Keys to Staying in Shape Through the Holidays," www.personalfitnessadvantage.com, December 9, 2004, p. 2.

27. Tara Parker-Pope, Health Journal column Contributing Editor, "The Diet That Works," *The Wall Street Journal*, Tuesday, April 22, 2003, p. R6.

28. Pope.

29. Donna Fish, "Worried About Your Child's Diet? You Should Be," *USA Today*, The Forum, Wed., July 20, 2005, p. 13A.

30. Tammy Kime-Sheets and Karen S. Mazzeo, "Establishing A Weight-Wellness Mindset," methods pamphlet and instructional tool given during presentations to Bowling Green State University, Ohio students in Tension Management Classes, and professional seminars for clients, Spring 1995.

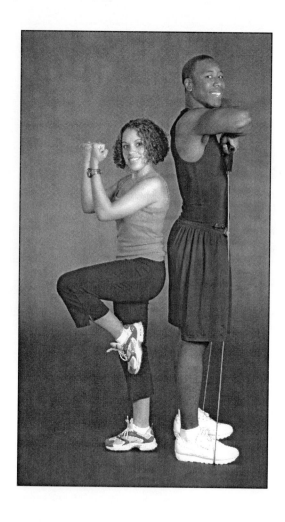

# *Websites!*

**Chapter 1**

*American Heart Association  http://www
.amhrt.org
*Bob Greene, noted exercise physiologist
working corporately with McDonald's
restaurants www.goactive.com
*American Medical Association
http://www.ama_assn.org
*American College of Sports Medicine
http://www.acsm.org
*American Council on Exercise
http://www.acefitness.org
*Polar Heart Rate Monitors® sylvia
.hom@polar.fi,polarusa.com

**Chapter 3**

*Hydropedes™ Glycerin Filled Insoles
www.hydropedes.com

**Chapter 8**

*Dynamix Music Services, (800) 843-6499,
(410) 918-1000,
www.dynamixmusic.com
*Muscle Mixes Music, (800) 526-4937, (407)
872-7576, www.musclemixes.com
*Power Music, (800) 777-2328, (801) 975-
7771, www.powermusic.com
*PRO Motion Music, (800) 380-4776, (972)
446-0388 www.promotionmusic.com

**Chapter 9**

*Walk4Life™ DUO® 2-Function Digital
Pedometers: www.Walk4Life.com

**Chapter 10**

*American Council on Exercise
www.acefitness.org (800) 825-3636
*Strength Training Nutrition
www.johnbernardi.com
*Doug Jackson, CSCS, ACE Personal Trainer,
Newsletter www.personal
fitnessadvantage.com
*Billy Hofacker, Fitness Professional,
Newsletter  http://www.howtogetlean
.com
*Jonathan Ross, Personal Trainer, Newsletter
http://www.aionfitness.com
*Brian Calkins, Personal Trainer, Newsletter
http://www.briancalkins.com
*Phil Kaplan, Personal Trainer, Newsletter
http://www.philkaplan.com
*Spri:™ www.spriproducts.com

**Chapter 12**

*American Massage Therapy Association
www.amtamassage.org
*The Kerr House: www.thekerrhouse.com;
info@thekerrhouse.com

**Chapter 13**

*Service program entitled, *Nutrition
Generator* is accessed from The Institute
of Medicine of the National Academies
of Science website  http://www.
1shoppingcart.com/app/?Clk=1012710
* www.dietdirectives.com
*National Eating Disorders Association
http://nationaleatingdisorders.org
*Eating Disorders Awareness & prevention:
www.edap.org
*Anorexia Nervosa and Related Eating
Disorders Inc.: www.anred
*Harvard University Eating Disorder Center:
www.hedc.org

**Chapter 14**

*U.S. Department of Agriculture, Dietary
Guidelines 2005
http.//www.health.gov/dietaryguidelines/
dga2005/document/html/chapter3.htm.
*American Medical Association
http://www.ama_assn.org (General
Health/Interactive Health Sections).
*Shape up America. Healthy Weight for Life
http://www.shapeup.org
*Weight Watchers http://www.
weightwatchers.com

CPSIA information can be obtained
at www.ICGtesting.com
Printed in the USA
FFOW04n1331220414
4954FF